Career Development
for Health Professionals

THIRD EDITION

Career Development for Health Professionals

Success in School & On the Job

Lee Haroun, MA (Education), MBA, EdD
Educator and Health Care Writer
Sunriver, Oregon

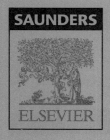

SAUNDERS

ELSEVIER

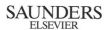

3251 Riverport Lane
Maryland Heights, Missouri 63043

CAREER DEVELOPMENT FOR HEALTH PROFESSIONALS: ISBN : 978-1-4377-0673-4
SUCCESS IN SCHOOL & ON THE JOB, THIRD EDITION

Notice

Knowledge and best practice in this field are constantly changing. As new research and experience broaden our understanding, changes in research methods, professional practices, or medical treatment may become necessary.

Practitioners and researchers must always rely on their own experience and knowledge in evaluating and using any information, methods, compounds, or experiments described herein. In using such information or methods they should be mindful of their own safety and the safety of others, including parties for whom they have a professional responsibility.

With respect to any drug or pharmaceutical products identified, readers are advised to check the most current information provided (i) on procedures featured or (ii) by the manufacturer of each product to be administered, to verify the recommended dose or formula, the method and duration of administration, and contraindications. It is the responsibility of practitioners, relying on their own experience and knowledge of their patients, to make diagnoses, to determine dosages and the best treatment for each individual patient, and to take all appropriate safety precautions.

To the fullest extent of the law, neither the Publisher nor the authors, contributors, or editors, assume any liability for any injury and/or damage to persons or property as a matter of products liability, negligence or otherwise, or from any use or operation of any methods, products, instructions, or ideas contained in the material herein.

Library of Congress Cataloging-in-Publication Data

Haroun, Lee.
    Career development for health professionals : success in school and on the job / Lee Haroun. – 3rd ed.
        p. ; cm.
    Includes bibliographical references and index.
    ISBN 978-1-4377-0673-4 (pbk. : alk. paper) 1. Medical personnel – Vocational guidance.
I. Title.
    [DNLM: 1. Health Personnel. 2. Career Choice. 3. Vocational Guidance. W 21 H292c 2011]
    R690.H377 2011
    610.69–dc22

                                                                           2009042181

Publishing Director: Andrew Allen
Acquisitions Editor: Jennifer Janson
Associate Developmental Editor: Kelly Brinkman
Publishing Services Manager: Hemamalini Rajendrababu
Project Manager: Deepthi Unni
Designer: Charles Seibel

Printed in Canada

Last digit is the print number: 9 8 7 6 5 4 3 2

To David, whose spirit and optimism
remind me daily that all things are possible.

Preface

This book is intended to help students in allied health care programs improve the quality of their own lives, get the most from their education, and make meaningful contributions to the lives of others. Specifically, the purpose in writing this book is to help students achieve the following four goals:

1. Successfully complete their educational programs
2. Think and act professionally
3. Find the right jobs
4. Attain long-term career success

Many students who begin health care studies with great enthusiasm drop out when they discover they lack some of the study, personal, and organizational skills necessary for academic and career success. This book shows students that becoming a health care professional begins *as soon as they start school*. In truth, many of the skills needed for academic success are the same as those needed on the job.

During my years working with postsecondary students, I learned that they want to begin their occupational studies as soon as possible. Showing students how study and other school success skills are directly related to job success in health care makes learning organizational and study skills more meaningful and easier to remember.

WHO WILL BENEFIT FROM THIS BOOK?

Students enrolled in all types of postsecondary health care programs, such as medical assisting, dental assisting, nursing, physical therapy assisting, x-ray technology, and health information technology, will benefit. The study and life skills presented are applicable to all types of health care occupations, and the on-the-job examples used throughout the book are drawn from a variety of health care settings.

This book is designed to be flexible and can meet a variety of needs. It can be used in a number of courses and learning contexts, such as the following:

- Orientation and study skills classes for new students
- Introductory health care courses
- Professional development courses
- Job search courses
- Academic refresher and review classes for math, writing, and communication
- A supplement to health care specialty courses to expand the coverage of oral and written communication skills; to provide a math review; to teach note taking, research, and test-taking strategies; and to enhance personal organization and problem-solving skills
- Independent study in which students are assigned to work on the development of specific skills
- A reference book for students to use, as needed, for help with their study, organizational, and job search needs

WHY IS THIS BOOK IMPORTANT TO THE PROFESSION?

The need for competent, thinking health care professionals continues to grow as health care remains one of the fastest growing industries in the United States. Helping students succeed in their educational programs has the greater benefit of providing society with the competent, caring employees needed to fill the growing number of positions available today . . . and tomorrow.

ORGANIZATION

Career Development for Health Professionals is divided into two major sections. The first section, consisting of Chapters 1 through 8, introduces students to the world of health care and presents the life-management and study skills essential for both learning in school and working successfully in a health care occupation. These include the following:

- Understanding what it takes to be a competent and caring health care professional
- Planning and preparing ahead for employment success
- Developing a positive attitude and effective personal organizational skills
- Taking good notes in class
- Reading for understanding and learning
- Conducting useful research
- Improving writing skills
- Preparing to take tests successfully
- Overcoming math anxiety
- Getting the most from lab classes and clinical experience
- Communicating and working effectively with others
- Applying problem-solving techniques
- Succeeding as an adult student
- Improving English language skills when English is the student's second language
- Developing strategies to overcome learning disabilities

Chapters 3 through 8 may be presented and studied in any order depending on the needs of the students. Chapter 2 introduces the concept of the resume as a tool that can be used to encourage success in school. Students can begin building their resumes early in their educational programs. Some instructors prefer to teach this chapter later as part of the job search process. This can be done without disrupting the flow of the book; however, students should not be assigned the "Building Your Resume" activities in the subsequent chapters.

The second section, consisting of Chapters 9 through 14, focuses on job search skills and how to achieve and maintain career success. These skills include the following:

- Locating job leads
- Creating an appealing resume
- Taking advantage of new trends, such as using the Internet and preparing a scannable resume
- Presenting oneself effectively and confidently at interviews
- Increasing the chances of being hired
- Becoming a valued employee
- Keeping career progress on course

Note that Chapters 9 through 12 focus on the job search and would be best presented in order. Chapters 13 and 14 apply to success on the job and are appropriate for use at any point in a professional development class or unit.

DISTINCTIVE FEATURES OF THIS BOOK

Emphasis on Connecting School and Health Care Careers

Examples are given throughout the text that show students how they will use personal management and study skills on the job.

CONNECTING SCHOOL AND CAREER

The process of becoming a health care professional began the day you started classes. In addition to providing you with opportunities to learn important technical skills, this process involves acquiring the **attitudes**, personal characteristics, and habits of a successful professional. What you think and do while in school will determine, to a great extent, the quality of the professional you will become. Students who demonstrate good work habits in school generally carry those same habits into the workplace. The opposite is true, too. Students who practice poor conduct in school tend to struggle on the job. You are faced with a great opportunity to determine your future. Your career has indeed started now.

The organizational and study skills presented in the first eight chapters of this book are designed to help you succeed in school. But they can also be applied to your professional and personal life. In fact, the term "study skills" is misleading, because these skills are not isolated sets of activities restricted to school situations. "Study skills" have many applications on the job. Let's look at four skills that will be discussed more fully in future chapters. Each one can be applied to your studies, your job search, and your future work in health care. The four skills, along with examples, are summarized in Table 1-1.

TABLE 1-1	Examples of Skill Applications	
School	**Job Search**	**Career**
	APPLICATIONS OF NOTETAKING SKILLS	
Take notes during lectures	Write down facts about job openings	Take notes at staff meetings
Write instructions during lab demonstrations	Find and write down information about the organizations with which you have interviews	Fill out medical history forms
Develop review outlines	Note times, directions, and other information about interviews	Accurately record telephone messages
	List facts learned during interviews	Make notes on patient charts
	APPLICATIONS OF TEST-TAKING SKILLS	
Take daily quizzes	Prepare for national and/or professional exams	Perform daily work accurately and completely
Review and take final exams	Present self successfully at interviews	Participate in annual performance evaluation with supervisor
Demonstrate practical skills	Answer interviewer's questions	It's all a test!

USING ABBREVIATIONS ON THE JOB

Abbreviations are used in health care work, so learning to apply them is an important skill. The following is an example of notes on a patient history form.[3]

Chief complaint: L shoulder pain p̄ playing basketball this AM.

Present illness: Soreness and immobility L shoulder ×8 hours; strained on collision w/ another player

IMPORTANT NOTE: Abbreviations used on medical records *must be standardized* (the same for everyone who adds information), so be sure to use only those that are approved by the facility in which you work. Also, some abbreviations are no longer allowed because they lead to confusion and medical errors. The Joint Commission and the Institute for Safe Medication Practices have both published lists of abbreviations that should not be used on the job.

Information and Skills to Encourage and Empower Students to Succeed

The book is written in a conversational, reader-friendly style. Each major skill, such as test taking, contains many suggestions from which students can choose what they think will work best for them. Specific examples are given so students can see how to apply what is presented in the book.

Tests can turn otherwise sensible individuals into quivering masses of anxiety. For many students, the grades earned on tests influence their feeling of self-worth. You may be worried about appearing stupid and wonder if you have the ability to learn. Or you may feel insecure about your test-taking skills. In reality, your own personal experiences may be helpful in dealing with tests and other stressful situations. Although there is no denying that tests are used as indicators of progress by both instructors and students, understanding more about tests and their purpose can help you control them rather than letting them control you.

UNDERSTANDING YOUR INSTRUCTORS

We have discussed how people have different learning and working styles. Another factor that can influence your academic success is teaching and classroom management styles. Instructors are individuals who have their own ideas about education, teaching methods, and the proper roles of teachers and students. Understanding what is important to your instructors will help you benefit fully from your classes. You will use these same skills to identify the characteristics of your future supervisors so you can work with them more effectively.

Specific Suggestions and Tips for Success

Suggestions for applying the information in the chapters are consolidated into lists called "Success Tips For …" to help students focus on finding methods that will work for them.

 POSITIVE SELF-TALK FOR THIS CHAPTER

1. I have worthy goals and am on track to achieve them.
2. I manage my time efficiently.
3. I am well organized and in control of my life.

BOX 3-2   Greg's Plan for Mastering a List of Medical Terms

- Goal: Over the next 10 weeks, I will learn the meaning, pronunciation, and correct spelling of 300 new medical terms.
- Plan: Learn 30 new terms each week. Study terminology 4 hours per week using flash cards, the workbook, tapes, and self-quizzes. Quiz myself at the end of each week.
- Deadline: 30 terms each week. Achieve goal of 300 words at the end of 10 weeks on (date).
- Resources: Text and workbook; CD that came with the textbook; additional tapes and CDs from the library; suggestions from instructors on best way to learn; medical dictionary.
- Visualization: I see myself in class receiving 100% on the medical terminology test. I see myself using medical terms correctly when talking with a coworker on the job.
- Affirmation: "I, Greg, am mastering medical language easily and on schedule."

Success Tips for Managing Your Time

☐ Consider your priorities and goals when you plan your schedule and decide how to spend your time.

☐ Write out a weekly schedule. Take a few minutes every week to plan ahead. This allows you to coordinate your activities with family members, plan ahead for important days (to avoid trying to find just the right birthday present on the way to the party), combine errands to save time, and plan your study time to avoid last-minute cramming.

☐ Schedule study time every day. This is your top priority! Give yourself a chance to succeed. Arrange not to be disturbed, and let friends and family members know that when you are at your desk, the time is yours.

☐ Schedule around your peak times. We all have individual body rhythms, specific times of the day when we feel most alert and energetic. Some people do their best work late at night. Others accomplish the most between 5:00 AM and 9:00 AM. Class and work schedules cannot always accommodate your needs, but when you have a choice, do the most challenging tasks during your best hours.

☐ Do the hardest thing first. When you have a number of things to do or subjects to study, try tackling the most difficult (or boring or tedious) one first, when you are freshest. Completing unpleasant tasks gives you a surge of energy by removing a source of worry and distraction from your mind and rewarding you with a sense of accomplishment.

☐ Be realistic about what you can accomplish and how much time tasks will take to complete. For example, thinking you can complete a research paper in one weekend can be a serious mistake because you may run into difficulties and end up with no time to spare. You will learn more about your work speed as you progress through your program. At the beginning, it is best to plan more time than you think you will need. On the other hand, take care not to spend more time than necessary on one project or assignment, causing you to neglect all others.

☐ Prevent feeling overwhelmed by breaking work into small segments. (The thought of writing this book was overwhelming until I broke it down into chapters, topics, and pages.) Plan deadlines for each segment, and put them on your calendar. Ask for help and cooperation from family members and friends.

☐ Learn to say "no." Your schedule cannot always accommodate the requests of other people. It's difficult, but sometimes necessary, to turn down demands on our time such as an invitation to a party or a request to help at the church rummage sale. An instructor who reviewed this book said the following response works very well: "I'm really sorry, but I won't be able to help. I wish you the best in finding someone who can."

☐ Use down time to your advantage. There are many pockets of time that usually go to waste, such as when waiting for an appointment or using public transportation. Use this time to study flash cards, write lists, review class notes, brainstorm topics for a research paper, review the steps involved in a lab procedure, or summarize the major points of a class lecture. (I did about half of the work toward my last college degree while sitting in airports and on airplanes!)

Assignments Targeted to Meet Specific Student Needs

Many of the exercises in the test ask the students to apply what they have learned to their own situation.

Prescription for Success 13-12
Increasing Your Job Satisfaction

1. What were your reasons for choosing a career in health care?
   _____
   _____

2. In what ways do you think you will receive satisfaction from your work?
   _____
   _____
   _____

3. How will you measure your success and satisfaction at work?
   _____
   _____
   _____

4. What can you do to make your work fulfilling?
   _____
   _____
   _____

Prescription for Success 11-1
Be Prepared

1. Select a facility where you might want to work.
2. Use the resources suggested in this chapter to learn as much as possible.
   What type of work do they do? _____
   What is their patient population or client base? _____
   What is the size of the staff? _____
   What are the duties and responsibilities of the job(s) for which you might apply?
   _____
   _____
   _____
   _____

   What is the mission of the organization? How does the organization describe its core values?
   _____
   _____
   _____
   _____

Building Block #2
EDUCATION

A list of all your education and training, with emphasis on health care training.

Start your list with the school you attended most recently. Include grade point average and class standing (not all schools rank their students by grades) if they are above average. Use the Resume Buildng Block #2 Education form, on page XX, as a motivator to do your best academically. OBJECTIVE:

_____
_____
_____
_____
_____
_____
_____
_____
_____
_____
_____
_____
_____
_____
_____
_____
_____
_____
_____

NEW TO THIS EDITION

New Chapter

A new chapter entitled "Strategies for Students with Special Situations" has been added to this edition. The chapter contains three sections, each one addressing the concerns of specific groups of postsecondary students: adults with multiple responsibilities, English-as-a-Second Language students, and students with learning disabilities. This chapter was added to encourage and provide specific help to students who face additional challenges in their quest for an education and a health care career. It is intended to be a supplement to the book and to be assigned to students who think that they can benefit from the information and suggestions it contains.

Topics in this chapter include:

Adult Students
Advantages of Being a Mature Student
Time Management—Advanced Techniques
Managing with Children in the House
Maintaining Personal Relationships
Combining Work and School
Overcoming Academic Weaknesses

English for the Non-Native Speaker
Improving Your English
Increasing Your Vocabulary
Idiomatic Expressions
Combining Sounds
Improving Your Reading Comprehension
Improving Your Spelling
Improving Your Grammar

Learning Disabilities
What Is a Learning Disability?
General Suggestions
Specific Strategies for a Variety of Common
    Difficulties

Accommodations
Learning Difficulties During the Job Search

Interviews with Health Care and Education Professionals

The author conducted interviews with a variety of professionals to bring students current, real-world advice. The individuals interviewed included a medical clinic human resource director, a postsecondary school career services' director, nurses, a medical assistant, a direct caregiver in a residence for the elderly and disabled, and the staff in a dental office.

Updated Job-Search Techniques

Hiring trends and methods are continually changing, especially in terms of electronic technology. This edition contains updated Internet search strategies, as well as the latest job-search websites. The section on job interviews has also been updated with more current typical questions and suggestions for succeeding in the increasingly popular behavioral interview.

Spanish Phrases

More health care–related Spanish phrases have been added to Appendix B to help health care professionals better respond to the needs of Spanish-speaking patients.

Internet Resources

Internet resources have been added to the "To Learn More" sections at the end of each chapter. Students are increasingly using the web as a source of information, and larger numbers of reliable sites, such as from university study centers, are becoming available.

LEARNING AIDS

- **Objectives** that help students focus on the most important chapter topics. They provide direction and serve as a checklist for students to assess their mastery of chapter material.
- **Key Terms and Concepts** that include definitions to ensure understanding of important concepts and ideas.
- **Quotes** to inspire, motivate, and promote thinking.

- **Boxes** to provide additional information or applications of chapter material. These include specific examples of how the skills presented are used on the job.
- **Tables** to present facts in an easy-to-read and an easy-to-understand format.
- **Personal Reflection—Journal Entry** questions that are opportunities for students to reflect on how the chapter content applies to them.
- **Prescription for Success** exercises that provide a wide variety of assignments for students to apply the ideas presented, collect additional information, and develop practical skills.
- **To Learn More**, at the end of each chapter, that lists books, articles, and websites that contain further information about the chapter topics.
- **Building Your Resume** exercises that enable students to use resume writing to positively guide their actions while in school and create a resume over time.
- **Internet Activities** that build research skills while taking advantage of student interest in the Internet and the vast number of resources available.

ANCILLARIES

Evolve Resources for the Student

- Chapter quizzes in which students apply what they have learned to themselves
- Internet activities to apply research skills and learn more about each chapter's content
- Weblinks to hundreds of websites that supplement the content of each chapter

Evolve Resources for the Instructor

- TEACH Instructor's Resource, including:
  - **Lesson plans** that include learning objectives; background information about the chapter; references to the book and other instructional materials; and ideas for discussion and critical thinking, class activities, and assessments.
  - **Lecture outlines** for each chapter to guide the presentation of major topics to students.
  - **PowerPoint slides** that include major topics and are coordinated with the lecture outlines.
  - **Instructor's Resource** with additional learning activities for students.
- **ExamView Test bank** with a variety of questions for each chapter to be used for student performance evaluation
- **Answer Keys** to Student Chapter Quizzes and guidance for Internet Activities

FOR STUDENTS

DEAR STUDENT,

I have devoted my professional life to working in education and helping students achieve their education and life goals. The purpose of this book is to provide you with tools to become your best and realize your dreams. It is filled with information and practical tips to help you succeed not only in school, but also on the job. It is not simply a book you will use in class but a useful self-help reference you can use in the years to come.

To make the best use of this book and the tools it contains, I suggest you try the following:

1. Trust yourself. You have the power and ability to succeed.
2. Be willing to try new ideas. If something in the book looks like "too much trouble" or even a little crazy, give it a try and see if it works for you.
3. Don't be overwhelmed by the number of ideas and suggestions in each chapter. They are intended to appeal to a wide range of learning styles, personal preferences, and student needs. You are not expected to do all of them but to choose the ones you think will work best for you.
4. Put forth your best efforts when doing the Prescription for Success exercises. Use them as opportunities to learn, not as "must-do's" to complete an assignment and get a grade.
5. Apply the ideas to your own life. The material is meant to be practical, not simply topics to read and discuss in class.

Start now to become a competent, caring health care professional who will enjoy a satisfying career while making a positive contribution to the lives of others.

Wishing you success
Lee Haroun

Acknowledgments

I would like to thank Patrick Wenrick, RHIA, Director of the Institute of Technology, Inc., and Director of the Coastal Education Institute in Tampa, Florida, for reviewing this text.

Contents

Your Career Starts Now

OBJECTIVES

The information and activities in this chapter can help you:

- Explain the meaning of the concept "Study skills are job skills."
- Give five examples of study skills that can help you succeed in school, obtain the job you want, and increase your worth as a health care professional.
- List three ways you can maximize your school experience.
- Describe how the principles of marketing can be applied to career preparation and the job search.
- Describe what employers and patients expect from health care professionals.
- Identify skills and attitudes you need to develop more fully.
- Develop a personal philosophy of work and identify your work preferences.

KEY TERMS AND CONCEPTS

Attitude: Your mental approach to any situation. It is under your control and can be either positive or negative.

Career Ladder: The organization of occupations or positions in a related field that requires progressively higher levels of skill and responsibility. Additional education or training is often needed to move up the ladder.

Certification: Recognition from a professional or government organization that you have specific knowledge and skills. Certification usually requires taking written and/or hands-on tests.

Clinical Experience: The term used in this book to describe supervised, unpaid work experiences performed by students in health facilities or offices to gain hands-on, practical experience. Other names for this experience include "clinical," "externship," "fieldwork," "internship," "practicum," and "preceptorship."

Commitment: Dedication to something, such as an idea, a relationship, or an organization.

Competency: Mastery of a skill; performing a skill in a manner that meets predetermined standards.

Confidentiality: The act of keeping something, such as medical records, absolutely private.

Consequence: The result, either positive or negative, of taking a certain action.

Empathy: An understanding of the experiences and feelings of another person gained by considering a situation from the other's point of view.

Ethical: Correct and moral.

Ethnic: Referring to the customs and behaviors practiced by a specific racial or national group of people as distinguished from other groups.

Habits: Ways of acting or thinking that are developed over time and become automatic, with little awareness.

Informational Interview: A meeting with someone who works in the career field in which you are interested. The purpose is not to obtain a job but to ask questions and learn as much as possible about the nature of the work.

Integrity: Behavior based on honesty, sincerity, and good intentions.

License: Legal approval given to professionals to ensure that only those who are properly trained can perform certain duties. Licenses are granted by governmental bodies and require applicants to meet specific educational requirements and to pass tests.

Per Diem: Work performed on an on-call basis.

Philosophy: The system of beliefs that forms the foundation of a person's view of the world and ideas about the meaning of life.

Prioritize: To rank a group of items or tasks in order of importance.

Reason: To organize facts so they make sense and/or help you draw correct conclusions.

Self-Esteem: The way people see themselves and the opinions they have about their appearance, competence, intelligence, and other personal characteristics.

Standard Precautions: Practices that prevent the transmission of disease through the microorganisms (germs) present in blood and other body fluids.

Sterile Technique: Special procedures used to create an environment that is free of all living microorganisms.

Vulnerable: Being physically and/or emotionally weakened and possibly dependent on others.

YOUR FIRST STEP ON THE ROAD TO SUCCESS

"Today is the first day of the rest of your life."

Congratulations! By choosing to study for a career in health care, you have taken the first step toward achieving a productive and satisfying future. You have made a significant **commitment** to yourself and your community. By enrolling in an educational program, you have demonstrated your ability to set your sights on the future, make important decisions, and follow through with action. You have proven you have the strong personal foundation on which you can build the skills and **habits** needed to ensure your success in school and in your career.

The purpose of this book is to help you succeed in this building process by sharing the knowledge and

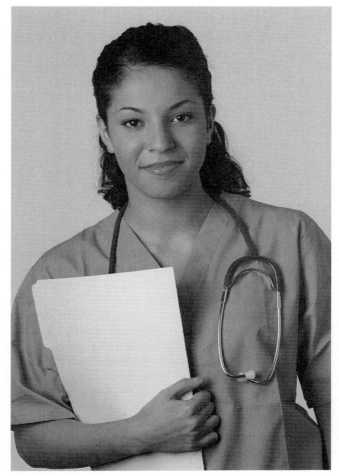

Figure 1–1   What you do now will influence your future success. Employers suggest treating school as you would a job. Dressing professionally, arriving to class on time, and completing homework accurately are a few ways to develop good work habits. What are other behaviors you can practice while pursuing your studies?

techniques that have helped other students achieve their goals. It is written with the hope that you will apply what you learn here to maximize your investment in education, secure the job that you want after graduation, and find satisfaction in your career as a competent and caring health care professional like the young woman in Figure 1-1.

CONNECTING SCHOOL AND CAREER

The process of becoming a health care professional began the day you started classes. In addition to providing you with opportunities to learn important technical skills, this process involves acquiring the **attitudes**, personal characteristics, and habits of a successful professional. What you think and do while in school will determine, to a great extent, the quality of the professional you will become. Students who demonstrate good work habits in school generally carry

TABLE 1–1	Examples of Skill Applications	
School	Job Search	Career
APPLICATIONS OF TIME MANAGEMENT SKILLS		
Plan study schedule Attend classes on time Meet deadlines for assignments Prepare for exams Balance school and job schedules Allocate time for family	Pursue job leads without delay Schedule interviews Arrive for appointments and interviews on time Send thank-you notes promptly Follow up in a timely way	Schedule and track patient appointments Balance work, family, and personal needs Allocate time for patient treatments Follow facility schedules Schedule time for continuing education activities
APPLICATIONS OF ORAL COMMUNICATION SKILLS		
Ask questions in class Answer questions in class Present oral reports Share information with classmates	Make telephone inquiries about job openings Introduce yourself to potential employers Ask questions of potential employers Present your qualifications at interviews	Participate in staff meetings Give instructions to patients Relay information to co-workers Give reports to supervisor
APPLICATIONS OF NOTE-TAKING SKILLS		
Take notes during lectures Write instructions during lab demonstrations List important ideas when reading Develop review outlines	Write down facts about job openings Find and write down information about the organizations with which you have interviews Note times, directions, and other information about interviews List facts learned during interviews	Take notes at staff meetings Fill out medical history forms Accurately record telephone messages Make notes on patient charts
APPLICATIONS OF TEST-TAKING SKILLS		
Take daily quizzes Review and take final exams Demonstrate practical skills	Prepare for national and/or professional exams Present self successfully at interviews Answer interviewer's questions	Perform daily work accurately and completely Participate in annual performance evaluation with supervisor It's all a test!

those same habits into the workplace. The opposite is true, too. Students who practice poor conduct in school tend to struggle on the job. You are faced with a great opportunity to determine your future. Your career has indeed started now.

The organizational and study skills presented in the first eight chapters of this book are designed to help you succeed in school. But they can also be applied to your professional and personal life. In fact, the term "study skills" is misleading, because these skills are not isolated sets of activities restricted to school situations. "Study skills" have many applications on the job. Let's look at four skills that will be discussed more fully in future chapters. Each one can be applied to your studies, your job search, and your future work in health care. The four skills, along with examples, are summarized in Table 1-1.

1. **Time management.** For busy people, time is one of the most precious possessions. Juggling class attendance and study time with family responsibilities, work, and personal time involves **prioritizing** and careful planning. Your success in school depends heavily on how well you organize your time.

An effective job search typically requires you to devote time each day to identifying leads, making appointments, attending interviews, and completing follow-up activities. You must allocate adequate amounts of time for these efforts and organize your time to avoid delays that could cost you employment opportunities.

Once you are on the job, effective use of time is critical in health care work. Many health care professionals are responsible not only for their own time, but also for planning other people's time. Medical assistants, for example, are often in charge of the physician's daily appointment scheduling, a task that can affect the profitability of the practice. Insurance coders and billers must submit claims on time to avoid rejections and financial losses. Nurses who have patient care responsibilities must plan a schedule that permits them to complete these during their shifts.

2. **Oral communication.** Strong communication skills are essential to success. Expressing yourself clearly is important for giving presentations, as well as for asking and answering questions in class. It is also necessary for establishing and

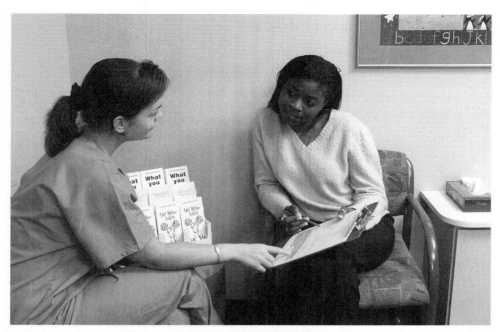

Figure 1–2   Good oral communication skills are essential for delivering effective health care. Patients must understand their condition and what they can do to promote their own health. Notice the body posture and eye contact this health care professional is demonstrating. What are other characteristics of good communication?

maintaining satisfactory relationships with your instructors and classmates.

A critical part of the job search process is the interview, in which you combine your ability to think clearly and use verbal skills effectively. Feeling confident about expressing yourself will enable you to present your qualifications in a convincing way.

All jobs today require good communication skills. This is especially true in health care because many positions involve constant interaction with others, including patients, co-workers, supervisors, and the general public. Interaction with a patient is illustrated in Figure 1-2. Physical and occupational therapy assistants are examples of the many health professionals who provide extensive patient education. The effectiveness of their explanations of exercises and self-care techniques influences the rehabilitation progress of their clients.

3. **Taking notes.** You may think of note-taking as being limited to use in lectures, but this skill is used extensively outside the classroom. During the job search, it will be important to accurately record information about job openings, as well as interview appointment dates and times and directions to facilities. After interviews, you may want to make notes about the job requirements, additional information you need to send to the prospective employer, and other important facts.

When you become employed, you will be expected to absorb a lot of new information about your facility's rules and procedures, the location of supplies and equipment, people's names, and many other details. You can use your note-taking skills to create a personal reference notebook, a resource that will increase your efficiency on the job. Note-taking is also an important health care job skill. Many professionals are responsible for interviewing patients and taking notes on special forms called *patient histories*. Another specialized form of medical note-taking is called *charting*. Charting means making notes on patient medical records, in either written or electronic form. The notes include information about symptoms, treatments, and medications prescribed. These medical records not only affect patient care, but they also are legal documents. They must be clear, accurate, and complete.

4. **Taking tests.** You may think you have escaped the dreaded test once you leave school, but testing is not limited to the classroom. The truth is that life is full of tests. Job interviews are a form of test designed to assess your ability to present yourself and your qualifications. To legally work in many health care occupations, such as licensed practical nurse, radiologic technologist, and physical therapist, you must pass a professional exam. Other occupations, such as medical assistant, have voluntary tests to obtain certification that improves your chances of getting a job. In fact, many employers hire only certified medical assistants.

Once on the job, you are in a sense, being tested every day. Although you may not think of your everyday tasks as tests, they are applications

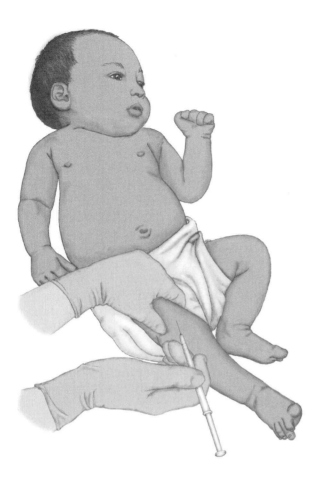

Figure 1–3   The mother of this infant wants to know that the health care professional giving the injection has "passed the test" and is qualified to safely perform this task. *(From James SR, Ashwill JW:* Nursing care of children: principles and practice, *ed 3, St Louis, 2007, Saunders.)*

of what you have learned, and your ability to perform them correctly will be noted by your patients, co-workers, and supervisor. The annual employee performance evaluation may be considered a type of test in which your supervisor writes a report about your work and then meets with you to discuss it. Learning to perform "when it counts" is a valuable skill and represents the ultimate ability to take and successfully pass a test. The mother of the infant in Figure 1-3 wants to know that the health care professional giving the injection has "passed the test" and is qualified to safely perform this task.

From these examples you can see that skills traditionally labeled as personal or school skills have valuable applications during the job search and on the job. Throughout this book you will continue to see how "school skills" are also valuable job skills.

Go to page 16 to complete Prescription for Success 1-1

MAXIMIZING YOUR EDUCATION

You are making a significant investment of time, effort, and money in your education. You can simply get by, doing only what is required to pass your classes, or you can fully benefit from this investment. A worthy personal goal is to do everything possible to become the best health care professional possible. Both you and your school have responsibilities to ensure that this happens.

Your Rights as a Student

"Making mistakes is inevitable. Not learning from them is inexcusable."

1. **Make mistakes.** You may think this sounds a little strange. After all, aren't you supposed to do the best you can, earning the highest grades possible? Yes, but many students see grades as ends in themselves, rather than as signs of having mastered the skills they will need in the future. Good grades do not guarantee mastery, nor do you receive grades for all the skills that will determine your future success.

   Many students want to know "what's on the test" so they can focus their efforts on learning only what they will be tested on. But think about it—can you possibly be tested on everything you will need to know and do to perform your job? If you were, all class time would have to be devoted to testing, leaving little or no time for learning! Studying only what you need to pass tests and earn grades may make you a "good student," but a good student is not necessarily a good health care professional.

   Compare your educational experience with learning to ride a bike. First, you use training wheels, go slowly, and tip over once in a while. Eventually you become a proficient cyclist, ready for the big race. School offers you a rehearsal for professional life, providing you with opportunities to learn from mistakes that would be unacceptable if you were to make them on the job. If you do not score 100% on an exam, it has still served you by allowing you to make mistakes and learn from them so you avoid making them on the job when the consequences are more serious. The health care worker in Figure 1-4 may have made mistakes when she practiced working with a classmate, but she learned from them and is now able to use correct techniques to help her patients.

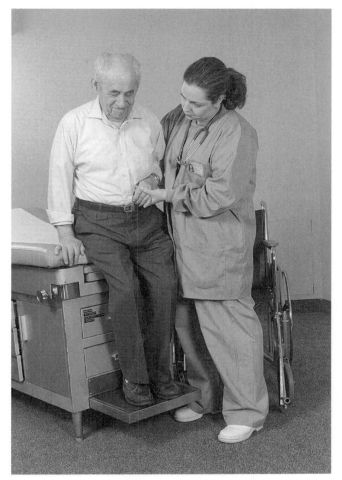

Figure 1–4 The time to learn—and even make a few mistakes—is while you are in school. You want to be competent on the job when you work with patients like this man, who depend on your knowledge. Perfecting your skills, as well as developing a caring and respectful attitude, will help you contribute to the well-being of all your patients.

2. **Ask questions.** You are attending school to benefit from the knowledge and experience of your instructors. Take advantage of this opportunity by being an active participant in your classes. Don't be an invisible student. Even if the textbooks and lectures are excellent, you may still need to ask for explanations, examples, and additional resources. If there is anything you don't understand, ask questions. Students aren't expected to understand everything the first time they hear or read it—maybe not even the second time. Consider this: there would be no need for you to attend school at all if you already knew the information presented in your program.

   Many adults are afraid of "looking stupid" and hesitate to admit they don't understand or are confused. However, failure to ask questions not only decreases the chances of maximizing your education, it prevents you from learning a critical health care skill—asking questions. Consider the serious consequences for professionals who are not sure of drug dosages or steps in a procedure but are afraid to ask their supervisors for direction. In these situations, risking the well-being of patients is indeed stupid, whereas asking questions demonstrates intelligence. Start learning now to be comfortable asking questions. If it is too difficult for you to speak up in class the first few times you have questions, start out by speaking with your instructor at the break, after class, or during office hours.

   Of course, you should not use questions to substitute for reading your textbook or studying assigned material before each class meeting. This results in the misuse of class time and is unfair to students who are prepared. A related on-the-job example is employees who arrive late and unprepared for meetings, thus wasting their co-workers' time. Develop habits that show consideration for others and will contribute now to the efficiency of the classroom and later to that of the workplace.

3. **Take advantage of school resources.** Every school wants every student who enrolls to graduate, and considerable resources are spent on services to support this effort. Find out now what services are available to you, the hours they can be accessed, and whether appointments are necessary. Two of the most important services that all students should become familiar with are the library (or resource center) and career services (sometimes called *job placement*).

   If you are having personal problems or academic difficulties, ask whether your school provides counseling and/or tutoring. Some schools refer their students to outside agencies that offer assistance for difficulties such as dealing with domestic abuse and finding reliable child care. Asking for help when you need it can make the difference between dropping out and graduating and becoming successfully employed.

   The school catalog is an often overlooked information resource that can help you succeed in school. Many students never take the time to read it and as a result are unaware of available resources. Even worse, they risk unknowingly breaking rules or missing important deadlines. Spend a few minutes becoming an informed student by reading the catalog and other printed information. On the job, you will likely be expected to read organizational handbooks and procedure manuals. Getting in the habit of reading informational literature is a good job skill.

 Go to page 16 to complete Prescription for Success 1-2

Your Responsibilities as a Student

1. **Attend all scheduled learning activities.** Health care educational programs feature a variety of learning opportunities including lectures, lab sessions, guest speakers, field trips, and hands-on experiences in health care facilities. Your instructor may also recommend additional activities outside of those organized by the school, such as watching a television documentary, attending a professional meeting, or visiting a medical supply company. These activities are designed to help you understand and master all the knowledge and skills necessary for your future work, as well as to provide exposure to your future work environment. You cannot afford to miss them. They are opportunities to develop the competencies essential for working in health care. Learning to perform essential tasks, such as the administration of injections, requires you to spend time and put forth effort under the guidance of your instructors. Now is the time for learning and making mistakes, not when you are faced with your first patient. Someday you will be performing tasks that affect the well-being of others, so it is essential that you fully participate in every learning activity offered in your program.

    Employers routinely request information about a student's attendance record. Good attendance is considered a valuable job skill because health care services are driven by time requirements. The success of a private physician's practice depends heavily on efficient patient scheduling and service. Hospitals have daily responsibilities for performing hundreds of treatments, procedures, and surgeries that must be completed in a timely way. In both settings, effective care can be provided only if the staff is available to do the work. Patients who need help should not have to wait because someone didn't show up. Start now to develop the habit of consistent and punctual attendance.

 Go to page 18 to complete Prescription for Success 1-3

2. **Apply your best efforts to learning.** As a student, you have the right to ask questions and make mistakes. At the same time, it is your responsibility to complete all reading, writing, and lab assignments and to participate actively in class. Instructors cannot cover everything you are expected to know. Learning will require effort on your part. The study techniques and suggestions for learning presented in the following chapters are intended to help you succeed as a student.

    In performing your work as a health care professional, you will encounter new situations in which you will apply what you learned in school. To be successful in those situations, you must now focus on your studies, work hard, and be persistent. Your willingness to do the "shoulds" when you would rather be doing the "wants" will be a major determinant of your success. You will not always feel like studying after a day that may include classes, a few hours on the job, and family responsibilities. Being a college student is not always easy. Keeping your long-term career goals clearly in mind will help you find the self-discipline to stick with it.

3. **Ask for help when you need it.** Instructors and administrators want to see their students succeed. Educators are interested in helping students complete their programs and graduate. At the same time, you must take responsibility for requesting assistance. Ignoring problems will not solve them; they usually only get worse. Don't wait until you are hopelessly lost in a class and cannot possibly be ready for the upcoming final exam before asking for help. Take charge of your learning and at the first sign of trouble, ask about tutoring, study groups, computer labs, and any other resources available through the school.

    If you experience problems of a personal or financial nature, refer to the list of school resources you prepared in Prescription for Success 1-2. Remember that asking for help when you need it is a sign of strength, not weakness, and it is one of the main actions that distinguish a graduate from a dropout.

    The flip side of asking for help is being willing to give it. Offer your assistance to others in the school community. Volunteer to hand out papers for the instructor. Give a student who lives in your area a ride to school. Tutor a classmate who is struggling with a subject you find easy. (This doesn't mean sharing your work; it means helping the other person understand and learn.) You have chosen a profession that is based on giving service, and this is a habit you can start practicing now in all areas of your life. Students who give of themselves are the type of people who become indispensable employees.

PLANNING FOR CAREER SUCCESS

The time to start thinking about your first job in health care is now, as you are starting your educational program. In the following pages, we look at how you can use job search tools, such as a resume, to help guide you to a successful career.

PERSONAL REFLECTION

What are some other ways you can take responsibility for your own learning so that you succeed in your health care program?

_____

_____

_____

_____

_____

BOX 1-1   Recent Job Postings

The following are the stated requirements from 2009 employment postings at a large clinic and a hospital.

URGENT CARE NURSE

- Computer skills are a must
- Team player with excellent communication skills
- Must have excellent organization skills and the ability to multitask in a very busy team environment

ONCOLOGY MEDICAL ASSISTANT

- Must be able to maintain confidentiality
- Ability to work quickly with attention to detail and accuracy
- Ability to provide excellent customer service
- Must be a self-motivated, task-oriented individual

And the Product Is...You!

Marketing is a multi-step process that begins with an idea for a new product and ends with the sale of that product. Mastering this process is essential for the survival of any business. Successful marketing is similar to successfully starting a new career. You—the combination of your skills, characteristics, and talents—are the product. To make sure you have the skills and qualities needed by employers, you must prepare appropriately for the workplace and learn to present yourself effectively during the job search.

The marketing process can be organized into a five-part plan called the "Five Ps of Marketing," as follows:

1. Planning
2. Production
3. Packaging
4. Presentation
5. Promotion

You can use the 5 Ps to develop your own personal marketing plan now, as you begin your health care studies, to help ensure future career success. We will discuss the first P, planning, in this chapter and the remaining four Ps in Chapter 2.

PLANNING: THE FIRST "P" OF MARKETING

"Give yourself a running start."

Studying the needs of customers is called _market research,_ and its purpose is to find out what customers want. Your customers will include your future employers and patients. Waiting until the end of your educational program to think about getting a job is like creating a product without doing market research. Designing and manufacturing a product that no one wants or needs doesn't make sense. Just like a business, you are investing time, effort, and money in the development of yourself as a product.

What Do Employers Want?

In recent years, employers in all industries have expressed concerns that entry-level workers are not adequately prepared for the modern workplace. Employers are looking for job candidates who not only are qualified technically, but who also bring essential supporting skills such as the ability to communicate effectively, work cooperatively with others, accept responsibility, and solve problems. These skills are especially critical in the health care industry because it is service-based and depends heavily on the quality of its personnel. This is even truer today as health care facilities strive to provide higher quality care and control costs. See Box 1-1 for a sample of the skills requested in February, 2009, job postings.

SCANS Report

In the late 1980s a commission appointed by the U.S. Secretary of Labor conducted a nationwide employer survey to determine the **competencies** needed by all entry-level workers. The resulting report, called _A SCANS Report for America 2000,_ was published in 1991. It organized lists of competencies that have become known as the SCANS Skills. (_SCANS_ stands for Secretary's Commission for Achieving Necessary Skills.) Even though this report has been out for a number of years, the skills listed are still relevant today. For example, "being responsible" remains an essential characteristic for an employee, especially in health care.

BOX 1-2 Highlights from the SCANS Report

Employers want workers who can do the following:
- Think creatively
- Make decisions
- Solve problems
- Continue to learn
- **Reason**
- Identify, organize, plan, and allocate resources
- Work with others
- Manage themselves
- Acquire and use information
- Understand complex interrelationships
- Work with a variety of technologies
- Be responsible
- Believe in their self-worth
- Demonstrate **empathy**
- Demonstrate **integrity** and honesty

BOX 1-3 Examples of the National Healthcare Foundation Standards and Accountability Criteria

Health care workers will:
- Apply speaking and active listening skills
- Summarize basic professional standards of health care workers as they apply to hygiene, dress, language, confidentiality, and behavior
- Exemplify professional characteristics
- Engage in continuous self-assessment and career goal modification for personal and professional growth
- Apply **ethical** standards in health care
- Demonstrate respectful and empathetic interactions with diverse age, cultural, economic, **ethnic,** and religious groups
- Recognize methods for building positive team relationships
- Apply behaviors that promote health and wellness
- Recognize technology applications in health care[1]

Earlier in this chapter you read about how the sets of skills commonly referred to as "study skills" can be applied to all areas of your life. Take a look at the SCANS Competencies in Box 1-2 and note that the same is true for them. For example, demonstrating integrity and honesty as a student means you set high standards for yourself and do your own work to complete assignments and take exams; as a job applicant, it means you present yourself honestly in job interviews and apply for only those positions for which you are competent; and as an employee, it means you never cut corners when working with patients and fellow staff members.

Go to page 19 to complete Prescription for Success 1-4

National Health Care Skill Standards

A project of special interest to future health care professionals is the National Health Care Skill Standards, a list of entry-level worker competencies. Box 1-3 contains examples that apply to all health care occupations. You can see that they are not limited to technical skills, such as taking blood pressure, but include the ability to communicate, maintain good attendance, and demonstrate responsibility. Some employers report that these so-called "soft skills" are as important as technical skills in the provision of good health care.

Did you notice how many standards mention the ability to communicate well? The lack of effective communication skills among health care workers is reportedly the leading contributor to patient dissatisfaction and personnel problems in health care facilities. Your future success can be greatly enhanced by your ability to listen and to convey information effectively.

Go to page 20 to complete Prescription for Success 1-5

Professional Organizations

Many of the professional organizations that represent specific health care occupations have statements outlining the characteristics needed to work in their fields. Box 1-4 contains examples from four associations. Note how certain characteristics, such as working well with people, appear in all of them.

Go to page 21 to complete Prescription for Success 1-6

What Do Patients Want?

"Patients do not care how much you know until they know how much you care."

Patients want to receive competent care delivered with consideration and respect. When seeking health care, people are often at their most **vulnerable.** They fear what might be discovered during a diagnostic test or that they will experience pain during a necessary treatment. The **self-esteem** of patients can be threatened by a feeling of powerlessness that often accompanies illness and injury.

BOX 1-4   A Word from Health Care Professional Organizations

AMERICAN ASSOCIATION OF RESPIRATORY CARE

"If you want to join this field, you must be sensitive to the needs of patients who have serious physical impairments. You must work well as a member of a team. You need superior communication skills to deal with other members of the health care team, your patients, and their families. The ability to pay close attention to detail and to follow instructions are prerequisites for practitioners. Because much of your work will center on the equipment you use, you should have an interest in learning the mechanics of medical technology."

AMERICAN ACADEMY OF PHYSICIAN ASSISTANTS

People who are considering becoming physicians' assistants should have the following characteristics:
- "Enjoy helping people
- Want to learn and grow

- Want a challenging and rewarding career
- Want responsibility
- Want to make a difference."

AMERICAN SOCIETY OF PODIATRIC MEDICAL ASSISTANTS

"Enjoy contact with people and have a willingness to help them...the ability to do neat and precise work... good manual dexterity...along with cooperativeness, good judgment, and a pleasant personality are valuable and necessary assets for a successful podiatric assistant."

AMERICAN PHARMACEUTICAL ASSOCIATION

"Qualifications:
- Professional demeanor
- Ability to respect **confidentiality** of patient data
- Strong communication skills
- Courteous attitude."

Many patients want to participate in making decisions about their care. They have the right, both ethically and legally, to be fully informed about their condition, treatment options, and possible outcomes. Health care professionals must give clear explanations in everyday language and offer patients the opportunity to ask questions and receive honest answers. At the same time, patients want and have the legal right to confidentiality. As a health care professional, you must guard the privacy of your patients. Without the patient's permission, nothing can be discussed with anyone other than the health care team members directly involved with the patient's care, and all files and paperwork must be securely stored and electronic records protected.

Changes in American society and increasing costs of providing medical care have brought special challenges for patients and for health care professionals. In the past, many people had the same physician throughout their lives. Doctor and patient belonged to the same community, and a sense of trust developed over the years. Patients today may see a different physician each time they visit their health care facility. They may face a serious illness or life-threatening situation in the care of a stranger, adding to the stress of an already difficult situation. Studies have shown that patients who belong to a caring, supportive community recover more successfully than patients who don't. Providing a supportive health care community can improve patient outcomes. As a health care professional, you can demonstrate a caring attitude that helps develop a bond of trust with patients by being attentive, listening carefully, and practicing empathy.

Health care professionals today face the challenge of working with patients from many different ethnic backgrounds, some of whom have beliefs about health care practices that differ from those of traditional Western medicine. Patients also come from many different economic and social groups. They may have lifestyles or personal beliefs with which you disagree. All patients have the right to be respected and to receive appropriate, high-level care, regardless of your personal opinions about them. Every patient deserves your best efforts.

Patients seek help in solving their health problems, but your responsibilities in meeting their needs go beyond performing a painless blood draw, giving effective breathing treatments, or sending out accurate bills for payment. You must be willing to combine a caring attitude with technical competence by treating each patient as worthy of your full attention. Studies have found that even if a health professional excels in one area, poor communication skills or the appearance of not caring can cause patients to view that person negatively.[2] Box 1-5 contains a list of important characteristics that patients seek in their health care providers.

The Patient Care Partnership

Health care organizations have formally recognized the rights of patients to receive proper care. The American Hospital Association has written a brochure for patients, entitled "The Patient Care

BOX 1-5   What Do Patients Want?

- Competent care
- Someone who listens
- Clear communication
- Courtesy
- Compassion
- Empathy
- Understanding
- Sincerity
- Respect

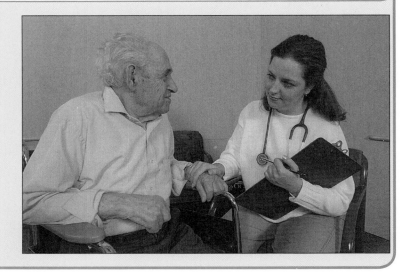

Partnership: Understand Expectations, Rights and Responsibilities," which is used by many health care facilities nationwide. These include, among others, the rights of patients to do the following:

- Be treated with compassion and respect
- Receive information about the benefits and risks of treatments
- Have their privacy protected
- Participate in making decisions regarding their care, including the right to refuse treatment
- Have their health goals and values taken into account as much as possible

Go to page 22 to complete Prescription for Success 1-7

What Do You Want?

"If you don't know where you're going, chances are you'll end up somewhere else."

In addition to exploring the needs of your "customers"—your employers and patients—an important part of planning is to identify what *you* want. You must consider your own needs and desires as you create your professional self. The clearer you are about your career goals and expectations, the greater the chance you have of achieving them.

Beginning now to think about your specific career goals and workplace priorities will keep you alert to appropriate employment possibilities as you go through your educational program. Take every opportunity during your studies to observe, ask questions, and read about your field. Then compare your findings with your own interests. Many fields in health care today feature newly

created positions and expanded responsibilities for traditional jobs. A wide variety of choices is available for new graduates. Being aware of these opportunities improves your chances of finding employment that matches your interests and preferences.

Developing a Philosophy of Work

Most of us spend a significant number of our waking hours on the job. How we spend that time determines, to a great degree, the quality of our lives. It makes sense, then, to think about what work means to you. Exploring your personal beliefs will help you increase the amount of satisfaction you get from your career. The following list contains a variety of reasons why people work[3]:

- Survive financially
- Define self
- Gain self-respect
- Demonstrate competence
- Gain power
- Help others
- Learn
- Experience variety
- Contribute to the community
- Experience enjoyment
- Fill time

People are generally happiest and most productive when their work provides them with more than material rewards. Some people are motivated by continual challenges, others value consistency, and still others are content with either condition as long as their work allows them to help others.

Health care is a complex, ever-changing field that offers both opportunities and challenges for those

Q&A with a Health Care Professional
Charlie McKnee

Charlie McKnee provides direct care to older adults in a long-term care facility. Charlie answers questions about beginning a career in health professions and his own experiences.

Q What would you say to someone who is starting a career in health care?

A First, I would say, "Congratulations, you've chosen a very honorable profession." As such, you're an honored and increasingly valuable person. People who take care of others for a living tend to be very giving. I think health care providers need to understand themselves and their own needs—and then take care of themselves, too. If they completely sacrifice themselves for the sake of others, this leads to burnout and their own health problems.

Q What can health care professionals do to take care of themselves?

A First, they need to understand their own importance and give themselves the respect they deserve. Realistically, patients aren't always able to show their appreciation because of their own problems. So health care professionals really have to recognize their own value—give themselves a pat on the back for work well done. They should also review their own strengths and limitations. They need to take care of their mental as well as physical health. My personal belief is that mental health comes before physical health, so I'm really big on this one.

Q It sounds like you have a holistic view of health, right?

A Absolutely. I really believe that as health care providers we should be aware of the emotional, spiritual, and social needs of our patients and residents. We leave too much out if we just focus on the physical. We need to see the multiple aspects of health if we are to truly experience love, concern, and purpose in our work.

Q Your specialty is working with older adults. Why do you find this work satisfying?

A I believe that older people have been stigmatized. Society says, "They're old, they have problems, they need our help." At the same time, many people kind of give up on them. They assume they are in decline and work from a disease model—that is, just taking care of any acute problems. I prefer to work from a wellness model. That means helping the people I work with to set goals and think about improving and being able to do more. Just sitting in a wheelchair—that shouldn't be how a person lives out their later years. I believe that older adults have many strengths. I like to do what I can to help them meet their potential. And to see what I—and we, as a society—can learn from them.

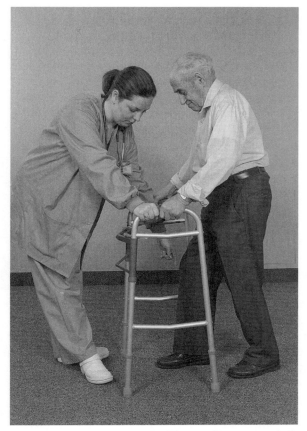

Figure 1–5   An occupation in health care allows you to help others improve their quality of life. This health care worker is helping a patient to overcome his physical limitations. Patients of all ages and conditions deserve your best efforts.

who choose to work in it. Here are some of the major sources of satisfaction you can expect.

1. **Meaningful work.** Good health is a basic need for both human survival and happiness. Working in a field that promotes health gives you the opportunity to make meaningful contributions to the well-being of others. Whether you provide direct patient care or perform supporting activities, your work directly affects patients, and the quality of your work can truly make a difference in their lives. A career in health care has purpose and value.

2. **Opportunity to serve.** People seek the services of health care professionals when they need help. They come with the hope that you can help them solve their problems, and they entrust themselves to your care. You have opportunities to enter both the physical and emotional space of others, sharing close personal contact. People who are ill or injured are often afraid and anxious. You, like the health care professional working with the patient in Figure 1-5, are in a position to influence their recovery.

3. **Career stability.** The need for health care will always exist, even if job titles change over time. The reorganization taking place in today's health

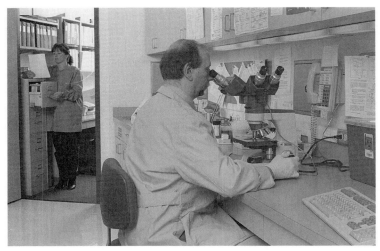

Figure 1–6 Advances in medical science are happening at an astonishing rate. Life-saving drugs, discoveries in genetics, increased knowledge of the role of DNA in body functions, and advances in cancer research are but a few examples. You can look forward to many changes in the coming years.

care delivery systems is causing continual shifts in the need for specific occupational positions. A decrease in the number of job openings for one position is often balanced by an increase in another. You may need to redefine your job in the future, but you will always have a solid knowledge base on which you can add the experience or training needed to qualify for new positions.

4. **Interesting work environment.** The world of health care is changing at a rapid rate, both scientifically and organizationally. Advances in our understanding of how the body works, along with discoveries about the causes and treatments of diseases, are reported almost daily. Computers have increased our capacity to collect and organize information and are sophisticated tools that are constantly being upgraded. Medical scientists like the one in Figure 1-6 are making discoveries at an astounding rate. You will witness advances in knowledge that extend and improve the quality of human life. The health care environment is never boring. There will be a steady stream of interesting information to learn, apply, and use.

5. **Opportunities for advancement.** The health care field provides many opportunities for upward mobility if you are willing to continue learning and adding to your skills. Many jobs offer opportunities for on-the-job learning that enable you to increase your value to your patients and employer, as well as your eligibility for promotion. In addition, many occupational specialties in health care present the chance for **career laddering**. Career ladders contain jobs within one occupational area that require different levels of knowledge and skills. The higher-level positions almost always require further education and additional **certifications** or **licenses,** which are official approvals for working

in a specific occupation. (You will learn more about these approvals in Chapter 2. Career laddering is discussed in more detail in Chapter 14.)

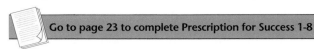

Go to page 23 to complete Prescription for Success 1-8

Work Preferences

It is also a good idea to begin thinking about the kinds of tasks you like to do and the working conditions you prefer. A wide variety of work settings exists for health care professionals. Being clear about your own preferences will help you choose and prepare for the most appropriate types of positions in your career area.

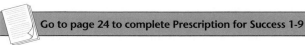

Go to page 24 to complete Prescription for Success 1-9

Alignment with Employers

Although it is important to try to meet your personal needs when seeking employment, you must also have realistic expectations. An essential activity in career planning is to compare your work preferences with the needs of potential employers to see how well they match. Students sometimes have unrealistic goals for the positions they hope to fill immediately after graduation. Recent graduates are qualified for entry-level positions. You can avoid frustration and disappointment if you understand the workplace and adjust your expectations. This way, you can maximize the benefits of your first work experiences in health care.

Formal training is only the beginning of your journey to developing competence as a health care professional. Your skills will continue to grow and be refined as you accumulate hands-on practice and everyday experience in the field. When starting a new career, it may be wise—even necessary—to trade your "perfect job" requirements for opportunities that lead to long-term career success. Consider looking for a first-time job in which you can do the following:

1. Gain self-confidence
2. Work with a variety of people
3. Acquire additional knowledge
4. Increase your skill base
5. Explore specialties within your field of interest
6. Network with other professionals
7. Demonstrate your abilities

Your first employer is giving you the gift of his or her confidence in your abilities. You will be entrusted with serious responsibilities that may include patient welfare, accuracy and confidentiality of important records, and other matters that influence the reputation and success of the facility. You will have a chance to prove your value by learning as much as possible, finding ways to help your employer and coworkers, and contributing to the overall success of the organization. Entry-level jobs, performed well, can be the first important step leading to positions that meet all your hopes for a fulfilling career.

Alignment with Your Profession

Health care professions vary in the type of work performed. You need to be aware of the daily tasks and working conditions of the occupation you have chosen. For example, respiratory therapy and radiology require the technical aptitude to work with complex equipment. Occupational therapy requires the ability to apply oral communication skills to teach patients and their families. Health information technology and insurance coding require accuracy and attention to detail when creating, filling out, and organizing medical records and forms.

You may need to consider tradeoffs to obtain a balance that offers maximum career satisfaction. For example, a recent nursing graduate who wants the excitement of a hospital emergency room and the convenience of a 9:00 AM to 5:00 PM weekday schedule may have a conflict. To avoid a mismatch between your expectations and the real world, learn as much as possible about the specific requirements of your future profession so you can rethink and reprioritize your requirements, if necessary.

Adjusting your short-term expectations doesn't mean giving up your long-term goals. In fact, purposeful planning now can help you arrive where you want to be in the future. If you discover that the specific type of job you want requires previous work experience, you can set short-term goals to serve as stepping stones to acquire that experience. Find out now what skills are emphasized in your target position and look for opportunities to learn as many of them as possible during your studies, **clinical experience**, and first job. For example, Rosa wants to work as a back-office medical assistant with a plastic surgeon, helping the physician with outpatient procedures. Her research shows there are only a few plastic surgeons in her area and they prefer to hire assistants with previous work experience. Rosa decides to look for a job with a general practitioner or pediatrician who does minor surgery in the office. Her short-term goals are to gain experience with **sterile technique**, **standard precautions**, surgical assisting, and patient care. While in school, she asks her instructor to recommend books and articles about plastic surgery and to allow her to spend extra practice time in the lab so she can reach a high level of competence with sterile technique, surgical instruments, wound care, and related topics.

Employees who are willing to meet the expectations of their employers are often rewarded with additional (and interesting) responsibilities and promotions. Some employers even create new positions so they can use the talents of their employees. For new health care professionals who are well prepared and who contribute enthusiastically to the success of their employers, entry-level jobs can serve as launch pads for career success. You, too, may benefit by having new and interesting responsibilities added to your job description, receiving a promotion, or having a job created that brings you satisfaction. Serving the needs of others can provide you with opportunities to meet your own needs.

Go to page 25 to complete Prescription for Success 1-10

Go to page 26 to complete Prescription for Success 1-11

Go to page 28 to complete Prescription for Success 1-12

Go to page 28 to complete Prescription for Success 1-13

SUMMARY OF KEY IDEAS

1. Your career as a health care professional starts now.
2. Study skills are also job skills.
3. As a student, you have both rights and responsibilities.
4. An effective health care professional needs more than good technical skills.

5. Preparing for a new career is like creating and marketing a new product.

To Learn More

About.com: Health Careers

http://healthcareers.about.com

This web page contains links to articles about choosing and succeeding in a health care career.

American Hospital Association: *The Patient Care Partnership*

www.aha.org/aha/issues/Communicating-With-Patients/pt-care-partnership.html.

This brochure contains an explanation of the rights of hospitalized patients.

Covey SR: *The 7 habits of highly effective people,* New York, 2004, Free Press.

This popular book lists seven principles that help individuals live effective lives. Students may find it helpful to learn about the seven habits, which are as follows:

- Habit 1: Be Proactive: Principles of Personal Choice
- Habit 2: Begin with the End in Mind: Principles of Personal Vision
- Habit 3: Put First Things First: Principles of Integrity and Execution
- Habit 4: Think Win/Win: Principles of Mutual Benefit
- Habit 5: Seek First to Understand, Then to Be Understood: Principles of Mutual Understanding
- Habit 6: Synergize: Principles of Creative Cooperation
- Habit 7: Sharpen the Saw: Principles of Balanced Self-Renewal

Explore Health Careers

www.explorehealthcareers.org

This noncommercial site contains general information about working in health care, as well as articles about specific careers.

Health Care Career Professional Organizations

All health careers have organizations that set standards and provide support and information for both students and working professionals. Many organizations are listed, along with contact information, in Appendix A.

National Consortium on Health Science and Technology and Technology Education

www.nchste.org

This website contains the foundation standards developed for health care students in all types of career programs. Reviewing these standards will give you an idea of what employers expect of their employees.

U.S. Department of Labor: *Occupational Outlook Handbook*

www.bls.gov/oco

This is a source of detailed information about hundreds of careers, including typical job descriptions, educational requirements, and average salaries. It is updated every 2 years.

REFERENCES

1. National Consortium on Health Science and Technology Education. "National Healthcare Foundation Standards and Accountability Criteria." www.nchste.org/cms/wp-content/uploads/2008/03/foundation_standards_ac_rev_01_08. (Accessed 2/13/09)

2. Anderson R, Barbara A, Feldman S: "What patients want: a content analysis of key qualities that influence patient satisfaction." www.drscore.com/press/papers/whatpatientswant.pdf (Accessed 2/9/09)

3. Binghang M, Stryker S: *Career choices and changes,* Washington, UT, 2005, Academic Innovations.

INTERNET ACTIVITIES

For active links to the websites needed to complete these activities, visit **http://evolve. elsevier.com/Haroun/career/.**

1. The *Occupational Outlook Handbook* (OOH), developed by the U.S. Department of Labor, is available online. Choose a health care occupation to review and list 10 facts you learn from the OOH profile.

2. Many of the general skills and characteristics employers seek when hiring new employees are described in an article featured by Quintessential Careers and a website listing the SCANS competencies. Read the article and list and then choose the 10 skills and characteristics you believe to be most important for succeeding in a health care career. Include your reasons for selecting each.

3. The National Healthcare Foundation Standards and Accountability Criteria are available from the National Consortium on Health Science and Technology Education. Read the 11 standards and the criteria listed under each one.

    a. Choose three accountability criteria under "Foundation Standard 2: Communications," and explain the importance of each in delivering high-quality health care.

    b. Review the accountability criteria under "Foundation Standard 4: Employability Skills," and explain how you can use this information now to begin to prepare for your career.

    c. Go to "Foundation Standard 8: Teamwork." Explain why, in your opinion, an entire standard is devoted to teamwork.

4. Do a Web search using the key words "marketing yourself." Explore some of the sites listed to read about the importance of self-marketing in planning and conducting a job search. Based on what you learn, write a short paper describing what you can do, as you begin your education, to make yourself more marketable.

5. Do a Web search using the key words "informational interview." Read about conducting an effective interview. List five techniques and 10 questions you can use to set up and conduct your interviews.

Skills for Success

Look over the examples of skill applications listed in Table 1-1. Use your own ideas to fill in the following table for reading and listening, two more skills critical to success in school, on the job search, and in your career.

Applications of Reading Skills

School	*Job Search*	*Career*
_____	_____	_____
_____	_____	_____
_____	_____	_____
_____	_____	_____

Applications of Listening Skills

School	*Job Search*	*Career*
_____	_____	_____
_____	_____	_____
_____	_____	_____
_____	_____	_____

Resource Treasure Hunt

When you need help, school services can seem like treasures. But to take advantage of everything your school has to offer, you must know about it. Take a tour of your school and record your findings for future reference. If your school does not offer all these services, find out if they are available elsewhere in the community.

Resource	*Services Provided*	*How to Access and When Available*
Advising or Counseling	_____	_____
Academic	_____	_____
Personal	_____	_____
Career Services	_____	_____
Job search assistance	_____	_____
School job fairs	_____	_____

Prescription for Success 1–2 *(Continued)*

Part-time jobs _____ _____

Resume preparation _____ _____

Interviewing skills _____ _____

Employer contacts _____ _____

Classes or workshops _____ _____

Financial Aid _____ _____

**Information Sources
and Referrals** _____ _____

Child care _____ _____

Financial help _____ _____

Transportation _____ _____

Other _____ _____

Learning Assistance _____ _____

Learning center _____ _____

Study skills _____ _____

Instructors _____ _____

Tutors _____ _____

Other students _____ _____

Study groups _____ _____

Refresher and basic skills classes _____ _____

Library _____ _____

Books _____ _____

Periodicals _____ _____

Internet Access _____ _____

Journals _____ _____

Reference assistance _____ _____

Other _____ _____

Continued

Prescription for Success 1–2 (Continued)

Professional Organizations (student chapters)   _____   _____

School Organizations   _____   _____

Special interest groups   _____   _____

Social clubs   _____   _____

Service clubs   _____   _____

Special Needs and Referrals   _____   _____

Alcohol abuse   _____   _____

Drug dependency   _____   _____

Family planning   _____   _____

Domestic abuse   _____   _____

Other   _____   _____

Volunteer Opportunities   _____   _____

Prescription for Success 1-3
Overcoming Obstacles

1. List any obstacles that might interfere with your school attendance (e.g., problems with child care).

   _____

   _____

   _____

   _____

2. What can you do now to overcome these obstacles (e.g., find backup for child care)?

   _____

   _____

   _____

   _____

   _____

   _____

Prescription for Success 1-4
Self-Assessment

How would you rate yourself on each of these general employment competencies? Fill out the following self-assessment guide as a first step in creating an action plan to fully develop the competencies most needed in the modern workplace. Check the column that best describes you.

	Often	*Sometimes*	*Seldom*
1. Creative thinking: I generate new ideas and come up with original approaches to everyday problems and situations.	_____	_____	_____
2. Decision making: I gather information, identify alternatives, consider **consequences**, select an alternative, and evaluate the effectiveness of the results.	_____	_____	_____
3. Problem solving: I recognize problems that need attention, identify possible solutions, create a plan, and carry out the plan.	_____	_____	_____
4. Continuous learning: I am interested in knowing everything I can that will help me succeed in my work and life, and I try to keep up with advances that will help me to do so.	_____	_____	_____
5. Reasoning: I understand the relationships among ideas and am able to apply them when learning and problem solving.	_____	_____	_____
6. Responsibility: I am dependable and complete any tasks I am given or for which I volunteer.	_____	_____	_____
7. Self-worth: I believe in myself and my ability to succeed.	_____	_____	_____
8. Empathy: I make an effort to understand the experiences and feelings of others and to see situations from their points of view.	_____	_____	_____
9. Self-management: I set personal goals, monitor my progress, and use self-discipline to ensure that I achieve them.	_____	_____	_____
10. Integrity: I guide my actions by a set of principles that defines right and wrong.	_____	_____	_____
11. Honesty: I tell the truth to myself and to others.	_____	_____	_____

Continued

Prescription for Success 1–4 (Continued)

- Review the ratings you gave yourself, and list any areas you believe need further development.

_____

_____

_____

- What can you start doing now to improve in these areas?

_____

_____

_____

Success Tip: Review your completed assessment and self-development plan periodically to see how you are progressing.

Prescription for Success 1-5
The Ideal Candidate

Imagine yourself as a busy pediatrician who runs a clinic in a low-income neighborhood. You need to hire a medical assistant. You have found a candidate who appears to have the necessary technical skills and experience.

1. What are five other characteristics you would want the candidate to have?

_____

_____

_____

2. Why did you choose these five characteristics?

_____

_____

_____

Now answer the following questions for yourself:

3. Explain how understanding the needs of employers can help you to better prepare for your future career.

_____

_____

_____

Prescription for Success 1–5 (Continued)

4. Which of your own personal qualities do you believe will be most valuable to future employers?

_____

_____

_____

Prescription for Success 1-6
Check Out Your Professional Organization

Find the website of the professional organization for your chosen occupation. (See the list of Web addresses in Appendix A.) Read through the material and look for answers to the following questions:

1. What kinds of personal characteristics are needed to succeed in this occupation?

_____

_____

_____

_____

2. Are there characteristics mentioned that also appear in the SCANS and National Health Care Standards examples? If so, list them here.

_____

_____

_____

_____

3. On the basis of what you read, in your own words describe an ideal person for this occupation.

_____

_____

_____

_____

_____

_____

Prescription for Success 1-7
And the Patient Is…You

Imagine you have just arrived at an urgent care facility with a suspected broken arm. You were out for an enjoyable Sunday afternoon, skating with friends, when you hit a hole in the pavement and fell. Your arm is very painful, and you are worried about your ability to work if you end up in a cast.

1. Describe how you would feel if you found yourself in this situation.

_____

_____

_____

_____

2. How would you hope to be treated by the health care professionals at the urgent care center?

_____

_____

_____

_____

3. What would be most important to you?

_____

_____

_____

_____

4. What would be least important to you?

_____

_____

_____

_____

5. Did you learn anything from this exercise that might influence your approach to working with future patients?

_____

_____

_____

_____

Prescription for Success 1-8
My Philosophy of Work

1. What meaning does work have for you?

_____

_____

_____

_____

_____

2. What needs do you want to be filled by your work?

_____

_____

_____

_____

_____

3. Why did you choose a career in health care?

_____

_____

_____

_____

_____

4. What do you hope to accomplish?

_____

_____

_____

_____

_____

5. What do you hope to contribute?

_____

_____

_____

_____

_____

What Do I Want?

Think about the characteristics you would prefer in your place of employment.

1. Type of facility
   Examples: large, small, urban (in the city), rural, inpatient (such as a hospital), outpatient (such as a clinic), home care

   _____

   _____

2. Type of population served
   Examples: economic status, age range, gender, ethnic groups

   _____

   _____

3. Work schedule
   Examples: steady employment with one employer; **per diem** (daily, contracted to different facilities); flexible, changing hours; fixed hours; frequent overtime; days only; evenings and weekends

   _____

   _____

4. Specialty
   Examples: emergency care, orthopedics (bones and muscles), hand therapy

   _____

   _____

5. Type of supervision
   Examples: closely monitored, work more independently

   _____

   _____

6. Work pace
   Examples: fast, moderate (There is no slow-paced work in health care!)

   _____

   _____

7. Amount of interaction with others (All health care professionals are part of a team, although some work more independently than others.)

   _____

   _____

8. Range of duties performed
   Examples: wide variety of tasks, concentrate on a few, somewhere in between

   _____

   _____

Prescription for Success 1-10
Conduct an Informational Interview

Conducting **informational interviews** gives you opportunities to learn more about the specific needs of employers in your career area, the skill requirements, and the everyday duties performed by professionals. Supervisors, as well as working professionals, are excellent sources of information. The goal of this type of interview is not to seek employment; it is to seek information. You may already know someone you would like to interview. If not, ask your instructor or the career services department (sometimes called *job placement*) at your school for suggestions. If you are a student member of a health care professional organization, this can be a good source of leads.

Once you have a contact, call and make an appointment. Explain that you are a student and want to learn more about your career area. Be considerate of the person's time, and if he or she is very busy, ask if you can schedule 15 or 20 minutes. Arrive a few minutes early and dress professionally. (Professional dress is discussed in Chapter 2.) Afterward, be sure to send a thank-you note to the person you interviewed.

Take along a list of prepared questions and a small notebook and pen. Here are some suggestions of questions for a supervisor:

1. What skills are most important to be successful as a _____?
2. What personal characteristics do you look for in a candidate seeking work as a _____?
3. What type of work is performed by a _____ in your facility?
4. What type of orientation or on-the-job training is given to new employees?
5. What is your best advice for someone who is interested in becoming a _____?
6. What learning and promotional opportunities are available for professionals who work in this field?

Examples of questions to ask a working professional include the following:

1. What are the typical duties of a _____?
2. What percentage of the day is usually spent on each duty?
3. Describe a typical day. (Is there a typical day? If not, describe a typical week.)
4. How many patients do you see in a day? How many tests do you perform? How many reports do you transcribe?
5. How much independent decision-making is required?
6. What is most challenging about your work?
7. What is most satisfying about your work?

To keep a record of what you hear, take brief notes during the interview or summarize the information as soon as possible afterward.

Write a summary of what you learned.

_____

_____

_____

_____

_____

_____

Continued

Prescription for Success 1–10 (Continued)

What else do you need to find out?

_____

_____

_____

_____

Describe anything you learned in the interview that surprised you.

_____

_____

_____

_____

On the basis of what you learned in the interview, describe anything you plan to work on while you are in school.

_____

_____

_____

_____

_____

Prescription for Success 1-11
Job Shadowing

Job shadowing means spending time with a professional as he or she works and performs typical duties. Many health care facilities offer programs to which you can apply. Typical requirements are a sincere interest in a health care career, a recent tuberculosis test, and willingness to sign a confidentiality form.

If you participate in a job shadowing program, take notes of what you observe and learn. Use the opportunity to ask questions like those in Prescription for Success 1-10. Keep records of the facility, the department, the dates you attended, and who you accompanied for future reference.

Name of Facility or Organization

_____

Address

_____

Prescription for Success 1–11 (Continued)

Phone _____

Name of Health Professional Shadowed

_____

Contact Information

_____

Name of Health Professional Shadowed

_____

Contact Information

_____

Name of Health Professional Shadowed

_____

Contact Information

_____

Dates and Times of Experience

_____

_____

_____

Total Number of Hours _____

Summary of What You Learned

_____

_____

_____

_____

_____

Prescription for Success 1-12
Paint an Occupational Portrait

Use what you learned from your research—informational interview, job shadowing, the National Healthcare Standards, the *Occupational Outlook Handbook* (see the To Learn More section of this chapter), and/or your professional organization—to write a summary report about your future career. Include the following:

1. Major responsibilities
2. Typical duties performed
3. Skills and personal characteristics required
4. Job outlook and salary information
5. Sources of continuing education
6. Promotional opportunities
7. What you find most interesting about the career

_____

_____

_____

_____

Prescription for Success 1-13
Are My Expectations Realistic?

Review the information you have gathered about your chosen occupation. Compare this information with your preferences and what you know about your personal qualities.

1. Do your preferences and personal qualities fit the occupation you have chosen?

_____

_____

2. How might you have to adjust your expectations?

_____

_____

3. What can you start doing now to ensure you are fully prepared for the requirements of your chosen occupation?

_____

_____

Your Resume Starts Now

OBJECTIVES

The information and activities in this chapter can help you:

- Begin to create a product—your professional self—that you can offer with confidence to prospective employers.
- Develop a professional appearance that is appropriate for the health care field.
- Use the contents of your future resume as a planning tool for managing personal and professional development.
- Take advantage of opportunities for personal and professional improvement.
- Start collecting items you can put in your professional portfolio.
- Begin professional networking activities.
- Start identifying potential references.

KEY TERMS AND CONCEPTS

Affirmation: A positive statement, said out loud, that you are or have something you want.

Civic Organizations: Groups that are devoted to improving the community.

Hygiene: Practices that contribute to cleanliness, good health, and the prevention of disease.

Networking: Meeting new people for the purpose of personal and professional development.

Optional: Not required.

Portfolio: An organized collection of items that provides evidence of your job-related skills and capabilities.

Proactive: Taking positive action before it is necessary or required.

Reference: A person who agrees to vouch for your professional skills and capabilities, such as a former supervisor.

Resume: A written document that summarizes your professional skills and capabilities.

Self-Fulfilling Prophecy: A statement that influences actions and therefore comes true.

Syllabi: Handouts prepared by instructors to let students know what they will learn, what the instructor expects from them, and how the students will be evaluated. Some instructors consider the syllabus to be a form of contract between them and their students.

Transferable Skills: Skills that can be applied to different types of occupations, such as organizing and tracking supplies.

Visualization: A technique in which you create detailed pictures in your mind of something you want to have or become.

PRODUCTION: THE SECOND "P" OF MARKETING

"You have to take life as it happens, but you should try to make it happen the way you want to take it."

—*Old German Proverb*

In Chapter 1, you read about the first step in the marketing process, planning. The second of the "5 Ps of Marketing" is production: using the information gathered from market research to design and put together a product that meets the needs of the customer. Your market research was finding out what patients and employers want and need from health care professionals.

Human beings have the unique ability to create their own lives. They can generate ideas, form mental images, and plan ways to achieve what they imagine. You have already generated the idea of becoming a health care professional and have completed the first step toward achieving that goal by enrolling in school. Whether you graduate and find satisfactory employment will depend, to a great extent, on your belief in your ability to succeed and your willingness to take the necessary actions to achieve your goals.

Henry Ford, who not only created fame and riches for himself but changed the history of transportation, is quoted as saying, "Whether you think that you can, or you can't, you are right." The tendency for people to get what they expect is known as the **self-fulfilling prophecy.** Our beliefs about ourselves—about what we can achieve—are more important than any other factor. Many prominent Americans, such as Abraham Lincoln and Thomas Edison, experienced many failures before finally achieving great success. Lincoln had business failures and lost elections before becoming one of our most famous presidents. And Edison conducted thousands of experiments before perfecting the electric light bulb, an invention that dramatically changed the world.

You can apply the principle of expecting success as you begin your career journey. All achievements begin as ideas, and what you picture mentally can become your reality. Positive images of you succeeding as a student act as powerful motivators. In addition to visual suggestions, your self-talk influences your success—or lack of it. We are continually holding conversations with ourselves that either give us encouragement ("I know I can pass this test.") or put us down ("I'll never be able to get this report finished."). By taking control of the pictures and words in your mind, you can apply their power to help you create the life you want.

A related and very powerful concept you can apply to your life is to act as if you already are what you hope to become. You can increase your chances of becoming a successful health care professional if you start approaching life as if you already were that person. Practice behaviors now that you know will be expected on the job. For example, because accuracy and efficiency are important characteristics for the health care professional, complete all class assignments as if the well-being of others depended on your accuracy. Working effectively with others as part of a team will be required in your work, so start using every opportunity to develop your teamwork skills. Cooperate with your classmates and instructors. Figure 2-1 illustrates how creating a mental picture of yourself as a health care worker can promote behaviors that lead to achievement of your career goals. Be **proactive** and look for opportunities to increase your personal and professional growth. Turn mistakes into lessons and learn from them. Approach personal difficulties as opportunities to learn and to grow. By the time you graduate, you will have become the health care professional you aspire to be.

Go to page 52 to complete Prescription for Success 2-1

Go to page 52 to complete Prescription for Success 2-2

PACKAGING: THE THIRD "P" OF MARKETING

Even an excellent product may not sell if it is poorly packaged. Companies know this and invest a lot of time and money to make their products visually appealing to customers. Appearance can make the difference between a product selling or collecting dust on the shelf. Most of us package ourselves to impress others or to fit into a specific social group. Americans spend billions of dollars annually on clothing, cosmetics, accessories, and hair care in an effort to create what we believe to be a pleasing appearance.

Appearance is especially important in the health care field because many patients form their opinions about the competence of health care professionals based on their appearance. Your effectiveness in meeting patient needs can be influenced by your appearance because patient satisfaction increases when health care professionals "look like they know what they are doing."

What is expected of the health care professional? How do you look competent, as the health care professional in Figure 2-2 does? There are several ways. The first is to be fairly conservative in dress and grooming. It is best to avoid fashion trends such as brightly colored hair, tattoos, and body piercing. At the same time, it is true that employers

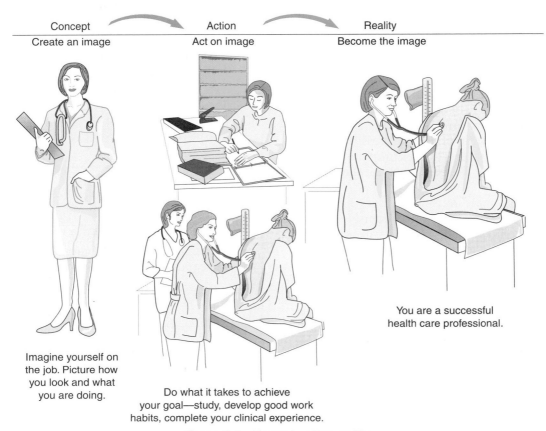

Concept	Action	Reality
Create an image	Act on image	Become the image

Imagine yourself on the job. Picture how you look and what you are doing.

Do what it takes to achieve your goal—study, develop good work habits, complete your clinical experience.

You are a successful health care professional.

Figure 2–1   Concept, action, reality.

are becoming more accepting of these trends. The problem is that some patients may interpret them as signs of rebellion, immaturity, and lack of common sense. Others are offended or even frightened by this type of appearance.

Even clothing that is not extreme may be inappropriate for work. Dressing for work is different from dressing casually for recreation or for social functions. What is perfect for a party may be totally out of place for a job interview or for the job itself.

A second consideration is to strive for an appearance that radiates good health. An important responsibility of the health care professional is to promote good health, and this is partly achieved by example. If you smoke or are overweight, putting you at risk for serious health problems, this would be a good time to adopt new healthy living habits. Other conditions such as teeth that need dental work, badly bitten fingernails, and dandruff indicate a lack of self-care, and this is inappropriate in a profession that encourages the practice of good personal health habits. The way you present yourself reflects your approach to life and your opinion of yourself. Failure to care for yourself can project a lack of self-confidence and can undermine patient faith in your effectiveness.

Third, the issues of cleanliness and **hygiene** are vitally important for professionals whose work

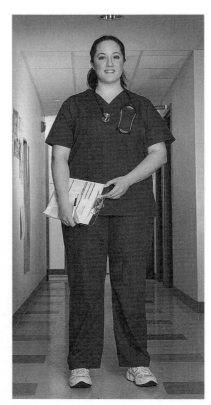

Figure 2–2   How does this health care professional's appearance project competence? (*From Bonewit-West K, Hunt S, Applegate E:* Today's medical assistant, *Saunders, 2009.*)

requires them to touch others. Patients literally put themselves in the hands of health care professionals and must feel assured that they will benefit from, and not be harmed by, any procedures performed. It is natural to want the professional to look clean and neat and be free of unpleasant odors. For example, although the hands of the dental assistant may be clean and gloved, dirty uniforms or shoes (or even shoelaces!) give an unfavorable impression to the patient, who may wonder whether proper attention was given to sterilizing the equipment and cleaning the work area.

Finally, professionals must consider the safety and comfort of both patients and themselves. Perfumes and scented personal products cannot be tolerated by many patients. Long fingernails, flowing hair, and large dangling earrings may be attractive and appropriate for a social event, but in a health care setting they can scratch patients, contaminate samples, get caught in equipment, or be grabbed by young patients. Safety on the job cannot be compromised to accommodate fashion trends. Some clothing customs are determined by one's culture, such as head coverings and flowing skirts. These customs may also have to be modified to ensure the safety of both you and the patient.

PERSONAL REFLECTION

1. Is there anything about my appearance I want to improve in preparation for work in the health care setting?

_____

_____

_____

a. Fashion trends

_____

_____

b. Health habits

_____

_____

c. Cleanliness and hygiene

_____

_____

d. Safety issues

_____

_____

2. How am I willing to change the way I dress, at least during working hours?

_____

_____

_____

3. What can I do now to create a professional appearance?

_____

_____

_____

Note: If you are not sure about any aspects of your appearance or grooming, speak privately with your instructor or someone else you trust. Dealing with these issues now will give you time to take care of them before you begin your job search.

PRESENTATION: THE FOURTH "P" OF MARKETING

Your **resume**, a written outline of your qualifications for work, is an important tool for presenting yourself and what you have to offer to prospective employers. The main purpose of a resume is to convince an employer to give you an interview, and in Chapter 10 you will learn how to write and organize an effective resume. The focus of the rest of this chapter is on learning about the content of the resume and how you can use it as a guideline to create your professional self. Starting to plan your resume now will help you do the following:

1. Recognize what you already have to offer an employer
2. Build self-confidence
3. Motivate yourself to learn both the technical and nontechnical skills that contribute to employment success
4. Identify anything you might want to improve about yourself
5. Know ahead of time what kinds of experiences will enhance your employability

6. Get a head start gathering information and collecting examples to demonstrate your value and skills

Your Resume as a Guide to Success

"Begin with the end in mind."
—*Stephen Covey*

Thinking about your resume at the beginning instead of waiting until the end of your educational program turns your resume into a checklist of "To Dos" for creating a product—your professional self—that you'll be able to offer with confidence to prospective customers: health care employers. The various components of a resume, listed in Box 2-1, are explained in this chapter, along with suggestions on how to make them work for you while you are still in school.

Building Block 1: Career Objective

The career objective is a brief description, often only one sentence long, of the position or job title you are seeking. In addition to describing the job you are seeking, you may create a brief statement of what you can offer the employer:

☐ Obtain a position as an administrative and clinical medical assistant where I can contribute by applying up-to-date skills

☐ Occupational therapy assistant in a pediatric facility

As discussed earlier, it is wise to have reasonable expectations for your first employment position. Set positive long-term goals, but be realistic when starting out. Your first job is your chance to work with real people who have real problems. The wider the range of jobs you are willing to accept when first entering the field, the better your chances of obtaining employment.

BOX 2-1   Resume Building Blocks

1. Career Objective
2. Education
3. Professional Skills and Knowledge
4. Work History
5. Licenses and Certifications
6. Honors and Awards
7. Special Skills
8. Volunteer Activities
9. Professional and Civic Organizations
10. Languages Spoken

As you go through your training, learn as much as possible about the various jobs for which you might qualify. You may be unaware of jobs that closely match your interests. It is not uncommon to rewrite objectives more than once before beginning the actual job search. Use the Resume Building Block #1: Career Objective form, on page 41, to begin defining the kind of job you want.

Building Block 2: Education

The education section contains a list of all your education and training, with emphasis on health care training.

Start your list with the school you attended most recently. Include grade point average and class standing (not all schools rank their students by grades) if they are above average. Use the Resume Building Block #2: Education form, on page 42, as a motivator to do your best academically.

Building Block 3: Professional Skills and Knowledge

Professional skills and knowledge refers to the skills and knowledge that contribute to successful job performance.

The way you organize this section when you actually write your resume depends on your educational program and the number and variety of skills acquired. You can list them individually if there are not too many (such as "Take vital signs") or as clusters of related skills (such as "Perform clinical duties").

Listing individual skills or clusters of skills is a good idea if your previous work experience is limited and you want to emphasize the recent acquisition of health care skills as your primary qualification. It is also helpful if you have trained for one of the newer positions in health care that is not familiar to all employers. For example, "patient care technician" is a relatively new type of multi-skilled worker who can be employed in a variety of health care settings. Even if you decide not to include a skills list on your resume, starting a list now will keep you aware of what you know and have to offer an employer. Employers report that many recent graduates do not realize just how much they really know, and therefore they fail to sell themselves at job interviews.

Find out if your school provides lists of program and course objectives and/or the competencies you will master. Some instructors give their students checklists to monitor the completion of assignments and demonstration of competencies. Other sources of information include handouts from your instructor, such as **syllabi** and course outlines; the objectives listed in your textbooks; and lab skill sheets. Develop your own inventory of what you have learned, using the Resume Building Block #3: Professional Skills and Knowledge form, on page 43, to begin a personal inventory of your skills. An additional benefit of tracking your progress is the sense of accomplishment you gain as you see the results of your hard work. You will be amazed by how much you are learning!

Building Block 4: Work History

The work history is a list of your previous jobs, including the name and location of the employer, your job title and duties, and the dates of employment.

You can benefit from this section of your resume even if you have no previous experience in health care. There are three ways to do this. The first is to review the duties and responsibilities you had in each of your past jobs. Which ones can be applied to health care work? Skills that are common to many jobs are called **transferable skills.** Take another look at the general skills listed in the SCANS report (see Box 1-2 in Chapter 1). Do you see any that you have used? Here are a few examples of both general and more technical skills common to many jobs:

- Work well with people from a variety of backgrounds
- Create efficient schedules that reduce employee overtime
- Purchase supplies in appropriate quantities and at competitive prices
- Resolve customer complaints satisfactorily
- Perform word processing duties
- Manage accounts receivable
- Provide customer service
- Provide appropriate care for infants and toddlers

Identifying transferable skills is especially important when you are entering a new field in which you have little or no experience. There is actually a type of resume that emphasizes skills and abilities rather than specific job titles held. It is called a "functional resume," and the format is described in Chapter 10. At this time, start compiling a list of possible transferable skills such as the ones illustrated by the cashier in Figure 2-3.

The second way to maximize the value of the work history section of your resume is to state what you achieved in each job. In a phrase or two, describe how you contributed to the success of your employer. When possible, state these achievements in measurable terms. If you can't express them with numbers, use active verbs that tell what you did. Here are some examples:

- Increased sales by 20%
- Designed a more efficient way to track supplies

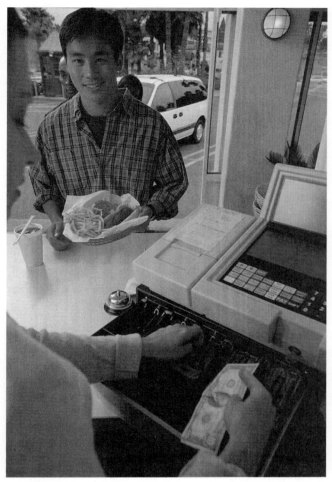

Figure 2–3 Many health care students have worked in jobs such as cashiering. How many skills are used in this type of work that can be applied to health care?

- Worked on a committee to write an effective employee procedure manual that is still in use
- Trained five employees to use office equipment correctly

A third way to add value to this section is to include your clinical experience. Although you must clearly indicate that this was a part of your training and not paid employment, it still serves as evidence of your ability to apply what you learned in school to practical situations. For many new graduates, this is their only real-world experience in health care. Students sometimes make the mistake of viewing their clinical experience as simply an add-on to their program—just one more thing to get through. They fail to realize the impact their performance can have on their career. Remember that clinical supervisors represent future employers. (In some cases they *are* future employers because some students are hired by their clinical sites.) Their opinion of you can help successfully launch your self-marketing efforts or cause them to fizzle, so commit to doing your best during your clinical experience. The inclusion of a successful clinical experience on your resume increases your chances of getting the job you want.

Use the Resume Building Block #4: Work History form, on page 44, to start compiling your work history.

Note: Do *not* be concerned if your work experience is limited or you can't think of any achievements. You may have finished high school recently or perhaps you spent several years working as a homemaker. Employers understand that everyone starts with a first job and you are receiving training to qualify you for work. And homemakers, as well as mothers and others who care for family members, gain experiences that are valuable to employers. Examples include caring for others, practicing time management, and handling family finances.

Building Block 5: Licenses and Certifications

Some professions require you to be licensed or have specific types of approval before you are allowed to work. Nursing is one example. Others include physical and occupational therapy and dental hygiene. Some professions have voluntary certifications and registrations, such as those earned by medical assistants. The kind of approvals needed vary by state and profession. Most licenses and certifications require certain types of training and/or the passing of a standardized exam. It is important that you clearly understand any professional requirements necessary or highly recommended for your profession.

Learn as much as you can now about the requirements for the occupation you have chosen. It is not advisable to wait until the end of your studies to start thinking about preparing for required exams. Ask your instructors about review classes, books, and computerized material. Check with your professional organization. (See the contact list in Appendix A) Become familiar with the topics on the exams, and plan your studies accordingly. Knowing the format of the questions (multiple choice, true-false, etc.) is also helpful. Increase your chances for success by preparing over time, the proven way to do well on exams. (Taking exams is covered in detail in Chapter 6.) Use the Resume Building Block #5: Licenses and Certifications form, on page 45, to start gathering information about certifications for your occupation.

Building Block 6: Honors and Awards

The section on honors and awards is an **optional** resume section. Your school may offer recognition for student achievements and special contributions. Community and professional organizations to which you belong may also give awards. Acknowledgments received for volunteer work can also be included in this section.

Investigate what you might be eligible for and use these rewards as incentives for excellent performance. Keep this in perspective, however. Awards should serve as motivators, not indicators of your value. They are nice to have but certainly not essential for getting a good job.

Use the Resume Building Block #6: Honors and Awards form, on page 46, to find out about the availability of and requirements for awards for which you might qualify.

Building Block 7: Special Skills

Special skills are those that don't fit into other sections but do add to your value as a prospective employee. Examples include proficiency in desktop publishing and the ability to use American Sign Language as the health care worker in Figure 2-4 can.

Research the needs of employers in your geographic area. Do you already have special skills that meet these needs? Would it substantially increase your chances for employment if you were to acquire skills outside the scope of your program—for example, becoming more proficient on the computer? If (and only if!) time permits, you might decide to attend workshops in addition to your regular program courses, do extra reading, or take a course on the Internet. Use the Resume Building Block #7: Special Skills form, on page 48, to record any skills that might supplement your qualifications.

Building Block 8: Volunteer Activities

Volunteer activities can be included on your resume if they relate to your targeted occupation or demonstrate desired qualities such as being responsible and having concern for others. If you are already involved in these types of activities, think about what you are learning or practicing that can help you on the job. If you aren't, consider becoming involved if you have a sincere interest and adequate time. Adult students face many responsibilities outside of class, and the additional activities mentioned in this chapter should be taken as suggestions, not must-dos. Mastering your program content should be your first priority. If applicable, use the Resume Building Block #8: Volunteer Activities form, on page 49, to investigate opportunities and record your service.

Building Block 9: Professional and Civic Organizations

Professional organizations provide excellent opportunities to network, learn more about your field, and practice leadership skills. Participation in **civic organizations**, groups that work for the good of the

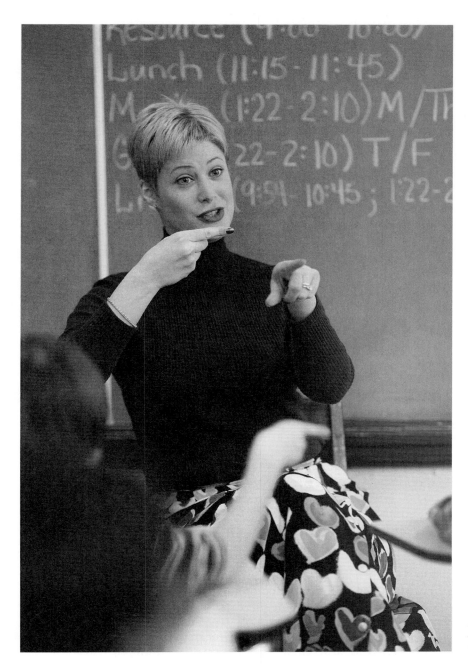

Figure 2–4 Many skills, such as sign language, enhance the value of the health care professional. What skills do you already have that you can use in your future work?

community, promotes personal growth and demonstrates your willingness to get involved in your community. Consider joining and participating actively in a professional or civic organization while you are in school. See whether your school or community has a local chapter. Use the Resume Building Block #9: Professional and Civic Organizations form, on page 50, to record your participation.

Building Block 10: Languages Spoken

In our multicultural society, the ability to communicate in a language other than English is commonly included on the resume. Find out whether many patients speak a language other than English in the area where you plan to work. Consider acquiring at least some conversational ability or a few phrases to use to reassure patients. Appendix B contains a list of useful Spanish phrases for the medical professional. If your school offers these languages as elective courses, they would be good choices. A patient benefits greatly, during the stress of illness or injury, when health care professionals know at least a few phrases of the patient's native language. Even speaking just a few basic phrases can increase your value to employers. Also consider learning about the customs, especially the ones related to health practices, of ethnic groups in your community. (Cultural differences are discussed in Chapter 8.) Use the Resume Building Block #10: Languages Spoken form, on page 51, if you have or plan to acquire knowledge of another language.

 Go to page 53 to complete Prescription for Success 2-3

Portfolios

Although resumes are the principal method for job seekers to present their qualifications to potential employers, portfolios are being used to supplement the resume. A **portfolio** is an organized collection of items that document your capabilities and qualifications for work. A portfolio can give you a competitive edge at job interviews.

Starting to plan your portfolio now can cast your class assignments in a new light. More than work you turn in to your instructor, they can serve as demonstrations of your abilities to an employer. Strive to perform consistently at your highest level, producing work that will represent you well.

As you complete each course, save assignments that might be suitable for your portfolio. Store them in a folder or large envelope so they stay in good condition. In addition to written assignments, there are nontraditional ways to showcase your abilities. The items you collect need not be limited to evidence of your technical skills. For example, it is appropriate to include documentation of other activities, such as organizing an event for charity. No standard list of items to put in your portfolio exists, although your school may have prepared a list for students. In any case, only accurate and neat work should be included. How to finalize the contents and assemble your portfolio for presentation is covered in Chapter 10. See Box 2-2 and Figure 2-5 for examples of portfolio contents.

PROMOTION: THE FIFTH "P" OF MARKETING

Think about how companies use promotional campaigns to give new products maximum exposure. They advertise—sometimes endlessly, it seems!—on television, in magazines and newspapers, and on the Internet to spread the word to as many consumers as possible about how the product will fulfill their needs. You will conduct a similar campaign when you conduct your job search. As with your resume and portfolio, you can begin to prepare now. Networking, references, and the job interview are the three main ways to promote yourself during the job search.

 Q&A with a Career Services Professional Melva Duran

Melva is the director of Career Services at Kaplan College in San Diego. Melva shares insight on how new graduates can get a first job in the health field and the salary they should expect.

Q You usually work with students as they graduate and begin their job search. Do you have any recommendations for students as they begin their training for a job in health care?

A I think it's important for them to consider what they need to earn in terms of dollars and what they can reasonably expect when they are beginning a new career. Ideally, they will have researched starting pay for the career they've chosen to train for before they actually start school. Even if they haven't, it's important for students to understand that it might take time to work up to either a higher position or pay raises as they gain experience.

Q Do you suggest that students develop a budget?

A Absolutely. They should track their expenses to see what they need for the basics. If they are changing careers, they may earn less for a while. Knowing what they are spending helps them see where they might cut back until they are earning more.

Q Do you have examples of students who have done this?

A Well, I recently had a student who was changing from a career in a financial institution to a career in medical billing. She had earned over $60,000 and was hoping to earn that much in the health field. I had to tell her that she would be starting out at about half that much—but that with hard work and promotions, she could earn well in the billing field. We discussed how she could set short-term goals and plan to live on less until she got established.

Q Are there ways that graduates can increase the amount they earn in first-time jobs?

A Wages do vary from one part of a city to another—and on the type of care offered and insurance accepted. As you know, reimbursement from private insurance, Medicare, and so on varies and influences what employers can pay. Websites such as salary.com can give graduates a general idea of salaries, but they are not accurate for specific geographic areas and working conditions. It is best for students to do their own direct research on employers rather than depending on the information they find on the Internet.

When the job market is good, a qualified graduate might want to research a variety of employers. Sometimes traveling extra distance to a job is worth it if the pay and benefits are higher than with employers who are closer to home. Work schedules, such as the night shift, that are a little less convenient may offer higher pay. This is why students should think about what they need so they can consider all the pros and cons of jobs that are available when they are ready to begin working.

BOX 2-2   Examples of What to Include in Your Portfolio

1. Assignments
   - Accurately filled out insurance form
   - Accounting forms
   - Perfectly typed or word processed letter
   - Lab reports
   - Sample medical history form, filled out
   - Charting entries
   - Research report
2. Certificates of completion or achievement
   - Verification of having completed courses, seminars, and workshops
   - Proof of skill mastery, such as cardiopulmonary resuscitation (CPR), first aid, or the Burdick electrocardiographic (ECG) procedure, or documentation of the number of successful performances of an important procedure, such as venipunctures, injections, and x-ray studies
   - Documentation of speed, such as for word processing or data entry
   - Recognition of special achievements, such as honor or merit roll or perfect attendance
3. Grade records or transcripts
   - Consider including these if your grades are above average. If they started out as average or even below average and then improved as you advanced through your program, you might use them to demonstrate your persistence and progress.
4. Employer reviews or evaluations
   - You can include these from your previous employment if they demonstrate attitudes or skills applicable to work in health care. A positive review from your clinical supervisor can be very valuable because it is recent and relates directly to health care.
5. Recognition of contributions
   - Thank-you letters
   - Verification of participation in activities such as walk-a-thons to raise money for worthy causes
6. Attendance record
   - Excellent addition if you have very good attendance
7. Honors and awards
8. Licenses or certifications (copies)
9. Photographs
   - Use these to document activities in which you had a major role, such as organizing a fundraising activity or planning and coordinating a school picnic.
10. Letters of recommendation

PERSONAL REFLECTION

What opportunities can I take advantage of now for professional networking?

_____

_____

_____

_____

_____

Networking

Networking, as we are using the word here, refers to meeting and establishing relationships with people who work in health care. It is an effective way to learn more about your chosen career. At the same time, it gets the word out about you and your employment goals. Examples of networking opportunities include professional meetings, career fairs, class field trips to health care facilities, and guest speakers who come to your school.

There are many ways to begin networking: at a professional meeting, introduce yourself to other members; after hearing a guest speaker in class, ask questions; at a career fair, ask a local employer for advice about what to emphasize in your studies. Be sure to follow up with a phone call or thank-you note to anyone who sends you information or makes a special effort to help you.

Another benefit of networking is building your self-confidence as you introduce yourself to people. You can improve your speaking ability and increase your ability to express yourself effectively. These are valuable skills you will use when attending job interviews. Start now to create a web of connections to help you develop professionally and assist you in your future job search and career.

REFERENCES

References are people who will confirm your qualifications, skills, abilities, and personal qualities. In other words, they endorse you as a product. Professional references are not the same as personal or character references. To be effective, professional references must be credible (believable) and have

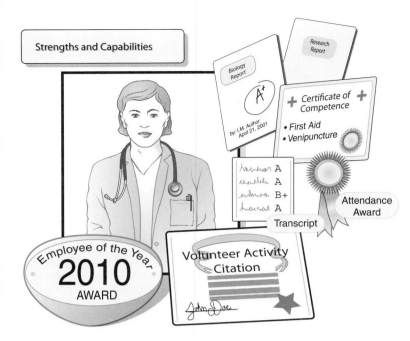

Figure 2–5 Start now to collect evidence of your qualifications for a job in health care.

personal knowledge of your value to a prospective employer. Your best references have knowledge of both you and the health care field. Examples include your instructors, clinical experience supervisors, and other professionals who know the quality of your work. Previous supervisors, even in jobs outside of health care, also make good references.

Recall the discussion in this chapter about becoming a health care professional by conducting yourself as if you already were one. Start now to project a professional image to everyone you meet, including your instructors and other staff members at your school. Become the person whom others will be happy to recommend.

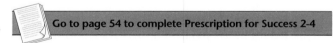

Go to page 54 to complete Prescription for Success 2-4

Job Interview

Job interviews provide the best opportunities to promote yourself to prospective employers. Interviewers often ask for examples of how you solved a problem or handled a given situation. Start thinking now about your past experiences and begin to collect examples from your work as a student, especially from your clinical experience, that will demonstrate your capabilities. It is not too early to start preparing so you can approach your future interviews as opportunities to shine, at ease and confident that you are presenting yourself positively, as the applicant in Figure 2-6 is. Job interviews are discussed in detail in Chapter 11.

⇨ SUMMARY OF KEY IDEAS

1. A professional appearance has a positive influence on patients.
2. The components of your resume can serve as a guide for career preparation and self–motivation.
3. It is not too early to start networking and preparing for your job search.

◀ Positive Self-Talk for This Chapter

1. I have many qualities of value to my future employers.
2. I have a plan for preparing to become a successful health care professional.
3. I am on my way to a great future.

To Learn More ◀◀◀

Covey SR: *The 7 Habits of Highly Effective People,* New York, 1990, Fireside.

This popular book lists seven principles that help individuals live effective lives. Students may find it helpful to learn about the seven habits:
- Habit 1: Be Proactive: Principles of Personal Choice
- Habit 2: Begin with the End in Mind: Principles of Personal Vision
- Habit 3: Put First Things First: Principles of Integrity and Execution
- Habit 4: Think Win/Win: Principles of Mutual Benefit
- Habit 5: Seek First to Understand, Then to Be Understood: Principles of Mutual Understanding

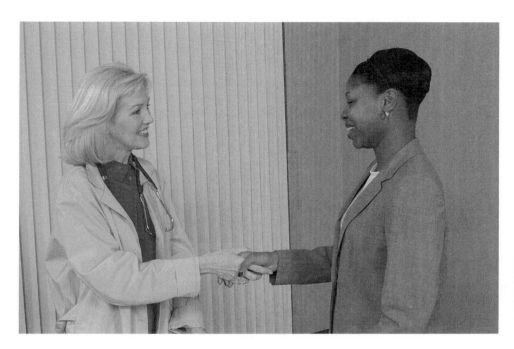

Figure 2–6 How is the job candidate on the right demonstrating self-confidence as she meets the employer? What can you start doing *now* to ensure you attend future job interviews with confidence?

- Habit 6: Synergize: Principles of Creative Cooperation
- Habit 7: Sharpen the Saw: Principles of Balanced Self-Renewal

Erupting Mind

www.eruptingmind.com

This website contains dozens of reader-friendly articles that offer self-improvement advice. The topics covered include self-esteem, success skills, and using mind power with affirmations and visualization.

Gawain S: *Creative visualization: use the power of your imagination to create what you want in your life*, Novato, Calif, 2002, New World Library.

This book, originally published in 1977, remains a classic in the use of visualization and affirmation to attain personal success. Creative visualization has been used in the fields of health, education, business, sports, and the arts. The author explains how to use mental imagery and affirmations to produce positive changes in one's life.

Key Career Networking Resources for Job Seekers

www.quintcareers.com/networking_resources.html

This website contains links to many articles and additional websites about career networking.

University of Mississippi Medical Center

Hospital Administrative Policy and Procedure Manual: Professional Appearance

http://hosped.umc.edu/docs/policies/(HADM.P-14) ProfessionalAppearance.pdf

See this website for an example of real-world requirements for health care employees.

INTERNET ACTIVITIES

1. A success-oriented website called "Affirmations for Success" contains information about using positive quotes, affirmations, and visualization. It also contains articles about self-esteem. Explore the website and choose an article or web page to summarize.
2. Use the search term "career networking" to find sites with information about this important job-search tool. What are five reasons to use networking? Include the names and addresses of the sites where you find the information.
3. Search "professional portfolio." Why is using a professional portfolio recommended in today's job search? Include the names and addresses of the sites where you find the information.

RESUME BUILDING BLOCKS

The forms included in this chapter for building your resume can be used throughout your educational program. The first part of each form is for use as you proceed through your classes. Some forms ask you to start collecting information; others give you ideas about activities to increase your employability; still others give you a chance to set goals to best take advantage of your education.

The second part of each form, entitled "Writing Your Resume," is to use later when you are putting together a resume for your job search. You will do this in Chapter 10, "Finalizing Your Employment Presentation Materials."

Resume Building Block #1
CAREER OBJECTIVE

Employers want to know what kind of job you are looking for. You need to know this, too! You may change your objective for your first job several times as you learn new subjects and get ideas from your lab and clinical experiences.

TO DO NOW

Write at least two sentences that describe your objective, as you see it now, for your first job in health care.

1. _____

_____

_____

2. _____

_____

_____

Add new ideas here:

-
-
-
-
-

WRITING YOUR RESUME

OBJECTIVE

_____

_____

_____

_____

_____

_____

Resume Building Block #2
EDUCATION

Your education is more than a list of schools you've attended. Take the steps to get all you can out of your training program.

TO DO NOW

List five things you can do to get the most from your education.

1. _____
2. _____
3. _____
4. _____
5. _____

Write three academic goals..

1. _____
2. _____
3. _____

WRITING YOUR RESUME

List the schools you have attended, starting with the most recent.

_____

_____

_____

_____

_____

_____

_____

_____

_____

_____

_____

Resume Building Block #3
PROFESSIONAL SKILLS AND KNOWLEDGE

TO DO NOW

Track the skills you are learning by keeping an inventory for each of your subjects. Fill in this form as you progress through your program. Here are some examples of the kinds of skills to include:

- Set up dental trays for common procedures
- Accurately complete medical insurance claim forms
- Create presentations using PowerPoint
- Teach a patient to use different ambulatory devices

COURSE TITLE	SKILLS ACQUIRED
1. _____	_____
2. _____	_____
3. _____	_____
4. _____	_____
5. _____	_____
6. _____	_____
7. _____	_____
8. _____	_____
9. _____	_____
10. _____	_____

WRITING YOUR RESUME

You can organize your professional skills and knowledge into clusters or write a list of individual skills.

_____

_____

_____

_____

_____

Resume Building Block #4
WORK HISTORY

TO DO NOW

List the jobs you've had in the past and start recording transferable skills and accomplishments.

JOB TITLE	TRANSFERABLE SKILLS	ACCOMPLISHMENTS
_____	_____	_____
_____	_____	_____
_____	_____	_____
_____	_____	_____
_____	_____	_____

WRITING YOUR RESUME

Remember that the different types of resumes (chronologic, functional, and combination), described in Chapter 10, will influence what information you include in your work history section.

WORK HISTORY

_____
_____
_____
_____
_____
_____
_____
_____
_____
_____
_____
_____

Resume Building Block #5
LICENSES AND CERTIFICATIONS

TO DO NOW

Describe the licensing and/or certification requirements for your occupation, if any.

_____

_____

_____

_____

_____

Are there voluntary approvals for which you can test or apply?

_____

_____

_____

_____

Are computerized, written, and/or practical exams required? What range of content is covered? How are the questions formatted (e.g., multiple choice, true-false)?

_____

_____

_____

_____

Are content outlines, review books, software, and/or practice exams available?

_____

_____

_____

_____

_____

Continued

Resume Building Block #5 (continued)

WRITING YOUR RESUME

LICENSE/CERTIFICATION/REGISTRATION (CHOOSE APPROPRIATE HEADING)

_____

_____

_____

_____

_____

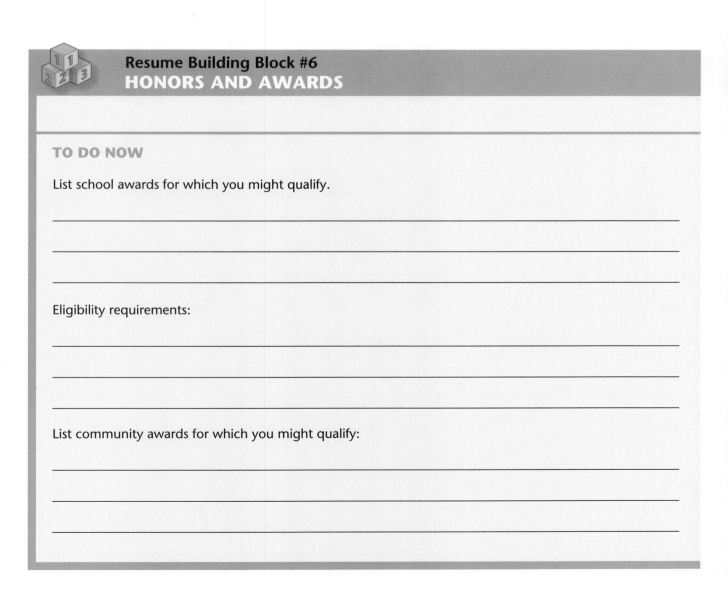

Resume Building Block #6
HONORS AND AWARDS

TO DO NOW

List school awards for which you might qualify.

_____

_____

_____

Eligibility requirements:

_____

_____

_____

List community awards for which you might qualify:

_____

_____

_____

Resume Building Block #6 (continued)

Eligibility requirements:

_____

_____

_____

List other awards for which you might qualify:

_____

_____

_____

Eligibility requirements:

_____

_____

_____

WRITING YOUR RESUME

HONORS AND AWARDS

_____

_____

_____

_____

_____

_____

_____

_____

_____

_____

_____

_____

Resume Building Block #7
SPECIAL SKILLS

TO DO NOW

Start recording special skills you think may be applicable to a job in health care.

SKILL	METHOD OF ACQUISITION	APPLICATION TO HEALTH CARE
_____	_____	_____
_____	_____	_____
_____	_____	_____
_____	_____	_____
_____		

WRITING YOUR RESUME

SPECIAL SKILLS

_____

_____

_____

_____

_____

_____

_____

_____

_____

_____

Resume Building Block #8
VOLUNTEER ACTIVITIES

TO DO NOW

List any volunteer activities you might use on your resume. Do you have time while you are in school for new or additional activities that are directly related to your career goals?

ACTIVITY	SKILLS ACQUIRED	PERSONAL QUALITIES DEMONSTRATED
_____	_____	_____
_____	_____	_____
_____	_____	_____
_____	_____	_____
_____	_____	_____
_____	_____	_____

WRITING YOUR RESUME

VOLUNTEER WORK AND COMMUNITY SERVICE

_____

_____

_____

_____

_____

_____

_____

_____

_____

Resume Building Block #9
PROFESSIONAL AND CIVIC ORGANIZATIONS

TO DO NOW

List any professional and/or civic activities you might use on your resume. Are there organizations you can join to gain experience and enrich your educational program?

ORGANIZATION	ACTIVITIES	SKILLS ACQUIRED
_____	_____	_____
_____	_____	_____
_____	_____	_____
_____	_____	_____

WRITING YOUR RESUME

PROFESSIONAL AND CIVIC ORGANIZATIONS

_____

_____

_____

_____

_____

_____

_____

_____

_____

_____

_____

_____

_____

Resume Building Block #10
LANGUAGES SPOKEN

TO DO NOW

Languages you speak other than English:

_____

_____

_____

Languages spoken by patients in your geographic area:

_____

_____

_____

Opportunities to learn another language (even a few phrases useful in the health care setting):

_____

_____

_____

WRITING YOUR RESUME

LANGUAGES SPOKEN

_____

_____

_____

_____

_____

_____

_____

_____

_____

Prescription for Success 2-1
Using Visualization

Visualization is a popular technique for harnessing the creative power of the imagination. If your goal is to become a medical assistant, for example, create a detailed mental picture of yourself working as a professional in a doctor's office or clinic. See yourself performing the tasks of your chosen occupation. Try the technique for yourself by following these steps:

1. Find a quiet, private place where you won't be disturbed.
2. Close your eyes.
3. Imagine yourself as a (member of the occupation of your choice).
   A. Create the details. Attempt to make the image as real as possible.
      1. What are you wearing?
      2. Who are your co-workers?
      3. What is the setting? A hospital? A physician's office? A business office?
      4. What are you doing? Interacting with a patient? Performing a procedure? Working on a computer?
   B. Create positive thoughts and feelings for yourself in the scene: You are competent. You work well with patients and co-workers. You like what you are doing.
4. Try to keep your scene going for a few minutes. Make it as specific as possible and keep filling in the details. The idea is to have a clear, firm image of yourself successfully carrying out the duties of your chosen profession.

Prescription for Success 2-2
Affirmations (Positive Self-Talk)

Filling your self-talk with positive statements is another technique for creating the future you want. These statements are called **affirmations**, and, like visualizations, they are based on the principle that we become what we first create in our minds. Here are a few examples:

- I, Rosa Maria, am a highly skilled dental assistant.

- I, Kenisha, perform my radiology duties with confidence.

- I, Jaime, conduct accurate laboratory tests.

- I, Andrea, am a competent, caring nurse.

- I, Pham, help patients with my therapeutic skills.

- I, Bill, am an efficient health information technician.

Note that each affirmation:

- is stated in the present tense

- includes your name

- is positive

Try writing a few affirmations on cards to carry with you or post them where you will see them every day. The important thing is to repeat them daily over a period of time.

Prescription for Success 2-3
How Much Do I Need?

Write down all of your regular expenses for a 3-month period. Include items that you are not paying now but can expect in the future, such as student loan payments.

Amount

Item	Month 1	Month 2	Month 3
Mortgage or rent	_____	_____	_____
Utilities	_____	_____	_____
• Gas and electricity	_____	_____	_____
• Television	_____	_____	_____
• Telephone	_____	_____	_____
• Online access	_____	_____	_____
• Garbage	_____	_____	_____
• Water	_____	_____	_____
Food	_____	_____	_____
Child care	_____	_____	_____
Student loan (future)	_____	_____	_____
Payments	_____	_____	_____
• Car	_____	_____	_____
• Credit card(s)	_____	_____	_____
• Other	_____	_____	_____
Transportation	_____	_____	_____
• Fares	_____	_____	_____
• Gas	_____	_____	_____
• Car repairs	_____	_____	_____
• Car registration and license	_____	_____	_____
Nonfood grocery items	_____	_____	_____
• Cleaning supplies	_____	_____	_____
• Paper goods	_____	_____	_____
Personal	_____	_____	_____
• Grooming	_____	_____	_____
• Haircuts	_____	_____	_____
• Clothing	_____	_____	_____
• Gifts	_____	_____	_____
Entertainment	_____	_____	_____
Total	_____	_____	_____

Continued

Prescription for Success 2–3 (Continued)

Add the three monthly totals and divide by three to calculate your average regular monthly expenses.
This is Monthly Amount A: $ _____
Now list expenses that occur less frequently.

Item	*Annual Amount*
Insurance	_____
• Homeowner's or renter's	_____
• Car	_____
• Health	_____
• Life	_____
• Other	_____

(*Note:* Health and disability insurance may be offered as employment benefits. This is discussed in Chapter 12.)

Property taxes	_____
Total	_____

Divide the total by 12 to get the average monthly amount needed for these annual expenses.
This is Monthly Amount B: $_____
Add Monthly Amounts A and B to see how much you need to cover your expenses:
$_____

Prescription for Success 2-4
Planning Ahead

1. Who do you already know who would be a good professional reference?

   _____

   _____

   _____

   _____

2. What can you start doing now to ensure you have access to at least four positive recommendations when you begin your job search?

   _____

   _____

   _____

   _____

Developing Your Personal Skills

CHAPTER 3

OBJECTIVES

The information and activities in this chapter can help you:
- Create a personal mission statement.
- Set achievable goals to help guide your life.
- Recognize the advantages of maintaining a positive attitude.
- Develop time-management and organizational strategies to improve your personal efficiency.
- Incorporate stress-reducing habits into your life.
- Identify and use personalized learning strategies.
- Improve your ability to retain information.
- Understand the benefits of having a mentor.

KEY TERMS AND CONCEPTS

Burnout: Physical and emotional exhaustion, often caused by overwork and feeling that one's efforts are not appreciated.

Efficiency: Getting the most done with the least effort and waste.

Insomnia: The inability to sleep well. It can be caused by worry, anxiety, or physical disorders.

Learning Styles: Different ways of taking in and processing information.

Mentor: A knowledgeable advisor or coach.

Mission Statement: A statement of one's fundamental beliefs that serve as the foundation for one's actions.

Peers: People with whom you have something in common, such as other students and co-workers.

Procrastinate: Put off doing something that needs to be done.

Relevant: Meaningful or important.

Stress: Physical and emotional reactions to life's events.

Values: Beliefs about what is important in life.

SETTING UP YOUR MISSION CONTROL

Starting on a new career path is a lot like launching a spacecraft. Both students and astronauts are entering new worlds, and for their missions to be successful, careful planning and preparation are required. Final destinations must be clearly defined so progress can be continually monitored and adjusted as needed to stay on course.

A helpful activity when planning a career launch is writing a **mission statement**, a statement of your basic beliefs and what you want to accomplish in your life. Stephen Covey, the author of personal success books, suggests mission statements as a way to identify what is really important to you. Individual mission statements are based on personal values. **Values** are our beliefs about what is important in life. They are the result of the teachings of family, school, religion, and friends as well as our experiences in life. Values provide a foundation for

making important life decisions, such as what we hope to contribute to the world, how we perform our work, and what we believe our obligations are to others and to ourselves.

A personal mission statement can help you choose an appropriate destination and then stay on track until you arrive. Many people, Covey points out, get sidetracked in life because they either lose sight of their basic values or fail to identify them clearly in the first place. Mission statements are usually written out, but there is no set format. You might want to write yours as a list, a series of paragraphs, or even a letter addressed to yourself. If you prefer, you can create a poster or collage, with each picture illustrating a value. Box 3-1 contains a sample mission statement written by Sarah, a medical assisting student.

Mission statements can serve as powerful motivators when you feel adrift or discouraged. For example, if you are committed to the well-being of your future patients, this value, rather than the need to

---

BOX 3-1   Sarah's Mission Statement

My decisions and actions will be based on my dedication to:
- Maintaining my health and that of my family
- Balancing my work and family life so that neither is neglected
- Doing my best to master the professional skills of medical assisting
- Serving the needs of all patients with whom I work

- Continuing to learn about my profession
- Being loyal to my family, friends, and employer
- Keeping a positive attitude
- Seeking to understand rather than to judge others

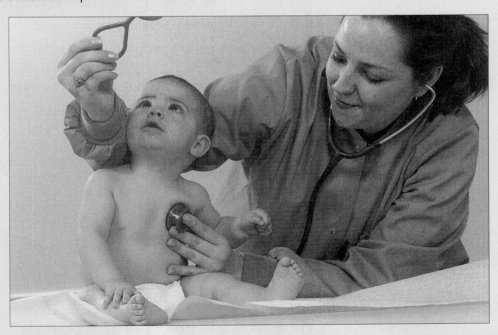

pass a test, should guide your studying. Suppose you have an anatomy test tomorrow morning. It is 10:00 PM and you have just finished a day filled with classes, work, and family responsibilities. Studying the skeleton becomes more meaningful when placed in the context of your dedication to helping future patients. You are not simply memorizing a collection of bones. You are learning about the source of Mrs. Jones's painful arthritis, and the more you know and understand about the bones and joints, the more you will be able to help her. Review Figure 3-1 to see the importance of focusing on what is really important to you—your major purposes in life.

Keep in mind throughout your program that your future patients will be directly affected by both what and how you are studying now, so you should be guided by your highest values. Here's another example: your mission statement includes the statement, "Provide high-quality care to all patients." You have an important exam for which you feel unprepared, and you are offered an opportunity to cheat. Cheating may take care of what you believe to be your most urgent need—getting a passing grade. But the consequences of this action—not learning the material and compromising your integrity—do not align with what should be your major goal of competently serving the needs of future patients. A well–thought-out mission statement functions as the control center that keeps guiding you in the right direction toward achieving what is most important to you.

Go to page 73 to complete Prescription for Success 3-1

GOALS—SIGNPOSTS ON THE PATH TO SUCCESS

"The purpose of goals is to motivate, not to paralyze."

—*Maureen Pfeifer*

Goals are based on your mission statement and serve as signposts, giving your life direction and measuring your progress on the road to success. You can use them to motivate yourself and mark your accomplishments. Effective goals have the following characteristics:

☐ They are based on your values and mission statement: The goals help you achieve what you believe to be important in life.
☐ They are reasonable: You may have to work hard, but you can accomplish them.
☐ They are measurable: You'll know when you have achieved them.
☐ They are clearly stated and written: Writing goals greatly increases your chance of reaching them.

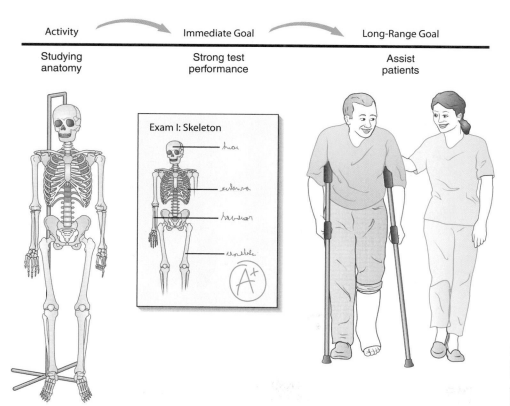

Activity	Immediate Goal	Long-Range Goal
Studying anatomy	Strong test performance	Assist patients

Exam I: Skeleton

A+

Figure 3–1 Keep your values and purpose in mind as a student. What you do now will influence your future effectiveness as a health care professional.

☐ They are worth your time: They are related to your career success, personal growth, and so on.

Here are two examples of well-stated goals for a health care student:

1. Over the next 10 weeks, I will learn the definition, pronunciation, and spelling of 150 new medical terms.
2. Within the next month, I will attend one professional meeting and talk with at least two people I have not met before.

Making Goals Work for You

Many people fail to achieve what they want in life because they fail to set clear goals for themselves. The first step, then, to is to spend some time deciding what it is you want to accomplish. The next step is to put together an action plan in which you outline what you need to do to reach each goal. Include reasonable deadlines for completing these actions. This is also the time to identify and locate any resources you might need to carry out your action plan. Examples of resources include people, materials, classes, equipment, and money. Greg, a medical transcription student, is taking a medical terminology course. Box 3-2 contains his plan to learn 300 medical terms.

Incorporate working on goals into your daily life. What can you do each day—even if it is something small—to move closer to achieving them? Long-term goals often get put aside in the scramble to meet everyday obligations, so it's a good idea to periodically review your goals to track your progress.

Long-Term Goals

Goals vary in the time and effort required to achieve them. Write your long-term goals first; then prepare short-term supporting goals. Link them together in a progressive series so each one supports the next. (See Figure 3-1.) For example, Jaime's long-term career goal is to become successfully employed as an x-ray technician in a large city hospital. Here is his plan:

- **Long-term goal:** Employment as an x-ray technician

BOX 3-2   Greg's Plan for Mastering a List of Medical Terms

- *Goal:* Over the next 10 weeks, I will learn the meaning, pronunciation, and correct spelling of 300 new medical terms.
- *Plan:* Learn 30 new terms each week. Study terminology 4 hours per week using flash cards, the workbook, CDs, and self-quizzes. Quiz myself at the end of each week.
- *Deadline:* 30 terms each week. Achieve goal of 300 words at the end of 10 weeks on (date).
- *Resources:* Text and workbook; CD that came with the textbook; additional tapes and CDs from the library; suggestions from instructors on best way to learn; medical dictionary.
- *Visualization:* I see myself in class receiving 100% on the medical terminology test. I see myself using medical terms correctly when talking with a co-worker on the job.
- *Affirmation:* "I, Greg, am mastering medical language easily and on schedule."

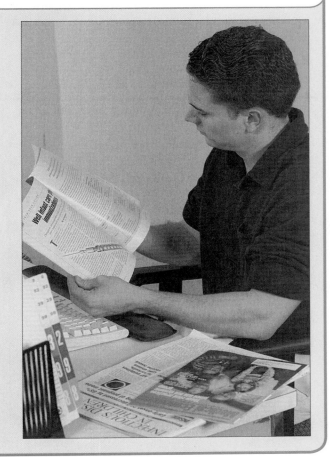

- **Supporting goals:** Graduate from an approved x-ray training program
  - Take a study skills course
  - Earn at least a B in all courses
  - Maintain perfect attendance for all classes
  - Complete all homework assignments on time
  - Receive a rating of at least "above average" on clinical experience
  - Pass the state licensing exam on the first try

As we discussed in Chapter 1, you may have to set short-term employment goals as a means of achieving your long-term ideal job goal. In Jaime's case, he discovers that the large urban hospital where he wants to work hires only technicians who have had at least 1 year of experience. Furthermore, they prefer technicians who are able to perform specialized x-rays not taught in most x-ray technology programs. So Jaime adjusts his goals as follows:

- **Long-term goal:** Employment in x-ray department at Grand Memorial Hospital
- **Short-term goals:** Receive a rating of "Excellent" on clinical experience
  - Improve communication skills
  - Work for at least 1 year in a facility that performs a variety of x-ray studies
  - Complete three specialized x-ray courses
  - Network with local professionals
  - Become active in the x-ray professional organization's local chapter

Jaime knows his clinical experience will provide valuable opportunities to demonstrate his hands-on competence as a technician. This will serve him well when he applies for his first job after graduation and will also supplement his work experience when he applies at Grand Memorial. His action steps to achieve his short-term goals include arranging reliable transportation (his old car is no longer dependable) so he can always arrive at his clinical site on time. By planning ahead, setting goals, and identifying appropriate action steps, Jaime has greatly increased his chances of achieving what he really wants.

Success Tips for Achieving Your Goals

☐ Visualize yourself achieving your goals.
☐ Use affirmations.
☐ Work on goals even when you don't feel like it. (Especially then!)
☐ Don't give up!

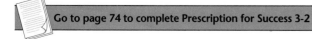
Go to page 74 to complete Prescription for Success 3-2

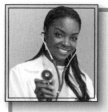

USING GOALS ON THE JOB

In addition to promoting your own growth and progress, the ability to set appropriate goals and take action to achieve them increases your effectiveness as a health care professional. Patients often benefit from goal setting, for example, when they are recovering from an illness or injury, arranging to pay a large medical bill, or attempting to follow a weight-loss plan. By developing your own goal-setting skills, you can share this knowledge and help patients plan the steps necessary to achieve their goals.

In some professional areas, such as physical and occupational therapy, goal setting is an integral part of the rehabilitation plan. Working with clients to set goals that are both realistic and challenging is an important part of therapy, and the same principles that work for personal goal setting can be applied in this area.

IT'S ALL IN THE ATTITUDE

"Man is not disturbed by the things that happened, but by the perception of things that happened."

—*Confucius*

Your attitude, the way you mentally look at things, can be your strongest ally or your worst enemy. It is more powerful than physical strength, is more important than natural talents, and has helped people overcome seemingly impossible difficulties. Many survivors of concentration and prison camps, for example, attribute their survival to having a positive attitude. The best thing about attitude is that it does not depend on other people or circumstances. It is yours alone, one of the few things in life over which you have complete control.

We hear about positive and negative attitudes to describe how people interpret things. Is the weather partly sunny or partly cloudy? Is a difficult class an opportunity to grow intellectually or a nightmare? Dr. Philip Hwang, a popular professor at the University of San Diego, tells his students he prefers to interpret a popular offensive gesture as "half a peace sign." He chooses his reaction, and this is the key to the power of attitude: we all can choose how we react to any situation.

"Well," you may say, "that doesn't make sense. If someone insults me or I'm having a bad day, it's natural to get angry or feel frustrated." It does seem natural because we are in the habit of responding negatively to situations that are annoying or upsetting. But how does this benefit you? In most cases, nothing is gained except bad feelings. For example, if you develop a negative attitude about a class ("I'll never learn how the endocrine system works," or "She really can't expect us to perform 20 perfect venipunctures after 2 weeks!"), you are working against yourself. Your attitude, whether positive or negative, will not change the circumstances. Your negative attitude, however, can make it more difficult, or even impossible, for you to understand the endocrine system or master venipunctures. A negative attitude is distracting, drains your energy, and interferes with your ability to concentrate. Choosing to approach life with a positive attitude releases you from the control of circumstances and frees you to focus fully on the priorities and actions that are in line with your mission and goals. Table 3-1 contains a list of suggestions for developing a positive approach to life.

Go to page 75 to complete Prescription for Success 3-3

TRIPPED UP BY YOUR THOUGHTS

"The only thing we have to fear is fear itself."
—*Franklin D. Roosevelt*

In Chapter 2 you read about how what we expect is often what happens—we get or become what we think! In fact, negative expectations can be just as powerful as positive ones, sometimes even more powerful. This is because our mental images, whether positive or negative, create our reality. It is important to understand that doubts and worries can actually bring about the outcome you fear. For example, Melinda thinks her supervisor dislikes her, so she avoids him and reacts defensively whenever he makes suggestions about her work. As a result of Melinda's behavior, chances are good the supervisor will have a problem with her. Tripped up by her thoughts, Melinda ends up creating what she expects and fears. Carl, pictured in Figure 3-2, uses a different approach.

The fact is, your attitude greatly influences your performance in school and your ability to secure and succeed in the job you want. Expect the best for yourself, and you are likely to get it.

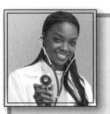

ATTITUDE ON THE JOB

Employers know that health care professionals with a positive attitude contribute to the success of their facility because attitude can promote the well-being of patients and improve the spirit of teamwork among the staff. Patients seek health care in times of need, and they bring with them an assortment of fears and doubts. They want hope and encouragement along with solutions to their health problems. Your cheerfulness, energy, and enthusiasm can assist in their recovery and increase their satisfaction with the care they are receiving. Your goodwill is an important part of the example you set as a role model. In short, your positive attitude can make a difference in the lives of those you serve. Happiness is contagious and is one thing we want to both give to and catch from others!

TABLE 3–1	Focusing on the Positive
Suggestion	**Ask Yourself**
Do an inventory of the good things in your life.	What do I have to be thankful for? Good health? Friends? Family? Decent living conditions? Opportunity to attend school? Ability to succeed in school and start a new career?
Keep things in perspective.	How important will this problem or situation be to me in 1 month? In 1 year?
Fix your sights on your mission and goals.	Should I distract my focus and waste energy on negativity? How will a positive attitude better help me get what I want and need?
Distinguish between what you can and cannot change, and concentrate your efforts on what you can change.	What action can I take? Which negative people and situations can I avoid? What changes can I make to improve the situation?
Find sources of help and inspiration.	Who can give me support? Who can give me advice? Do I have problems, such as depression or substance abuse, that may be helped with professional assistance?
Visualize the satisfaction you can receive by overcoming a difficult situation.	How will this contribute to my personal growth? What can I learn from this?
Challenge your negative beliefs.	Is this belief based on facts or on false perceptions and old ideas?

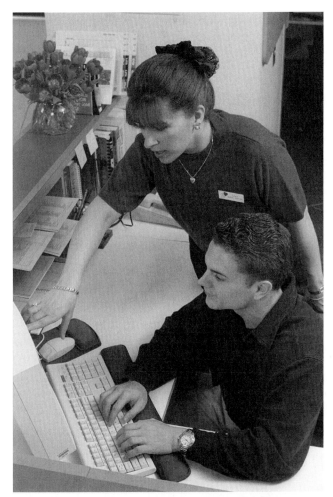

Figure 3–2 Carl was annoyed last week when he made an error inputting data. He thought it over and decided to use his mistake as an opportunity to learn from his supervisor, Gabriela. Do you have any current problems you can convert to learning opportunities?

MAKE TIME WORK FOR YOU

"Plan your work and work your plan."

Your success in life depends, to a great degree, on how you manage your time. Learning to use it to your advantage requires planning and self-discipline, but the payoffs are well worth the effort. One fact of life is true for everyone: there will never be enough time for everything you want to do. There are ways, however, to use your time more effectively. Two key strategies are prioritizing and practicing efficiency. Prioritizing means deciding what is most important and taking care of those tasks first. Your goals should determine your priorities. What do you most want to accomplish? Are you spending enough time and energy on activities that will help achieve your goals? For example, if your goal is to graduate from a medical lab technician program with honors, are you spending the necessary time

attending class, studying, and developing the work habits required of a lab technician? Or are phone conversations with friends and television viewing taking up a lot of your time?

Efficiency means planning and making the best use of time—getting the most done with the least effort. Examples of inefficiency include running to the grocery store to pick up a forgotten item, spending time looking for misplaced homework, and stopping for gas when you're already late for class rather than filling up the tank the day before. It's easy to feel very busy and yet be inefficient. Pay attention to how you spend your time. A short break from studying to "rest your eyes" can stretch into an evening of lost hours in front of the television set.

Keeping a calendar is an important part of good time management. Many types of calendars and planners, such as PDAs (personal digital assistants) that include everything from calendars to phones, are becoming very popular.[1] They allow you to store lots of information, including your schedule, telephone numbers, and other reference information. Many now enable you to access the Internet. Paper planners also work very well, and some people even prefer them over the electronic variety. The important thing is to select the best kind for you—one you will use. It should be convenient to carry with you and should have room to list several items for each date.

Collect all sources of important school and class dates: schedules, catalogs, and class syllabi. Mark important items on your calendar, including dates of quizzes and tests; due dates for assignments, projects, and library books; school holidays (for both you and your children); and deadlines for turning in required paperwork, such as financial aid and professional exam applications, and for paying fees. Add important personal dates: birthdays of family members and friends, deadlines for bills and taxes, doctors' appointments, and back-to-school nights for your children. If you work, note dates you need to remember: company potluck party, performance review, project deadlines. Colored ink is a good way to mark events you don't want to miss, like the day your professional exam is given! Again, the important thing is to create a planning tool that works for you.

 Go to page 77 to complete Prescription for Success 3-4

Success Tips for Managing Your Time

☐ Consider your priorities and goals when you plan your schedule and decide how to spend your time.

☐ Write out a weekly schedule. Take a few minutes every week to plan ahead. This allows you to coordinate your activities with family members, plan ahead for important days (to avoid trying to find just the right birthday present on the way to the party), combine errands to save time, and plan your study time to avoid last-minute cramming.

☐ Schedule study time every day. This is your top priority! Give yourself a chance to succeed. Arrange not to be disturbed, and let friends and family members know that when you are at your desk, the time is yours.

☐ Schedule around your peak times. We all have individual body rhythms, specific times of the day when we feel most alert and energetic. Some people do their best work late at night. Others accomplish the most between 5:00 AM and 9:00 AM. Class and work schedules cannot always accommodate your needs, but when you have a choice, do the most challenging tasks during your best hours.

☐ Do the hardest thing first. When you have a number of things to do or subjects to study, try tackling the most difficult (or boring or tedious) one first, when you are freshest. Completing unpleasant tasks gives you a surge of energy by removing a source of worry and distraction from your mind and rewarding you with a sense of accomplishment.

☐ Be realistic about what you can accomplish and how much time tasks will take to complete. For example, thinking you can complete a research paper in one weekend can be a serious mistake because you may run into difficulties and end up with no time to spare. You will learn more about your work speed as you progress through your program. At the beginning, it is best to plan more time than you think you will need. On the other hand, take care not to spend more time than necessary on one project or assignment, causing you to neglect all others.

☐ Prevent feeling overwhelmed by breaking work into small segments. (The thought of writing this book was overwhelming until I broke it down into chapters, topics, and pages.) Plan deadlines for each segment, and put them on your calendar.

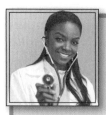

TIME MANAGEMENT ON THE JOB

A growing concern in the United States today is providing health care in a cost-effective manner. As a consequence, efficient scheduling and the use of time are increasingly important for health care facilities. A major expense for any employer is paying employees, which translates to paying for the time they are on the job. Using your time efficiently at work will contribute to the overall financial success of the organization.

A specific application of time management on the job is patient scheduling. In a clinic or doctor's office, scheduling may be performed by the receptionist or administrative medical assistant. The first part of this important responsibility is to properly schedule appointments for smooth patient flow as illustrated in the accompanying figure. The second part is working throughout the day to coordinate office activities and ensure that, with the exception of emergencies, everyone is kept on schedule. Waiting to see the doctor is reportedly the most common patient complaint and gives the impression the office does not value the patient's time. And constantly playing "catch up" is stressful for the staff. Good time management creates a better work environment and increases the quality of customer service.

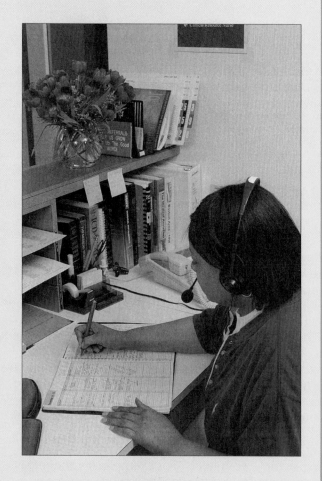

Ask for help and cooperation from family members and friends.

☐ Learn to say "no." Your schedule cannot always accommodate the requests of other people. It's difficult, but sometimes necessary, to turn down demands on our time such as an invitation to a party or a request to help at the church rummage sale. An instructor who reviewed this book said the following response works very well: "I'm really sorry, but I won't be able to help. I wish you the best in finding someone who can."

☐ Use down time to your advantage. There are many pockets of time that usually go to waste, such as when waiting for an appointment or using public transportation. Use this time to study flash cards, write lists, review class notes, brainstorm topics for a research paper, review the steps involved in a lab procedure, or summarize the major points of a class lecture. (I did about half of the work toward my last college degree while sitting in airports and on airplanes!)

Go to page 78 to complete Prescription for Success 3-5

DEFEATING THE PROCRASTINATION DEMON

To **procrastinate** is to put off doing what needs to be done. Procrastinating can cause late assignments, failed tests, poor recommendations, and increased stress. Yet many of us fall victim to this self-defeating habit. Although it's natural to delay what we perceive to be difficult, tedious, or overwhelming, there are steps you can take to break the habit (Figure 3-3).

The first step is to identify the reason for your procrastination. What is holding you back? Are you afraid of failing? Do you believe you lack the ability to do what needs to be done? Does the task seem so unpleasant you cannot motivate yourself to start it? Is the project so large you feel overwhelmed and are the victim of "overload paralysis"? Once you have identified the reason, examine it carefully. Is it true you don't have the ability? Can the job be broken down into manageable portions? Can you match completing the task to a meaningful long-term goal?

The next step is setting a time to start, even if you simply work on planning what you are going to do. Accomplishing even a small amount can inspire you to keep going. Look for ways to break large projects into manageable pieces and plan deadlines for each. Develop a controlled sense of urgency (not panic!) to encourage yourself to meet self-imposed deadlines.

If you find yourself stuck, identify sources of help, such as your instructor, your supervisor, or a friend. Perhaps you need additional materials or more information to get started. Try using affirmations such as, "I am capable of understanding how the nervous system functions. My presentation to the class will be interesting and well organized." Visualize yourself completing the work. Experience the feeling of satisfaction. Finally, focus on your future. Think about how completing the work will help you achieve your goals to graduate and get a good job.

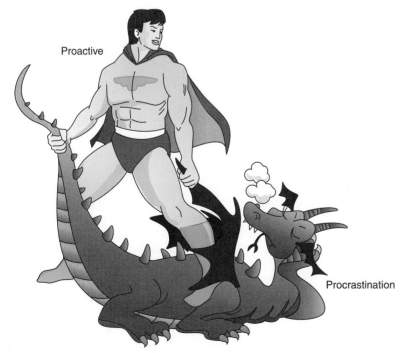

Proactive

Procrastination

Figure 3–3 Procrastination can cause stress and can result in work that doesn't show you at your best. Working to defeat this "demon" will free up the energy spent on worrying about getting your work completed.

Go to page 79 to complete Prescription for Success 3-6

PERSONAL ORGANIZATION: GETTING IT ALL TOGETHER

"A vital key to success is learning to work smarter, not harder."

The purpose of personal organization, like time management, is to make life easier. Organizational techniques build consistency and predictability into your daily routines, saving you time and energy. Surprise-filled adventures are great for vacation trips, but efficiency is a better way to ensure academic and career success. Hunting for your keys every morning and arriving late for class is a waste of your time and a sign of inconsideration for your instructor and classmates. On the job, lack of organization can reduce patient satisfaction. No one wants to wait while the massage therapist scurries about to gather clean sheets or the relaxation tape she wanted to play.

Organization, however, should never be an end in itself. It doesn't mean keeping a perfectly tidy house, with clothes arranged according to color and season. It does mean surveying your needs and developing ways to avoid unnecessary rushing, repetition, and waste.

Success Tips for Getting Organized

☐ **Write lists.** Most people today, especially students, have too many things on their minds to remember grocery lists, all the day's errands, who they promised to call, which lab supplies to take to class, and so on. Scraps of paper are easy to lose. Commercial organizers and planners, both paper and electronic, give you a place to record phone numbers, addresses of stores, recommendations from friends, ideas you think of throughout the day, and so on.

☐ **Carry a big bag.** A typical student's day may include classes, work, shopping, and errands such as returning a video. Start each day—either in the morning or the night before—by checking your calendar and to-do list to see what you need to take with you. If you go directly to class from work, pack your books, binder, uniform, and other necessary supplies. Take along a healthy snack to avoid having to raid the vending machines. Always carry your planner or calendar.

☐ **Stock up.** Running out of milk, shampoo, or diapers can lead to a frustrating waste of time and energy. Even worse is discovering at 11:30 PM, while finishing a major assignment due in the morning, that your printer cartridge is empty and you don't have another. (Cartridges seem to be well aware of deadlines and choose to dry up accordingly!) Keep important backup supplies on hand. A handy way to monitor these is to keep a shopping list on the refrigerator and instruct everyone in the household to list items as they run low. You can note needed study supplies on the same list.

☐ **Give things a home.** Keeping what you need where you can find it can save countless hours of search time. It will also prevent redoing lost assignments or paying late fees on misplaced bills. If your study area is a dual-use area such as the kitchen table, try keeping your books and supplies in one place on a shelf or in a large box where everything can stay together. This way you can set up an "instant desk" when it is time to study. Organize your class notes and handouts by subject in a binder. Color-coded files work well for keeping ongoing projects and notes from previous classes in order.

☐ **Keep things in repair.** Life is easier if you can depend on the car and other necessities. If money is tight, focus on keeping the essentials in working order and look for ways to economize elsewhere.

☐ **Cluster errands.** Modern life requires trips to the grocery store, the mall, the children's school, the post office—you name it, we go there! Save time and money by doing as much as possible on each trip. Look for shopping centers that have many services to avoid running all over town.

☐ **Take advantage of technology.** If you are connected to the Internet, take advantage of opportunities to shop, pay bills, and perform other tasks online. If you don't a have a PDA, investigate the use of one.

☐ **Handle it once.** If you find that mail, bills, announcements, and other paperwork accumulate in ever-growing piles, try processing each item as it comes in. Sort the mail quickly each day and do something with each piece: discard the junk, pay the bills (or file them together for payment once or twice a month), answer letters with a short note, read messages and announcements, and place magazines in a basket to be looked over when you have time. Handle other papers that come into the house—permission slips for the kids, announcements from work— the same way.

☐ **Get it over with.** Certain unpleasantries, like parking tickets and dental work, come into everyone's life. It's easy to spend time worrying about them. A good strategy is to get them over with as quickly as possible: pay the ticket or make an appointment with the dentist. Seek help if you need it, and do your best to take care of what needs to be done. Procrastinating and worrying can drain your energy and interfere with your concentration.

☐ **Plan backups.** Prearrange ways to handle emergencies: a ride to school if the car breaks down, child care to cover for a sick babysitter, a study buddy who will lend you notes if you miss a class. Backups are like insurance policies—you hope you won't need them, but if you do, they're good to have. And whenever possible, plan backups for your backups!

If getting organized seems like a waste of time, too much work, or just "not your style," consider the alternative: using even more time and energy in unproductive ways that result in frustration and inconvenience. You can start now to help yourself get it together at the same time you develop organizational skills that are valuable in all health care occupations.

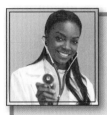

ORGANIZATION ON THE JOB

A typical job description for a medical assistant includes many organizational duties that correspond closely with the success tips listed in this section:

1. Sort and handle the mail daily. (Handle it once.)
2. Monitor warranties on equipment, and call for maintenance and repair. (Keep things in repair.)
3. Inventory and order administrative, laboratory, and clinical supplies. (Stock up.)
4. Organize and store supplies and equipment. (Give things a home.)
5. Complete all tasks as directed by the physician. (Write lists.)

WHAT IS THIS THING CALLED STRESS?

We hear a lot about stress these days. One friend says, "I'm so stressed over this exam." Another exclaims, "I just can't take any more of this stress." **Stress** refers to our physical and emotional reactions to life's events. These reactions can either help us or hurt us, depending on the circumstances. "Good stress" motivates us when we are called on to perform outside our usual comfort zone. For example, if you witness a car accident and stop to help the victims, your body probably experiences certain reactions: your heart rate speeds up, your blood

pressure rises, and the blood vessels in your muscles and the pupils of your eyes dilate. These changes increase your energy, strength, and mental alertness so you can best deal with the situation.

You can draw on these natural reactions to help you in important, although less dramatic, situations such as taking a professional licensing exam, giving a speech in class, or planning your wedding. This is making use of good stress to maximize your performance. The excitement experienced when you pass the exam and start a new career or get married and begin a new life with the person you love is also a form of good stress.

Pressure and unresolved worries experienced over long periods of time can create "bad stress." When the physical responses to stress are repeated over and over, with no resolution or action taken, they can actually decrease your ability to cope with life's ups and downs. In a sense, your body wears itself out as it continually prepares you to handle situations that are never resolved. Signs of long-term stress include **insomnia,** headaches, digestive problems, muscle tension, fatigue, frequent illness, irritability, depression, poor concentration, excessive eating and drinking, and use of illegal substances. It's easy to see that these don't work in your favor and are likely to increase your stress level. It's possible to get caught in a vicious cycle of ever-increasing stress that leads to feelings of hopelessness. Your mental images become dictated by worry and fear and may bring about, as previously discussed, the very thing you fear.

Sources of Stress

The first step in dealing with long-term stress is to identify its source. The following list contains some of the common sources of stress (stressors) for students:

- Financial difficulties
- Family problems: unsupportive partner, abuse, children's behavior, overdemanding parents
- Poor organizational skills
- Inability to manage time; having too much to do
- Lack of self-confidence and poor self-esteem
- Feeling unsure about study skills and ability to learn
- Loneliness
- Health problems, pregnancy
- Believing that instructors are unfair or don't like them
- Poor relationships with **peers**
- Believing the assignments and tests are too difficult or not **relevant**
- Difficulty following school rules and requirements

The second step in handling stress is to examine the source to see whether it's based on fact or fiction. For example, if you worry about failing your courses because you are not "smart enough," this may be based on a false belief about yourself. It is very likely you are intellectually competent. But believing you aren't can create stress that discourages you from even trying. After all, what's the point of making a significant effort if you're going to fail anyway? (The self-fulfilling prophecy at work!) A better approach is to seek guidance from your instructor or student services.

Finally, look for a practical solution. What are your options? Can you distance yourself from the stressor (for example, a negative friend who constantly asks why you are returning to school at your age)? Can you get help to resolve the problem (free financial counseling for budget and credit problems, tutoring in a difficult subject)? Can you empower yourself (math refresher course, speed-reading tapes)? The important thing is to face the stressor and look for ways to take control. Convert bad stress into good stress by using it as a signal that you may have issues that can prevent you from achieving your goals and attaining the success you want and deserve. Then take action to deal with the issues.

Success Tips for Handling Stress

The very nature of being a student and working in health care brings a certain amount of ongoing stress that cannot be avoided entirely. Many of the practices that promote good health are excellent for relieving stress: exercise, adequate sleep, eating properly, and avoiding excess caffeine. Here are some other things you can try:

☐ **Practice mentally.** If your stress is caused by an upcoming event such as a job interview, you can anticipate and mentally practice the event. Athletes use this technique to prepare for the big game. They "see" themselves performing the perfect tennis serve or making the foul shot. Employ your stress to motivate you to prepare in advance.

☐ **Use time-management and personal organization strategies.** Try the techniques suggested in this chapter to help you take control of your life. Work on eliminating the conditions that have you feeling like you're racing downhill with no brakes.

☐ **Seek the support of others.** People do better when they have the support of others. Studies have shown that students who have just one other person who really cares whether they graduate are more likely to finish school than

those who have no one. Seek the help of trusted friends, family members, classmates, or school personnel.

☐ **Perform relaxation exercises.** Meditation, yoga, deep breathing, and muscle relaxation, described in Box 3-3, can relieve physical discomfort and promote emotional well-being.

☐ **Engage in physical exercise.** Even a short walk can be a very effective stress reducer. Find something you enjoy doing and make a little time for it on a regular basis.

☐ **Adjust your attitude.** Focus on your goals, acknowledge all progress, and concentrate on the benefits you will receive.

☐ **Keep your sense of humor.** Look at the humorous side of life and its events. Laugh therapy has been found to strengthen the immune system and positively affect health.

☐ **Use school and community resources.** Refer to the chart you prepared in Prescription for

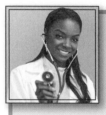

STRESS ON THE JOB

Good stress can serve the health care professional by providing extra energy and increased mental alertness to handle emergency situations properly, provide competent patient care, and maintain a busy schedule. Your success in assisting a fallen patient, performing first aid, and getting through a hectic day of processing medical bills are examples of using good stress. "Bad stress," however, can have negative results, so it is important to incorporate stress-reduction techniques into your daily work life. Tragic results of excessive buildup of stress among health care workers include **burnout**, addiction to painkillers, and alcoholism. Start now to learn effective stress management, so you can convert stress from an enemy to an ally.

Learning to handle stress will benefit not only you, but your future patients as well. Illness and injury are major stressors, and an important part of patient education is helping patients deal with both physical and emotional stress. At the same time, stress can be the cause of illness. Research has shown that the majority of visits to the doctor are based on stress-related conditions. If the health care staff is showing signs of stress, this can trickle down to patients, and this is certainly the last thing they need.

Success 1-2. Helpful information may be available from student services, your religious organization, or the local community center.

☐ **Make use of this book.** Chapters 3 through 8 contain many suggestions for developing effective study and life skills. Try them out and use the ones that work best for you.

PERSONAL REFLECTION

1. Do you believe you may be experiencing long-term stress?

   _____

   _____

   _____

2. If yes, what are the signs?

   _____

   _____

   _____

3. Can you identify the cause or causes?

   _____

   _____

   _____

4. List at least three strategies you will try for dealing with stress:

   _____

   _____

   _____

LEARNING FOR LIFE

Learning means much more than getting by in school and remembering information long enough to pass tests. It means storing information mentally and mastering hands-on skills that you can retrieve and use when you need them on the job. Furthermore, it means being able to apply what you have learned to solve problems and make informed decisions. For example, if you are learning about the circulatory system, you are not simply memorizing

| BOX 3-3 | Relaxation Exercise |

Eliminating muscle tension helps relieve anxiety and fatigue. Try this simple exercise to help you release this tension and prevent headaches and other pain.

1. Sit comfortably in a place where you won't be disturbed. Choose a chair that supports your back and allows you to place your feet flat on the floor.
2. Close your eyes.
3. Begin at your toes and tense each group of muscles. Hold for a few seconds and then release. Work from the bottom of the body to the top, tensing and relaxing each area. Pay special attention to the shoulders and jaw muscles, common areas of tension.
4. As you proceed, focus on the feelings of tension and then letting go.
5. When you finish, sit quietly and say to yourself, "I am relaxed."

the parts of the heart and the path of blood through the body. You are acquiring information to help real patients who have heart problems. If you are studying a form of therapy, your study of the muscular system will have practical applications. Your purpose for learning is far more important than simply studying to earn a grade. Your future patients and clients will depend on your knowledge, and they deserve your best efforts to learn now.

How Do You Learn Best?

If you ever have trouble following your instructors' lectures or find that your class notes are a confusing jumble, you are not alone. It is possible that you learn better when instruction is presented visually or through hands-on experience. Research has demonstrated that people learn in different ways, called **learning styles**, and that by identifying your own preferred learning styles you can be more successful in your studies. The three learning styles most commonly discussed are grouped by the senses used when acquiring and processing new information: auditory, visual, and kinesthetic (hands-on). Table 3-2 contains a description of each of these styles.

There are other learning preferences, in addition to the styles related to our senses. Table 3-3 describes six other approaches to learning.

None of us learns in just one way. And it is important to understand that there is not a "best way" to learn. Just as we have different personalities, we have different combinations of learning styles. The purpose of discovering your preferred learning styles is to help you study more effectively. Sandra,

TABLE 3–2	Three Major Learning Styles	
Learning Style	How Student Learns Best	Examples of Effective Learning Activities
Auditory	Through *hearing*. Remembers information from lectures and discussions better than material read in textbook. Prefers music over art and listening over reading. Understands written material better when it is read aloud. May spell better out loud than when writing. Misses visual cues. Prefers doing oral rather than written reports.	Lectures, CDs, tapes, music, rhymes, speaking
Visual	Through *seeing*. Remembers information presented in written or graphic form better than in lectures and discussions. Often needs people to repeat what they have said. Takes notes when oral instructions are given. Prefers art to music and reading to listening. Understands better when the speaker's face is seen. Prefers doing written rather than oral reports.	Reading, pictures, diagrams, charts, graphs, maps, videos, films, chalkboard, overhead projections
Kinesthetic (hands-on)	Through *doing*. Remembers information acquired through activities. Reads better when moving lips and saying words silently or moving finger along the page. Enjoys moving around while studying. Likes to touch things, point, use fingers when counting or calculating. Prefers doing a demonstration rather than an oral or written report.	Lab activities, skills practice, experiments, games, movement, building models

TABLE 3–3	More Approaches to Learning

DEDUCTIVE VERSUS INDUCTIVE	
Deductive	**Inductive**
Deductive learners prefer to learn facts before forming generalizations (the big picture). They prefer to first memorize dates, study individual events, and know the details. When learning about the circulatory system, for example, they would rather study the various parts of the system before learning how they all work together to circulate the blood.	Inductive learners want to see and understand the big picture which they use as a framework for learning the details. When learning about cells, for example, they would want to know the purpose and function of the cell before learning the individual components.

LINEAR VERSUS GLOBAL	
Linear	**Global**
Linear thinkers learn best when material is organized in a logical sequence. They like to do things in order, building on material previously learned.	Global thinkers like to work with all the facts, regardless of the order. They are interested in forming relationships within the material.

INDIVIDUAL VERSUS INTERACTIVE	
Individual	**Interactive**
Individual-type learners prefer to work on learning tasks alone. They like to figure out all aspects of assignments and projects on their own.	Interactive-type learners like to work with another student or in groups. They want to share their ideas and hear the ideas of others.

a nursing student, has found the following methods to work best for her:

1. Receive new information from a class lecture (auditory)
2. Review by studying notes alone (individual)
3. Concentrate first on memorizing the important facts (inductive)

 Go to page 79 to complete Prescription for Success 3-7

Developing Learning Strategies

Identifying your preferred ways of learning does not mean you will avoid the others. This would be impossible in a health care program that includes both theoretical and practical knowledge and skills. And individual instructors use a variety of approaches to teaching. Some will match your learning styles; others won't. For example, when teaching students how to take a blood pressure reading, the instructor might introduce the topic with a lecture (auditory), give a reading assignment (visual), demonstrate and describe the procedure (auditory and visual), assign a worksheet (individual), and have partners practice on one another (kinesthetic and interactive). In her lecture, she might list the individual steps first (inductive) or explain the purpose and significance of blood pressure before explaining how to take it (deductive). The good news is that you can learn in a variety of ways and benefit from your strongest methods while developing your weakest. Table 3-4 gives examples of study techniques for learning the names and locations of the major bones. Figure 3-4 shows students using a variety of learning strategies.

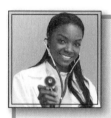

LEARNING STYLES ON THE JOB

The ability to provide good patient education is an increasingly important skill for today's health care professionals. Shorter hospital stays have resulted in patients and their families being responsible for care that was once provided by nursing staff. Patients must be taught about home care and signs of complications.

Many of the major health problems affecting patients today are influenced by lifestyle factors, such as weight, exercise, smoking, and stress. In fact, the three leading causes of death in the United States, cancer, heart disease, and stroke, are strongly influenced by personal habits. Teaching patients about self-care and healthy habits is easier and more effective when you understand that people learn in different ways. Health care professionals may need to provide information in a variety of ways, including oral explanations, pictures and written materials, and hands-on demonstrations of procedures.

Go to page 81 to complete Prescription for Success 3-8

DOWN MEMORY LANE

Memorizing is not the same as learning, but it is an important component of the learning process. Although you may be able to rely on your short-term memory to complete assignments and pass tests, it is the material stored in long-term memory that will serve you throughout your studies, when taking your professional exam, and afterward on the job.

There are many ways to improve your memory and better retain the material you study.

The way to start is by making sure you understand the new material. Experiments have shown it is much more difficult to remember nonsense syllables or lists of unrelated numbers than material that has meaning. In other words, it is very difficult to remember what you don't understand in the first place. So ask questions in class, look up words you don't know, and read difficult passages several times.

Repeat, repeat, repeat. The very best way to retain new material is repetition over an extended period of time. In fact, the length of time information is remembered is often in direct proportion to the length of time over which it is learned. Review new material as soon as possible after you first encounter it and continue to review it on a regular basis, at least weekly.

Use strategies based on your learning styles. If you are an auditory learner, listen to or say new math formulas over and over. Visual learners can post the formulas on the bathroom mirror. And kinesthetic learners can try writing each new formula 10 times. Use your imagination. Studying does not necessarily mean working quietly at a desk. Create rhymes or funny images. Make up movements associated with each item you have to remember. One method, called "pegging," has you place imaginary pegs on walls around the house. On each one, "hang" a fact or idea you must remember. As you walk through the house each day, review the material on each peg.

Look for ways to relate new information to your own experience by connecting it to something you already know. When you study something new, start by making a list of what you know—or would like to know—about the topic.

Success Tips for Improving Your Memory

☐ **Relax.** Your ability to store and remember things does not work well when your body is tense and your mind is distracted with worry. Try doing a relaxation exercise before starting a study session.
☐ **Remove distractions.** Studying for mastery requires concentration. Find a place where interruptions are limited and where you can use your chosen techniques. (For example, auditory learners who plan to use singing and tapping should probably not study in the school library!)
☐ **Break up your study sessions.** Most people can't concentrate fully for very long periods of time. The great thing about reviewing over time, rather than at the last minute, is that you can take time for short breaks.

TABLE 3-4	Developing Learning Strategies That Work for You
Learning Style	**Examples of Learning Strategies for Learning the Names of the Bones**
Auditory	Say the names of the bones out loud. Listen to a CD of the names and locations of each. Make your own CD of the names and locations. Create a song, rhyme, rap, or jingle. Silly is good because it helps you remember. ("There are fourteen phalanges in my little handies.") Clap or tap out a rhythm as you repeat the words. Make flash cards and say the words and/or definitions out loud. Create sound-alike association. Remember, silly is okay. ("The cranium holds the brain-ium.")
Visual	Look at photos or drawings of the bones as you study their names. Label a drawing of the skeleton. Color the bones on a drawing. Create mental pictures of associations (a crane lifting a huge cranium). Put up a labeled drawing of the skeleton where you will see it often—the bathroom mirror, your bedroom wall, near your study desk. Make flash cards with a picture of the bone on one side and the name on the reverse.
Kinesthetic	Point to or touch each bone as you learn its name. Use drawings, a model (inexpensive anatomic models are sold in toy stores), or your own body. Make two flash cards for each bone: one with the name, the other with the location. Mix the cards, then study by sorting and matching each set. Stand, move, or walk around as you study. Associate movements as you learn. For example, lift and bend your arm when studying the humerus, ulna, and radius. Write the name of each bone several times.
Deductive	Start by learning the name and location of each individual bone.
Inductive	Start by looking at the whole skeleton. Look at the relationships and connections between bones. Consider how the bones contribute to body function.
Linear	Study the bones in a structured order, such as by area (arms and legs) or from top to bottom (shoulder to hand).
Global	Study from a labeled diagram that includes the entire skeleton or all the bones of a given area.
Individual	Use the suggested learning techniques by yourself. Set goals for how many bones you'll learn each day. Create a reward system for yourself.
Interactive	Form a study group with classmates. Ask a friend or family member to quiz you. Organize a group or class competition.

☐ **Overlearn.** Continue to review and repeat material you already know. This helps to firmly lock it into long-term memory.

☐ **Quiz yourself.** Make up your own quizzes. Review one day and take the quiz several days later to evaluate your retention.

 Go to page 82 to complete Prescription for Success 3-9

THE PERILS OF CRAMMING

Cramming is a well-known student activity consisting of frantic last-minute efforts, sometimes fortified with coffee and junk food, to finish assignments or prepare for tests. The major problem with cramming is that it serves only the immediate goal of meeting a school deadline. True learning rarely occurs. The conditions required for learning, such as the opportunity for repetition over time, are absent. Most of what is crammed is forgotten within a few days—or

hours! Work in health care demands a higher level of competence than you are likely to achieve as a result of cramming. Do your future patients deserve your best efforts to learn, or are the bits you may remember after a night of cramming good enough? This is an important consideration for students who claim that cramming works well for them because they can study only at the last minute when the deadline is close. This is true only if passing the test is their only goal.

Another problem with cramming is it leaves you with few options. If you are writing a paper the night before it is due and you discover that the information you have is inadequate (and the Internet is not available), you have no time to consult other sources. If you are studying for a test and realize there are several points you don't understand, it's too late to ask the instructor to explain them.

Finally, cramming adds more stress to an already busy life in which you may be balancing various

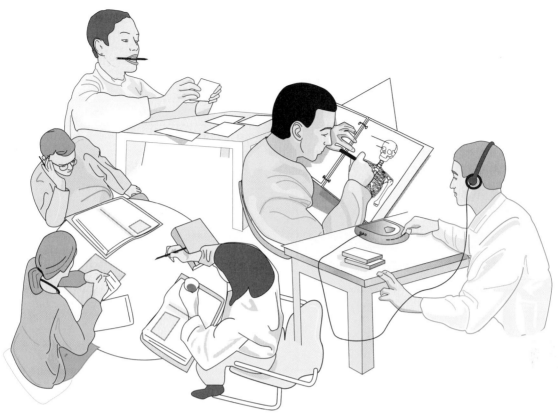

Figure 3–4   Identify and use the study techniques that work best for you.

responsibilities. If it costs you a night's sleep, it can deplete your energy, and it can interfere with your ability to concentrate. You end up creating a non-productive cycle consisting of a continual game of catch up and the danger of creating ongoing stress.

The reality is that things happen, you get behind, and you run out of time. Almost every student occasionally finds it necessary to cram. Here are some tips to make the best of a bad situation[2]:

1. Don't beat yourself up and waste energy feeling guilty. You'll only distract your attention from what you have to do. Just make a mental note to change your study habits to avoid the need for future cramming.

2. Do a very quick visualization in which you see yourself accomplishing what you need to do in the time you have available.

3. Minimize all distractions. For example, see if you can find someone to watch the children.

4. Focus on the most important material. What is most likely to be emphasized on the test? What are the main requirements of the assignment?

5. Use the learning and memory techniques described in this section. Draw on your learning style to help you learn the necessary material.

6. Try to stay calm. Physical tension distracts from mental effort. Breathe deeply, stretch, and do a quick relaxation exercise.

MENTORS MAKE A DIFFERENCE

"People seldom improve when they have no other model but themselves to copy."

—*Oliver Goldsmith*

A **mentor** is an advisor you choose for yourself, someone who has the experience and background to give you sound advice about your studies and career. This is a person you respect and see as a positive role model. Your chances of succeeding are greatly increased when someone you respect cares about your progress. This has been proven in both school and business settings. Where can you find such a person? It can be an instructor, school staff member, administrator, or someone who works in health care. You might find a graduate of your school who is working successfully. It is important to choose someone with whom you feel comfortable.

Once you have identified a person you would like to have as your mentor, ask for an appointment. Let him or her know you want to talk about mentoring. At the meeting, explain that you are pursuing a career in health care and would like this person to serve as your mentor and give you guidance. Ask how much time he or she has to meet with you. You should meet or talk with your mentor periodically to ask questions, stay motivated, and learn more about becoming a health care professional. Mentors who work in health care can give you information about the current state of your targeted occupation, suggest what you should emphasize in your studies, and introduce you to other health care professionals. If the first person you approach does not have the time or is not interested, don't be discouraged. Continue your search—it will be worth the effort!

PERSONAL REFLECTION

What would you look for in choosing a mentor?

_____

_____

_____

Who do you know who might be a good mentor?

_____

_____

_____

What can you do to find a mentor who works in health care?

_____

_____

_____

SUMMARY OF KEY IDEAS

1. Let your goals be your guides.
2. Never underestimate the power of attitude.
3. If managed well, time can work for you.
4. Work smarter, not harder.
5. You can use stress to work for instead of against you.
6. Learning how to learn will increase your ability to learn.
7. A mentor can help you succeed.

Positive Self-Talk for This Chapter

1. I have worthy goals and am on track to achieve them.
2. I manage my time efficiently.

3. I am well organized and in control of my life.
4. I use effective study strategies based on my learning styles.

To Learn More

Chapman E: *Life is an attitude!* Menlo Park, Calif, 1992, Crisp Publications.

Elwood Chapman has been an "attitude guru" since the 1950s. This is the latest in his bestselling books on how to control your outlook on life by beating negativity, eliminating doubts, and setting positive goals. The book is short and very easy to read.

Covey S, Merrill AR, Merrill RR: *First things first,* New York, 1995, Simon and Schuster. (Also available on a CD.)

This book connects your mission statement and goals with time management. Rather than describing ways to get more done, it explains how to do what you decide is the most important. Covey teaches a method of categorizing tasks to help you focus on what is really important, not just on what is urgent. As he puts it, "Doing more things faster is no substitute for doing the right things." Important items are identified by focusing on a few key priorities and roles that will vary from person to person, then identifying small goals for each role each week, in order to maintain a balanced life.

Felder RM, Soloman BA: Learning styles and strategies. Available at: www.ncsu.edu/unity/lockers/users/f/felder/public/ILSdir/styles.htm.

This article, written by a professor and an advisor at North Carolina State University, categorizes and describes a variety of learning styles along with strategies for effective learning.

Hansen K: *The value of a mentor.* Available at: www.quintcareers.com/mentor_value.html.

This article includes tips on finding and benefitting from a mentor as you pursue your career goals.

Lakein A: *How to get control of your time and your life,* New York, 1989, Penguin Group (USA).

Although first published 30 years ago, this book is still a classic. Many consider it to be *the* authoritative source on which all other time-management books are based. Lakein explains the importance of prioritizing tasks and learning to work smarter, not harder.

Mind Tools. Available at: http://mindtools.com.

This website contains hundreds of helpful articles about important life and career skills, including time management, memory improvement, and stress management.

REFERENCES

1. *Saunders Health professional's planner,* Philadelphia, 2002, Saunders.
2. Ellis D: *Becoming a master student,* ed 12, Boston, 2009, Houghton Mifflin.

INTERNET ACTIVITIES

For active links to the websites needed to complete these activities, visit **http://evolve. elsevier.com/Haroun/career/.**

1. Use the search terms "setting goals," "achieving goals," and "achieving personal goals" to locate information about using goals successfully. Assume the role of a "success coach" and use what you learn to write a short article for students.

2. Using the search term "effective time management," find five facts or suggestions on time management not covered in this chapter.

3. Search for information about the benefits of having a positive attitude. An interesting organization dedicated to teaching people to believe in themselves is the Positive Attitude Institute. Review their website and use the information you find to write a short report on how a positive attitude can contribute to school and career success.

4. MedlinePlus, a public health information website sponsored by the National Library of Medicine, has many links to scientific and health organizations. Review the articles on stress and write a report about its effects on health.

Explain how this information can benefit both you and your future patients.

5. Search for information about learning and memory using search terms such as "learning strategies," "learning techniques," and "improving memory." Find and describe three techniques you would like to try that are not included in this chapter.

BUILDING YOUR RESUME

1. Review the Resume Building Block #1 form at the end of Chapter 2. Think about how your goals relate to the career objective you are creating.

2. Review the Resume Building Block #2 form in Chapter 2. How can identifying your learning styles help you get more from your education?

3. Do you have good time-management and/or personal organization skills you can apply to a health care job?

Prescription for Success 3-1
Create Your Own Mission Statement

Develop a mission statement for your life as a student and future health care professional. Use the following questions as a guide for what to include. You may write out your mission statement or express it in another way, such as with drawings, pictures taken from other sources, your own photographs, or any other medium that works for you.

1. What do you most admire in other people?

_____

_____

_____

_____

2. How do you want to be remembered by people who matter to you?

_____

_____

_____

_____

Continued

Prescription for Success 3-1 (Continued)

3. Who do you most respect? Why?

_____

_____

_____

_____

4. If you could accomplish only three things in life, what would they be?

_____

_____

_____

_____

5. What makes you happiest? Why?

_____

_____

_____

_____

6. Which activities give you the greatest sense of purpose and satisfaction?

_____

_____

_____

_____

Exercise adapted from Covey S, Merrill AR, Merrill RR: First things first, New York, 1995, Simon and Schuster.

Prescription for Success 3-2
Name That Goal

1. Write a goal and two action steps to help you achieve your goal.

My goal: _____

Deadline: _____

Action step 1: _____

Prescription for Success 3-2 (Continued)

Deadline for action step: _____

Resources I will need: _____

Action step 2: _____

Deadline for action step: _____

Resources I will need: _____

2. Explain how your goal relates to your mission statement and supports your values.

_____

_____

_____

3. Create a visualization to help you achieve your goal. Briefly describe it here.

_____

_____

_____

4. Write two affirmations to help you achieve your goal.
   a. _____

   b. _____

Prescription for Success 3-3
It's All How You Look at It

Scenario 1
Your medical terminology class is more difficult than you expected. You must memorize long lists of words and word parts and take quizzes twice a week. To make matters worse, the instructor is quite strict and does not seem very sympathetic. For each of the following options, indicate whether it reflects a positive or negative attitude. Then describe the probable outcome of each attitude.

Attitude or Action	Positive?	Negative?	Probable Result of Having This Attitude
Be angry with the instructor and his "ridiculous" expectations.	_____	_____	_____
Focus on the fact that learning terminology relates to your goals of becoming a health care professional.	_____	_____	_____
Complain to your classmates about the unfairness of the situation.	_____	_____	_____

Continued

Prescription for Success 3–3 (Continued)

Organize a study group with your classmates.   _____ _____ _____

Meet with the instructor privately and ask for study suggestions.   _____ _____ _____

Look for ways to apply your learning style (discussed later in this chapter) to learning the terms.   _____ _____ _____

Skip class whenever possible because it doesn't really do any good to attend.   _____ _____ _____

Create and say affirmations stating you are mastering the vocabulary.   _____ _____ _____

Don't waste your time studying because you won't remember the words anyway.   _____ _____ _____

Think about how you will use medical terminology on the job.   _____ _____ _____

Scenario 2
You are working as a physical therapist assistant for a home health agency. Overall, you like your job and enjoy helping patients in their homes to regain mobility and strength after surgery and injuries. However, one of your clients is a teenager who is recovering from a cycling accident. You find her very difficult to work with. She is rude and seems to resent your efforts to help her. List six ways of handling this situation, and label each as being either a positive (effective) or negative (ineffective) reaction.

1. _____

_____

2. _____

_____

3. _____

_____

4. _____

_____

5. _____

_____

6. _____

_____

Prescription for Success 3-4
Where, Oh Where, Does the Time Go?

Keep a record of your activities for the next week. Make a chart that breaks each day into 1-hour blocks. At the end of the week, fill in the following table and answer the questions that follow.

Activity	*Number of Hours*
Attending class, labs, other school activities	_____
Cooking and household chores	_____
Shopping	_____
Entertainment, time with friends	_____
Exercise	_____
Job	_____
Sleeping	_____
Studying and doing homework	_____
Telephone	_____
Television	_____
Time with loved ones	_____
Other	_____

Are there activities that are mostly a "waste of time"?

_____

_____

Are there tasks you could delegate to others or put off until you finish school?

_____

_____

Are there tasks you believe you could do more efficiently?

_____

_____

_____

Continued

Prescription for Success 3–4 (Continued)

Are you spending enough time studying?

_____

_____

_____

If not, what can you do to make more time for your studies?

_____

_____

_____

_____

_____

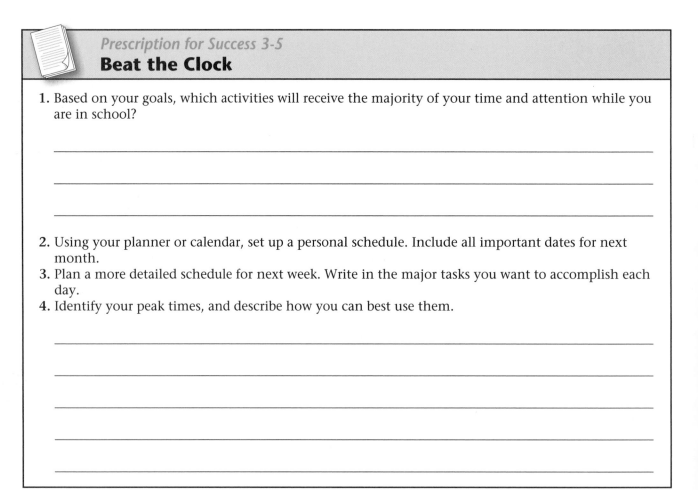

Prescription for Success 3-5
Beat the Clock

1. Based on your goals, which activities will receive the majority of your time and attention while you are in school?

_____

_____

_____

2. Using your planner or calendar, set up a personal schedule. Include all important dates for next month.
3. Plan a more detailed schedule for next week. Write in the major tasks you want to accomplish each day.
4. Identify your peak times, and describe how you can best use them.

_____

_____

_____

_____

_____

Prescription for Success 3-6
Defeating the Demon

Note: Students who never procrastinate may skip this exercise.

1. What have you been putting off doing?

_____

_____

2. Why do you think you have been procrastinating on this task?

_____

_____

_____

3. Which of the techniques listed in this chapter do you think would help you most?

_____

_____

_____

4. Develop a plan to get started, including the date you will begin.

_____

_____

_____

Prescription for Success 3-7
Learning Styles Inventory

Check the boxes for the statements with which you agree or that best describe you. When you finish the three checklists, total your score for each. The checklist with the highest number of points is likely to be your strongest or preferred learning style.

Auditory Checklist

☐ I follow oral instructions better than written ones.
☐ I enjoy listening to music more than looking at art.
☐ I would rather listen to a lecture than read the material in a textbook.

Continued

Prescription for Success 3–7 (Continued)

☐ I prefer to listen to the news on the radio rather than read the newspaper.
☐ I spell better out loud than when writing words out.
☐ When I read, I sometimes confuse words that look like other words.
☐ I remember things the instructor says better than what I read.
☐ I don't copy well from the board.
☐ I enjoy jokes told orally more than cartoons.
☐ I like games with action and noise more than quiet board games.
☐ I understand material better when I read it aloud.
☐ Sometimes I make errors in math because I don't see the sign or I read the numbers or directions incorrectly.
☐ I am often the last one to notice something new that requires observation—for example, if a room is painted or a wall display is changed.
☐ Reading a map is difficult for me.
☐ I like to use my finger as a pointer when I read. Sometimes when reading I get lost or skip lines.
☐ I often sing, hum, or whistle to myself.
☐ I frequently tell jokes, tell stories, and make verbal analogies to demonstrate a point.
☐ Matching tests are difficult for me, even when I know the answers.
☐ I often talk to myself when I'm alone.
☐ I sometimes need to have diagrams, graphs, or printed directions explained orally.
☐ *Score (total of all checked items)*

Visual Checklist

☐ I often have to ask people to repeat what they have just said.
☐ The best way for me to remember something is to picture it in my head.
☐ I typically prefer information to be presented visually on the board, PowerPoint slides, etc.
☐ I often find myself "tuned out" in class when the instructor is talking.
☐ Sometimes I know what I want to say, but I just can't think of the exact word.
☐ I am good at drawing graphs, charts, and other visual displays.
☐ I take notes during lectures so I can look at them later to review what was said.
☐ I can usually follow written instructions.
☐ I can understand maps and use them to find my way.
☐ I have difficulty understanding instructors or speakers when their backs are turned and I can't see their faces.
☐ Other people sometimes accuse me of not listening to them.
☐ I'd rather show someone how to do something than explain it in words.
☐ I prefer board games to games that require listening.
☐ I have trouble remembering things that are announced unless I see them written or write them down myself.
☐ Sometimes I confuse words when I am speaking, especially words that sound similar.
☐ When trying to recall the order of letters in the alphabet, I have to go over most of it from the beginning. For example, recalling whether "j" comes before or after "g."
☐ I would choose art over music activities.
☐ I do better when the instructor demonstrates how to do something instead of just explaining it in words.
☐ I often forget things I've been told, such as phone messages, unless I write them down.
☐ I often draw pictures or doodle on the edges of my notes, on scrap paper, etc.
☐ *Score (total of all checked items)*

Kinesthetic Checklist

☐ I read better when I say the words quietly to myself.
☐ I often draw pictures or designs when taking notes in class to help me concentrate and remember the lecture.
☐ When I shop I frequently touch the items displayed for sale; when I walk through a room, I tend to touch the furniture.

Prescription for Success 3–7 (Continued)

☐ I often count on my fingers.
☐ I like to smoke, eat, drink, or chew gum while I study.
☐ I am comfortable being touched by others. I often hug others or touch them when I'm speaking to them.
☐ I learn best by doing an activity, rather than reading or hearing about it.
☐ I enjoy hobbies that involve making things.
☐ I like to be able to move around as I learn. For example, moving about in the classroom helps me concentrate on the lesson.
☐ I would rather do a demonstration than give an oral or written report.
☐ I fidget a lot, such as tapping my pen or jiggling my leg.
☐ I usually prefer to stand while working.
☐ I use my hands more than the average person to communicate what I'm trying to say.
☐ I'm pretty coordinated and good at sports.
☐ I'm always on the move.
☐ I tend to talk and eat faster than most people.
☐ I would rather participate in an activity, such as a ballgame, than watch it.
☐ It's hard for me to sit still for long periods of time.
☐ I work well with my hands to make or repair things.
☐ I enjoy labs more than lecture classes.
☐ *Score (total of all checked items)*

Prescription for Success 3-8
Make Your Learning Styles Work for You

Apply what you know about learning styles to create five strategies you believe would help you learn the name and purpose of 25 vitamins (or other material for a class you are taking).

1. _____

2. _____

3. _____

4. _____

5. _____

Prescription for Success 3-9
Memory Test

Choose something you want or need to memorize, such as facts for an upcoming quiz. Use the memory techniques to help you learn and remember the material.

1. Which techniques did you choose?

_____

_____

_____

_____

_____

2. How did they work for you?

_____

_____

_____

_____

3. Which ones seemed to work best?

_____

_____

_____

_____

_____

Strategies for Students with Special Situations

Note: This chapter is different from all others in this text because it is written to help only those students who have specific challenges. The chapter is divided into three distinct sections for Adult Students, English-as-a-Second-Language Students, and Students with Learning Disabilities, each with its own set of objectives, exercises, and learning resources. Not all students will need to read all three sections; some students will not need any of the sections. It is up to individual students and their instructors to determine which topics might be useful to them.

OBJECTIVES

For adult students, the information and activities in this chapter can help you:
- Recognize how your experiences as an adult can help you succeed as a student.
- Confront and manage fears you may have about returning to school.
- Develop advanced time-management skills.
- Create relationships with family and friends to support your role as a student.
- Review and strengthen your academic skills.

For English-as-a-second-language (ESL) students, the information and activities in this chapter can help you:
- Identify areas of weakness in your reading and writing ability.
- Learn strategies to improve your English.
- Review grammatical points that frequently present problems for non-native speakers of English.

For students with learning disabilities, the information and activities in this chapter can help you:
- Better understand the nature of learning disabilities.
- Identify your own learning difficulties.
- Explore strategies and devices that help compensate for learning difficulties.

KEY TERMS AND CONCEPTS

Abbreviation Expanders: Computer programs that allow a user to create, store, and reuse abbreviations for frequently used words or phrases.

Academic Abilities: Specific subject abilities and skills such as reading, writing, and calculating.

Adult Student: A student who is over 25, who has been out of high school for at least 5 years, and who may have dependents and be employed. (Also called a *mature student.*)

Base Form of a Verb: The infinitive without the word "to." Examples: read, study, learn.

Clause: A group of words containing a subject and a verb. The group may or may not form a complete sentence.

Consonant: All the letters in the alphabet *except* A, E, I, O, U, and sometimes Y.

Context: The words surrounding an unknown word that may give you clues to its meaning.

Determiner: Words used in front of nouns to indicate whether you are referring to something specific or something of a particular type.

Eye-Level Reading Ruler: Plastic ruler specially designed to help individuals with visual and reading disabilities.

Gerund: A word ending in *-ing* that is derived from a verb but that functions as a noun.

Guided Imagery: Refers to various types of meditation and relaxation exercises that involve mental images of pleasant scenes and/or negative thoughts leaving the mind.

Helping Verb: Verb that adds to the meaning of the main verb in a sentence. Helping verbs are used to create verb tenses and express meanings such as expectation, permission, and probability. Examples: have, be, may, do will, can, must. (Also called *auxiliary verbs.*)

Idiomatic Expression: Words used together that have a different meaning from the dictionary definition of the individual words.

Infinitive: The basic form of a verb that does not indicate a subject or tense. It is preceded by the word "to."

Irrational: Without cause; unreasonable.

Learning Center: A dedicated section of a school that offers help with academics and study skills.

Mature Student: A student who is over 25, who has been out of high school for at least 5 years, and who may have dependents and be employed. (Also called an *adult student.*)

Modals: Verbs used with other verbs to express ideas such as possibility, intention, obligation, and necessity. Examples: can, could, may, might, must, should, will, would.

Motivated: Having enthusiasm or a purpose for doing something.

Past Participle: The form of a verb that is used to form the perfect tenses. This form typically ends in *-ed,* although many common verbs are irregular.

Personal Digital Assistants: Handheld computers that store information, access the Internet, calculate, and can include a wireless phone.

Phrasal Verb: Verbs that can be combined with prepositions to create phrases that mean something different from what the verb means by itself.

Prefix: A letter or a group of letters attached to the beginning of a word to add or alter its meaning.

Prepositions: Words that show relationships, such as direction, place, time, and cause, between other words in a sentence.

Present Participle: The form of a verb, ending in *-ing,* that is used to indicate continuous action.

Scan: Read quickly to find something specific.

Self-Advocacy: Seeking solutions to your problems, taking steps to solve them, and asking for help when you need it.

Skim: Read quickly to explore or review.

Study Group: A group of students who meet together on a regular basis to study, work, and support one another's learning.

Study Skills: Skills used for learning and mastering material.

Suffix: A letter or a group of letters attached to the end of a word to form a new word or to alter the grammatical function of the original word.

Support Group: A group organized to help its members with specific types of problems.

Syllable: The shortest part of a word that can be pronounced as a unit. For example, *contamination* has five syllables: con-tam-i-na-tion.

Transcript: Official record of classes taken and grades earned.

Tutor: A person who helps others learn specific subjects or skills in a one-on-one or small-group setting.

Vowels: The following letters: *A, E, I, O, U* and sometimes *Y.*

Yoga: Practices for health and relaxation that include breath control, meditation, and the adoption of specific body postures.

ADULT STUDENTS

PORTRAIT OF THE ADULT STUDENT

Just what is an **adult student** or a **mature student?** There are a variety of definitions, depending on the source. Generally, students are considered to be mature if they have one or more of the following characteristics:

- Have been out of high school for at least 5 years
- Are over the age of 25
- Work either full- or part-time
- Have children or other dependents

COME JOIN THE CROWD

"Through education, you hope to give a new direction to life."

—Linda Simon

If you've been out of school for a number of years, you may be quite nervous about the idea of returning to school. Something you should know is that returning to school after a few—or even many—years is becoming much more common these days. In fact, the crowd of older students is getting larger. Some sources report that up to 50% of all college students are over the age of 25. The world is changing rapidly, and education is increasingly important for securing good jobs and moving up in careers. This is especially true for health care careers.

Continuing your education will ultimately add to the quality of your life—and to the lives of those around you. But you may be experiencing a number of fears and wondering if you have made the right decision. It is not unusual for adults to have a variety of concerns about their ability to succeed as students. Table 4-1 lists common fears, along with suggestions for overcoming each one.

One proven way to deal with fears is to share and discuss them with others, especially those who are in the same situation. It can be comforting to know that other students have the same concerns. You will find that you are not the only one feeling the way you do and that your fears are not **irrational**. Talking with someone else, however, should not simply be an "ain't it awful, this is tough" gab session. Rather, use it as an opportunity to help each other focus on the positive, exchange ideas for managing difficulties, and share resources. Examples of such resources include the following:
- Trading childcare
- Carpooling
- Teaching each other, such as computer skills
- Sharing class notes when one of you is absent

According to Al Siebert, an expert in helping adult learners, "Creating a personal **support group** and issue-specific learning teams is the most effective thing you can do to help assure your success in college."[1] This makes sense because research has shown that social support—relationships with other people—has powerful positive influences. For example, people with good social support have been shown to have reduced stress, improved resistance to disease, and improved recovery from illness.

Once you have graduated, consider maintaining your support group as you navigate the job search and the first few months on the job. You will likely encounter new challenges, and sharing these experiences can help smooth the road during these times.

Another suggestion for overcoming fears is to grit your teeth and face them head on. Ask yourself if the fear is based on reality. Then think about ways you can deal with it: ask for help; take a class; use the suggestions in this book. Do your best to get through what needs to be done and then reflect on

TABLE 4–1	**Common Fears of Adult Students**
Fear	**Suggestions for Overcoming**
My brain is rusty and I won't be able to learn quickly.	Think of it this way: your brain may not have been in school, but if you have been working and/or raising a family, your brain has had plenty of workouts! You have simply been using it in different ways, but they all involve thinking and learning.
I won't be able to compete with younger students.	You actually have certain advantages over younger students. These are described in the next section of this chapter.
My **academic abilities** are not that great. I didn't do well in math/science/English, etc.	This book can help you review basic skills and overcome special fears such as math anxiety. See Chapters 5, 6, and 7. Take advantage of any resources available at your school such as the **learning center** and **tutors**.
I don't have a computer or Internet access.	Computers have become quite affordable. If purchasing one is not an option, check with your school and the public library. Most have computers that students and the public can use.
I don't know how to use computers like the kids do.	Technology does have a way of moving on, and it's not uncommon to feel left behind. (The manual for the car I bought last year was 506 pages long!) If possible, take a computer class. Your school may have them. If not, they are often available for free or at a small charge at public libraries, adult schools, and community centers. There are also many good books and websites for beginners.
I might not be able to do it all—work, study, and raise a family.	This is a problem faced by many students. See the suggestions in this chapter as well as the sections in Chapter 3 on time management and personal organization.
My family will feel neglected.	There are actions you can take to help prevent you family from feeling this way. This chapter contains many specific ideas.
People in my life will try to sabotage my efforts.	People who truly care about you will support your efforts to improve your life. It may be that they feel threatened or left out. This chapter contains suggestions you can try to gain their support.
The thought of taking tests worries me.	Taking tests is a skill discussed in detail in Chapter 6.
Instructors might not like older students.	Actually, many instructors believe that older students are more motivated and committed.

Adapted from: Siebert A, Karr MK: *The adult learner's guide to survival and success,* ed 6, Portland, 2008, Practical Psychology Press.

your success. Over time, with each new triumph, your fears will decrease.

ADVANTAGES OF BEING A MATURE STUDENT

It is quite possible that you have a number of advantages over more traditional students—those who are entering college directly from high school or who have been out for only a couple of years. Perhaps you left school to get married and raise a family, join the military, or go to work. If so, you have almost certainly accumulated a wealth of experience that will help you as a student. In fact, it is likely that as an older adult you have acquired many skills you can apply at school. Examples of these are listed in Table 4-2. In fact, many educators believe that lessons learned from life are the most valuable.

Certain life experiences are especially helpful for health care students. If you are a parent, for example, you have undoubtedly taken your children to the doctor. You understand how important it is to have faith in those who are caring for your loved ones. You yourself may have had health problems. These experiences can motivate you to do your best in school to become a truly qualified health care professional.

Okay, now you're feeling more confident about being a mature student. At the same time, adult students who find themselves with instructors and classmates younger than themselves should take care not to assume a know-it-all attitude. Adults who

TABLE 4–2	Skills Acquired through Life Experience
Skill	**Application in School**
Meeting deadlines	Turning in assignments on time
Handling several activities at the same time	Coordinating studying, caring for children, and completing household tasks
Interacting and working with others	Developing working relationships with instructors; getting along with other students
Solving problems	Determining the best ways to learn; balancing adult responsibilities so you can study; completing assignments that require solving problems
Adapting to new situations	Adjusting to being in school; adapting to the role of student
Having patience and knowing that situations will improve over time	Staying with your studies even if the going gets tough

are used to being in charge at home—and perhaps even on the job—can find it difficult to become a student and follow the directions of others. You may believe that you have more practical experience than the instructor and many of the other students. At times like this, it is especially important to focus on your goal of becoming a competent health care professional. Recognize the need to learn from individuals who, although younger, have health care experience and knowledge. On the other hand, don't hesitate to share your experiences when these are appropriate for the topics being presented in class. Offer your comments courteously, and take care not to dominate the discussion.

MEETING NEW CHALLENGES

"Believe in yourself and take things one day at a time.

—Al Siebert

The greatest challenge faced by most adult students is the matter of time—having enough of it! Adults have multiple responsibilities that may include running a household, caring for children, and holding down a job (Figure 4-1). They may even include helping elderly parents and holding volunteer positions in the community. Balancing these demands can be stressful, even overwhelming. At times your responsibilities may seem like acceptable excuses for being

---

PERSONAL REFLECTION

1. Which of the life skills listed in Table 4-2 do you believe will most help you in your role as a student?

   _____

   _____

   _____

2. Can you think of others that you can apply to help you succeed in school?

   _____

   _____

   _____

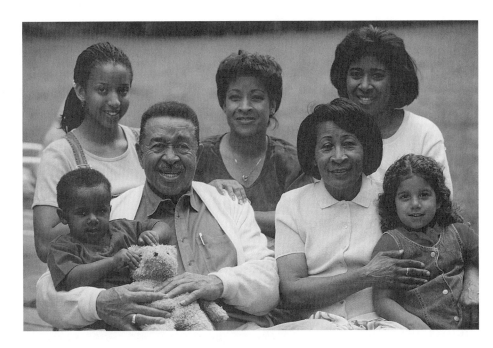

Figure 4–1 Although school and your studies must be high priorities, your family is an essential part of your life. Do your best to include them in your plans and achievements. (*From Gerdin J:* Health careers today, *ed 4, St Louis, 2007, Mosby.*)

late to class, or even absent. You may feel that your instructors are not caring or understanding if they don't accept your excuses. But you must remember that the goal of health care education is to prepare you for a career. You will have important responsibilities, and your employer and your patients will count on you to know what you are doing. Being prepared to serve requires being in class regularly. If instructors were to let students slide through school because they have good excuses and good intentions, the instructors would be doing a disservice to their students and to the future employers and, most important, the future patients of these students.

Time Management—Advanced Techniques

This section is called "Advanced Techniques" because good time management is especially important for adult students. The fact is there are only 24 hours in a day. When you combine typical adult responsibilities with attending class and studying, no day will seem long enough to take care of everything that needs to be done. Adding the role of student may require some major adjustments and new strategies.

As discussed in Chapter 3 in the section on time management, prioritizing is the key to effective use of time. Recall that prioritizing means determining which tasks are most important and then making sure that they are completed. Start by determining which activities are critical to your success as a student, and focus on these. If you are a parent and/or a spouse, maintaining these relationships will also

be high on your list of priorities. For example, when time is short, spending an hour with a child may be more important than dusting and vacuuming the house or performing volunteer activities. The fact is you may have to temporarily put off some of your customary activities. Attending school—and putting in the necessary time to study—is a big commitment and will almost certainly require some sacrifices. You may have less time for social and volunteer activities and household chores. See which of these can be put off, without endangering the health of you or your family, until after you graduate.

In addition to the ideas presented in Chapter 3, adult students may benefit from the following suggestions:

- Let family members and friends know your schedule. Consider putting up a large calendar where everyone can see it. Mark the dates when assignments are due and you have tests so everyone knows when you will be especially busy. Include events that are important to others as well, such as a child's music recital.
- Work with your family to delegate tasks. Organize a family meeting to discuss your need for study time and to assign age-appropriate chores. Have follow-up meetings to evaluate how things are going and make any needed adjustments to schedules and tasks.
- Schedule dedicated fun time with your family. Plan activities together that everyone enjoys. Aim for days that follow a major exam or project due date.
- Treat your studies as you would a job. After all, you wouldn't just leave your job to visit with a

friend or stay on the phone for an hour catching up on the latest news.

- Plan to study each day, even if some days it is for only a short period. Don't wait until you have long periods of uninterrupted time—this luxury may happen rarely, if at all! (I have learned that 20 minutes here and there eventually results in a book.)
- Add 15 minutes to each day, either by getting up earlier or staying up later. This will actually add 91 hours a year to your waking—and hopefully productive—hours.[2]

Managing with Children in the House

Being a parent presents special challenges for adult students, especially if you are a single parent. In spite of comments throughout this book about committing yourself to your studies, the truth is that your children are your top priority. If they are young, finding appropriate childcare is critical. Even with a good provider, you should develop a backup plan to cover emergencies. For example, preschools can close during severe weather, individual caretakers can become ill, or your child can get sick and be required to stay home.

Your children's school and the adults who care for them should be able to reach you in an emergency. Be sure they have your school's phone number. If your instructors require that you turn off cell phones during class (not an unreasonable request), ask the administration about their policy for taking emergency calls and notifying students in class.

Handling childcare issues now is excellent preparation for later when you are employed. Although employers understand true emergencies, they cannot tolerate employees who regularly miss work because of child-related issues. Health care providers must make patient care and achieving work goals their highest priorities.

Your children may be upset by changes in your schedule, absences from home, and limitations in the time you have to spend with them. It can help if they know where you are spending your time and what you are doing. Ask your school for permission to show your children the classrooms, labs, and other areas. Explain how you are learning new things to help others and to help them have a better future. Explain to your children why you are in school. Show them a picture of a health care professional, and tell them about your future job. Make it a habit to tell them about your day in school, something interesting that happened, and what you learned (Figure 4-2).

Make time for each child to do activities you enjoy doing together, talk about their concerns, and

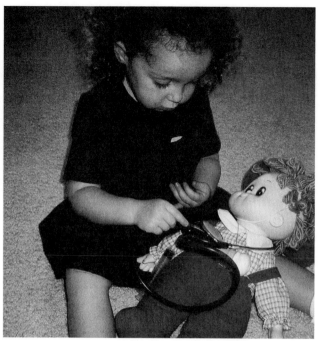

Figure 4–2 Make an effort to involve your children in your education. Here a child plays with a stethoscope to learn more about what Mommy is learning in school. (*From Gerdin J:* Health careers today, *ed 4, St Louis, 2007, Mosby.*)

let them know how much they mean to you. Focus on them during this time so they feel included and loved. Neighbors of mine have a busy family with two working parents and four school-age children. They eat dinner together whenever possible, and during the meal each person is allotted 2 minutes (they set a timer) to give a presentation about their day. The message is that each person, even the 6-year-old, has something of value to contribute.

When your children help around the house, show appreciation. Even if the beds aren't made perfectly or dinner isn't as nutritious as you would like, let them know that you are grateful for their efforts. Al Siebert offers the following ideas[1]:

- Say "thank you."
- Buy or fix their favorite food.
- Give hugs and kisses.
- Give treats or little gifts.
- Leave nice notes for them; send cards.
- Tell them about something interesting at school.
- Speak highly of them to others.
- Let them feel that your success is their success.

Finding quiet time to study can be challenging when children are present. Here are a few suggestions:

- If your children are old enough, work on homework together.
- Have young children "help" you by drawing, coloring pictures, filling in sticker books, or performing other "desk work."

- Try turning your study time into a positive experience for the kids by saving their favorite videos, toys, and other activities for the times when you are busy.
- Set up a special place for children to play quietly while you study. Childproof a room in the house where older children can play while you study.
- Set a timer for quiet periods. If children know there is an end to the quiet time, they may be more willing to oblige.
- Let children help you study, such as by showing you flashcards or asking you questions. Exchange babysitting services with friends and family members, arranging to help them out when your study load is lightest.

Working with your children in these ways can be a win-win situation. Not only will you accomplish more, but you serve as a positive role model for your children. They will see your behavior as a disciplined, goal-oriented person who enjoys learning and self-improvement.

Explore combining resources with other students. For example, see about organizing a study group with classmates who have children. Contribute to a babysitting fund, and hire someone to watch all the children while you study together. Or you might exchange childcare with one other student, trading off watching the children for an afternoon. For older children, investigate activities such as day camps, sports teams, and craft classes. Organizations such as churches and community centers offer these at reasonable prices. There may also be opportunities for single parents who are continuing their education.

Finally, if it becomes necessary, try studying before and after classes in the school library. You may accomplish more there in shorter periods of time than if you are at home with constant interruptions.

Maintaining Personal Relationships

Adults have many relationships with others. These may include aging parents, a spouse or significant other, friends, and co-workers. Becoming a student can put a strain on these relationships because you will have less time to devote to them. In addition, your new status as a student may cause others to feel frustrated, jealous, or even threatened.

Include people who are important to you when making your educational plans. Let them know what you are doing and why—how pursuing a career in health care is going to contribute to the quality of your life, the quality of your family, and even to the welfare of the community. Assure them

that you will schedule time with them, and let them know how you are doing. Consider throwing a going-back-to-school party. Invite friends and family and tell them about your plans, what you'll be studying, and the great future you anticipate working in health care. Let them know how important this is to you and ask for their support.

When adult students are interviewed, married women report more difficulties in their role as "caretaker of family needs" when they assume the role of student.[1] It can be hard for a spouse or significant other to accept your new status as a student. They may worry you will leave them behind or not have time for them, or they may be jealous of your opportunity. Here are some things you can try if you find yourself with an unhappy spouse[1]:

1. Ask your spouse what is really bothering him or her. It will be easier to deal with if you are both clear on the nature of the problem.
2. Focus on the future. Emphasize that attending school is temporary.
3. Discuss how your studies can benefit your relationship.
4. Schedule time together to do something you both enjoy.

Being pulled in many directions can be stressful for everyone, and it is important to make a special effort to include family members in your decisions. If behavior problems develop, such as being upset and refusing to talk, allow some time for adjustments. If the reactions of others are extreme, it may be necessary to seek help such as family counseling. If this is financially difficult, check with your school about free or low-cost services in your community.

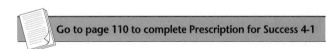

Go to page 110 to complete Prescription for Success 4-1

When you do spend time with others, try to minimize complaining. That is, don't go on and on about how difficult you are finding a subject, how a certain instructor gives difficult tests, how stressed you feel, and so on. These issues should be addressed with people at your school who can help you with these problems. It's best to focus on the positive when visiting with friends. The same advice applies at home. If there is already some stress over your attending school, the last thing you need to do is cast a dark cloud over everything when you are home. Describing how tired you are, how difficult your classes are, how unfair your instructors are will take away from the time you do have to spend with loved ones.

Personal relationships can cause problems as you begin your studies. At the same time, strong support systems can increase your chances for success. This is not surprising because studies have shown that social support is associated with good mental health and the ability to handle stress. There is even some evidence that social support positively influences physical health. For example, the survival rates of individuals who have heart attacks are higher in those with the greatest emotional support.[3,4]

Your personal support system may extend beyond your immediate family and can include anyone who encourages you and supports your goals: your health care provider, spiritual advisor, and members of your place of worship and other groups to which you belong.

There are three basic types of social support, and you can benefit from each:

1. Emotional: provided by people who make you feel loved and cared for and increase your sense of self-worth
2. Instrumental: provided by those who help you with specific tasks such as childcare, household tasks, and transportation
3. Informational: provided by instructors and others who give you information you need in order to succeed as a student[5]

Don't hesitate to ask for support: explanations from your instructor, encouragement from your spouse. Show appreciation and let people know how important their help is to you. And don't forget to give back—even if you are busy, you can offer to provide these same kinds of support to others. In fact, giving of yourself is a valuable characteristic of the health care professional.

 Go to page 111 to complete Prescription for Success 4-2

Combining Work and School

Working takes time, but according to government surveys, many working students believe that employment helps them with their coursework; more than half think it helps them prepare for a career.[6] If possible, work as few hours as is financially possible. Working full-time while attending school is doable, but it is very difficult for most people.

Either way, try to enlist the support of your employer. Discuss your educational plans and see if there are ways you can tie school assignments to your work. Take care not to use work time inappropriately. At the same time, if you are seeking a new job, see if you can find a position that would permit studying while working, such as receptionist or security guard. (This would be with the employer's permission and without performing poorly.)

 Q&A **with a Health Care Professional**
Kim Fruge

Kim is a manager and caregiver in a care home for older and disabled adults. She shares her experience going back to school as an adult student with a family and full-time job.

Q When did you return to school to study medical assisting?

A Six years ago. I was married with grown children—they were 20 and 21 at the time—and had worked many years in retail. When I decided to make a change, I was a scan supervisor. That means I was supervising the coding and pricing of items in a large grocery store.

Q Why did you decide to change careers and return to school?

A I never really liked working in retail, but it was something I could do without any education beyond high school. I had always wanted to work in something where I could work directly with people, helping them in some way. I loved raising my kids and we always had their friends around the house. So I checked around and found out I could earn my certificate in medical assisting in a reasonable amount of time.

Q How did your family react when you decided to return to school?

A When I first decided to go back to school, my family thought I was crazy! They didn't think I would do it. But after I started talking about it and what I would achieve, they were 100% behind me. Then, after I started, they thought I would give up. But when they saw how well I was doing and the grades I was getting, they started encouraging me and trying to help me in any way they could. They helped me to study and to research. My son was still living at home. Actually, both my son and daughter helped me with homework and quizzed me. My daughter helped me with math.

When accomplishments were done, they were very happy for me and patted me on the back. My son's friends were so nice—they would call me, help me study. Then my children's friends came to my graduation. They were so proud of me and what I had done because I graduated with a 3.8. And that was after 20 years of not being in school!

with a Health Care Professional—cont'd
Kim Fruge

Q Did you find returning to school difficult?

A Oh, yes. I was still working 40 hours a week at the store, from 4 am to noon or sometimes 2 pm. I'd go home for a quick nap and then go to class. My classes met Monday through Friday for 5 hours a night, so my schedule was intense. Including my externship, this all lasted about a year.

After not being in school for all those years, trying to learn how to study again was really hard until I found a way to make it easier for myself. I discovered flashcards and that really helped me. I made my own flashcards for whatever we were studying. I learned about these when we used them for medical terminology. Then I started making them for facts and questions in all my subjects. I don't think I could have made it through without those flashcards.

I did get discouraged sometimes—with pharmacology, for example. I had trouble learning to convert ratios so I could calculate medications. Math was always my worst, worst subject. I didn't think I would have to worry about math studying medical assisting, but I was wrong about that!

Q What helped you most when you had problems with math?

A Actually, my husband, Jimmy, was great about helping. He could explain things in words I understood. Also, my instructors were wonderful. I always stayed after class and got as much help as possible. I always asked lots of questions. I would get help from Jimmy at home and then ask my teachers. Talking with my teachers really helped. I'm a hands-on learner, so once I saw it on paper, I could do it. So ask for help when you need it!

Q What other advice do you have for adults who are returning to school?

A Set your goals and work to achieve them. Study hard. Do lots of research. Make sure you have the time to spend on school. You have to make this a priority. Always tell yourself what the outcome will be—what you will achieve by doing this. Do lots of research on things you don't understand. I spent lots of my time in the library trying to understand certain things. I did extra practice, too. I did lots more blood draws than were required to make sure I got it.

Q How did you handle time management?

A Very carefully! I stayed on a schedule that worked best for me and my family. I spent all my spare time studying, getting ahead on courses—doing extra homework ahead of time as much as possible because I always liked to be ahead of where we were, always doing extra credit to learn and better understand.

Q How did you handle the pressure of balancing so many activities?

A I look deep breaths and told myself, "I am smart enough to do this." I said that to myself at least once a week. I had pressure to make sure I got all my classwork done. And at work the pressure was making sure I met all my deadlines. As scan coordinator, I had to be sure the prices were all up to date.

Q How did you balance your job and school?

A The other employees and my boss were really great. I got their support when I started school. For example, when I did my externship from 8 to 5, I worked at the store on the weekends. They were all really good about accommodating me and my scheduling needs.

Overcoming Academic Weaknesses

You may have had difficulties during your previous educational experiences. This is very common for students of all ages who are pursuing career training. You may be a practical person who learns best through hands-on activities. If so, a health care career is a good choice because much of the work is hands-on. At the same time, health care requires a knowledge of what you are doing. Therefore academic skills are needed for the reading, writing, and studying necessary to learn important background information.

If your academic and **study skills** are not what they should be, the first step is to acknowledge this. There is nothing to be embarrassed about. In fact, it is a sign of strong character to recognize our weaknesses and seek the means to make improvements. It is very important to seek help as soon as you realize you need it. Many health care programs move along quickly. You may have only 1 month or a few weeks in a class. You cannot wait until just before the final exams to seek help. There are a couple of good reasons for this. First, it may simply be too late to catch up. Second, even if you are able to pass the class, have you really learned what you should? Have you mastered the information and skills you need to perform your future health care duties?

If you believe that your academic skills are not strong, plan to spend a little time each day working on them. For example, spend 15 or 20 minutes working on math skills or spelling. Over time, you are likely to acquire the skills needed to master your classes.

There are many ways to strengthen your study and academic skills, including the following:

1. Read the information and try the suggestions presented in this book. They include everything from understanding what you read to overcoming math anxiety to writing a well-organized paper. See Chapters 5, 6, and 7.
2. Investigate learning resources at your school: learning center, review courses, tutors, writing lab.
3. Look for helpful classes open to the public in your area: computer literacy, basic skills, using the Internet.
4. Organize a **study group** with other students.
5. Most important, don't hesitate to ask your instructors for help. They have chosen to teach because they want to share what they learned working in the health care field. They want successful graduates—in other words, they want their students to succeed!

Many adults have trouble admitting when they don't know something or when they need help. But think of it this way: you are paying for your instructors to help you learn. That is their job, and seeking this help is one way to ensure that you are getting what you pay for, just as you would with any service. One difference with education, of course, is that you must do your part, too, by reading assignments, attending class, and doing the homework.

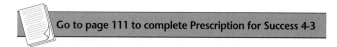
Go to page 111 to complete Prescription for Success 4-3

Achieving academic success is important. At the same time, a common cause of stress among adult students is striving for perfection. You may feel that because you are older, you should do as well as or perhaps even better than younger students. You may believe that others expect more of you. However, just as age doesn't mean your brain is rusty, neither does age equate with intelligence and ability. If your previous experiences in school were not all positive, don't stress yourself out thinking you must earn an A in every class. Your goals should focus on learning and preparing yourself for your health care career.

If you are paying for your education yourself, you may see grades as a reflection of the value you are receiving for your money. Again, focus on your goals and purpose in attending school. Your future performance on the job, not your **transcript**, is the product you are paying for. Doing it all perfectly—studying, working, parenting—is not possible for anyone, so decide what is most important and work to achieve balance.

Go to page 112 to complete Prescription for Success 4-4

ENGLISH-AS-A-SECOND-LANGUAGE STUDENTS

ENGLISH FOR THE NON-NATIVE SPEAKER

English may be your second—or even third or fourth—language. This may be because you grew up in a family that spoke another language. Or you may have moved to the United States from another country. In either case, you probably speak English pretty well—perhaps very well. However, you may have concerns such as the following:

- I'm not always sure which verb tense to use. In fact, I could use some help with many parts of grammar.
- English spelling is difficult. How can I remember words that have so many letters that aren't even pronounced?
- I have an accent and am self-conscious about speaking.
- I'm worried about doing writing assignments in school or having to write on the job.

These are natural concerns when English is not your first language, and they, along with other language difficulties, will be discussed in this chapter. First, let's look at some of the advantages of knowing more than one language. You may have heard the term "global economy," which is evidence of just how interconnected the countries of the world have become. You also know that the people of the United States come from a variety of countries and cultures. Large numbers of people living in the United States do not speak English well. Some do not speak it at all. Knowing at least two languages can be a real advantage in this environment. This is especially true in health care. Think about how frightening it can be for patients who are being treated by someone with whom they can't easily communicate. If you speak a language that is spoken by many people in your area, this is a valuable and helpful skill. You have something extra to offer your future employers.

If you speak a Romance language, such as Spanish, you may be surprised to find that some medical terms you will be learning are similar to everyday words in your language. (Even if the spelling is different, the sounds are similar.) Table 4-3 contains several examples of terms that speakers of Spanish might find easier to learn than students who speak only English.

Go to page 113 to complete Prescription for Success 4-5

IMPROVING YOUR ENGLISH

"Surround yourself with English; practice it, study it, and you will learn it."

—*Kathy Ochoa Flores*

To be successful at improving your English, it is important to be **motivated.** This means that you *want* to improve your English communication skills. Working on language skills takes time and effort, as well as taking risks, so it really helps to be clear about why you want to improve.

TABLE 4–3	Medical Words and Everyday Spanish	
Medical Term or Word Element	**Related Everyday Spanish Word**	**Meaning**
mandible	mandíbula	jawbone
costa, costal	costilla	rib
pulmonary	pulmón	related to the lungs
brachi/o	brazo	arm
oste/o	hueso	bone
ot/o	oído	ear
quadr-	cuatro	four
axillary	axila	pertaining to the armpit

The best way to improve any skill, and this includes communicating, is to practice. Although this is the best way, it is not always easiest. For example, you may speak a language other than English with the people with whom you spend most of your time. Perhaps your parents don't speak English. You may be more comfortable with friends who speak your language and understand your cultural background. But if you are serious about improving your English, you will need to seek opportunities to use it. Here are some suggestions:

- Make friends with classmates who speak only English. Invite them to have coffee and use the time to practice speaking English. This is a good way to learn slang and informal conversational English (Figure 4-3).
- Organize or join a study group in which the majority of the members speak English. Use this time to work on vocabulary related to your studies.
- Speak up in class if you have questions. If this is too difficult at first, ask to speak with your instructors outside of class.
- Talk with everyone you can, such as people you do business with: clerks in stores, the librarian, the receptionist at the doctor's office.

It can be scary speaking English with people you don't know, especially if you are self-conscious about your speaking ability. It is especially hard for adults who worry about looking dumb. But this is the best way to learn. The first chapter said that students have the right to make mistakes. This is also true for people who are learning to speak English well—they have the right to make mistakes. In fact, you must give yourself permission to make mistakes. Think about it this way: if you only repeat what you already know and don't try new things, you won't

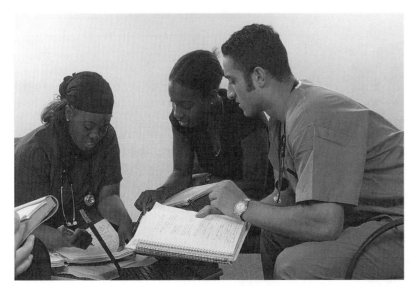

Figure 4–3 Become friends with native English speakers with whom you can study and practice your English. (*From Young A, Procter D:* Kinn's the medical assistant, *ed 10, St. Louis 2007, Saunders.*)

learn anything new. English instructors believe that their best students are the ones who are willing to take risks. They are not afraid to make mistakes and don't worry about using perfect grammar, vocabulary, and pronunciation. When they make mistakes, they are not discouraged. Instead, they learn from their errors. Good students visit with other people (not during class when the instructor is speaking, of course!), ask and answer questions, and interact as much as possible or as much as they can. If your instructors have you work in groups, this is an excellent way to practice. Health care involves working with others, and interacting with your classmates is excellent practice for this on-the-job skill. If you sit quietly in class everyday, you will lose many (good) opportunities to learn and practice.

You might try practicing at home. If you have family members who are interested, try teaching them new English words and phrases. Teaching others is an excellent way to learn and reinforce what you know.

Language teachers agree that to learn or master another language, you need to spend some time— even if it is only 20 minutes—studying or practicing every day. They believe this is more effective than working on it once a week for several hours. Teachers also recommend that you set reasonable goals and try to make your language studies fun.

The following sections cover topics that can be difficult for learners of English. They are *not* intended to provide an English course. Rather, the purpose is to provide encouragement, suggestions about how to improve your English, and examples of common problems in areas such as pronunciation, spelling, and grammar. For more in-depth study, you might take an intermediate or advanced English class, explore the websites listed at the end of this chapter, or spend time practicing with native English speakers. The important thing is to find what works best for you and then "go for it."

Increasing Your Vocabulary

The English language has more words than any of us—even teachers and textbook writers—will ever know. Depending on how you count them (for example, are "talk" and "talking" one word or two?), there are more than 250,000 words in English! And new ones are added every day. To just get along in English, you should know about 2000 frequently used words. To succeed in college, that number grows to 10,000 to 15,000 words.[7]

Here are a few suggestions for increasing your vocabulary:
1. Set a goal of learning a certain number of new vocabulary words each week. While you

---

PERSONAL REFLECTION

What are some reasons you want to improve your English?

_____

_____

_____

_____

_____

How would better English help you in school?

_____

_____

_____

_____

In your future career?

_____

_____

_____

_____

_____

_____

---

are studying health care, you might want to concentrate on terms related to your future career.
2. In a notebook or on your computer, list new words as you encounter them. Write the word, its definition, and a sentence using the word. Write something personal to make the word your own.[7] Use the new words, in both oral and written forms, as often as possible.
3. If you are a visual learner, make posters of your new vocabulary and post where you will see them every day. Use pictures and drawings when appropriate.

4. If you are an auditory learner, record your new words along with a sentence for each one. Listen to the recording over the following weeks.
5. Study word lists such as vocabulary, key terms, and the glossaries in your textbooks.
6. Find other basic English word lists, such as those on the websites listed at the end of this chapter.

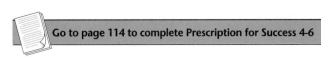

Go to page 114 to complete Prescription for Success 4-6

Idiomatic Expressions

Idiomatic expressions exist in many languages and can present difficulties to language learners. This is because they consist of words that when used together have meanings that are different from the dictionary definitions of the individual words. Because these expressions are commonly used in English, consider adding these to your vocabulary learning goals. A good list is available at www.using english.com/reference/idioms.

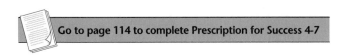

Go to page 114 to complete Prescription for Success 4-7

Improving Your Pronunciation

Pronunciation can be a problem, especially if you learned English as an adult. Once our habits are established and the muscles in our tongue and mouth become accustomed to making the sounds of our first language, it becomes more difficult to form "foreign" sounds. A problem for some people is distinguishing between similar sounds. For example, I knew a gentleman from Peru who could not hear the difference between the words "duck" and "dock." If you can't hear the difference, it is nearly impossible to pronounce them differently.

If you can be understood easily, you may not need to worry too much about having an accent. Some people find accents interesting, even charming. If you are working on developing an "American accent," it is a good idea to model your speech after television newscasters. This is because they speak what is considered standard or neutral American English rather than one of the many regional ways of speaking found throughout the United States.

Perhaps even more important than the pronunciation of individual words is how they are combined into sentences and on which words and **syllables** (parts of words) the stress (emphasis) is placed. Using a rhythm that is different from the way Americans speak makes speech difficult to understand. Therefore listening carefully to native speakers and practicing entire sentences are important parts of pronunciation practice.

Combining Sounds

A common custom in spoken English is to link words together when there is a **vowel** sound between them. An example is the sentence "I want an apple." If each word is pronounced carefully and separately, this results in a "foreign" accent. Spoken by a native speaker, this sentence sounds like "I wannanappul." The words are run together, and the letter "t" disappears. Another example is "Would you like an apple?" which becomes "Would juh likeanappul?" Consider the following examples:

1. "An elephant" sounds like "a-nelephant" or "uh-nelephant"
2. "An orange" sounds like "a-norange or "uh-norange"

You may not realize it, but many languages do this. French is especially full of linked sounds in which whole parts of words seem to disappear. When spoken quickly and naturally, Spanish does the same thing. We grow accustomed to understanding our own language. It's just more difficult when we don't know a language well.

Here are a few more examples of English pronunciation challenges:

- The common use of the sound "uh" for vowels: mother—m*uh*ther; the—th*uh*; complicated—complicat*uh*d.
- The letter "t" pronounced as a "d" when the word requires a faster sound: little—liddle; anatomy—anaduhmy; thirty—therdy. (Note, however, that "thirteen" retains the "t" sound. This is because the word parts before and after the "t" in "thirteen" are longer than in "thirty.")
- Many words are pronounced differently than they are spelled: have to—haffto; bright—brite.
- Some words are spelled the same but pronounced differently to convey different meanings: "read" is pronounced "reed" when meaning the present tense and "red" when meaning the past tense.
- Combinations of consonants. In many languages, there are vowels between consonants that give kind of a running start to the tongue. For example, the word just used—"start"—begins with two consonants, s and t. When first learning English, speakers of some languages may say "e-start"—they need that extra first vowel to get the word going.

As you can see, English pronunciation is not easy to learn by studying the language's written form. So just how do you learn to speak this language well? The answer is *by listening and practicing.* The best way is to spend time communicating with native English speakers who don't slow or simplify their speech. They also must be willing to correct your mistakes. Their being too nice to say anything will not help you to learn. Practicing this way may sound challenging, but trying to learn English speech from rules is much more difficult. There is just no way to list and memorize all the different combinations of words and sounds. And it certainly is a lot more fun to work with someone else.

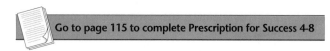
Go to page 115 to complete Prescription for Success 4-8

Improving Your Reading Comprehension

Reading has the advantage of time—you can take your time and read a sentence over and over. You can also stop and look up new words in the dictionary. At the same time, this can create a problem. This is because you may be tempted to look up every word you don't know and end up spending hours reading. English-language professor Kathy Flores recommends that students read an entire assignment first without stopping.[7] Your purpose during this first reading is to look for the main ideas. This can be difficult to do if you are constantly stopping to look up words. Here are some suggestions for completing this first reading[8]:

1. Ignore words that seem unimportant.
2. Use the **context** to guess the meaning.
3. **Scan** for specific information.
4. **Skim** for general information.
5. Read in units or chunks of words.

When reading textbook assignments, review any key terms given at the beginning of a chapter. This will highlight the vocabulary that the author considers to be most important for understanding the chapter. Second, read the learning objectives. These will help you identify what is most important and what you should be looking for as you read.

Once you have finished the first reading, write a list of the main ideas as you understood them. Then read the chapter again, this time listing and looking up the words you don't know. Later you can practice the words by writing sentences and using your preferred learning method, such as using flashcards. This is especially important if these are key words for the subject you are studying.

Improving Your Spelling

Spelling is difficult for both native and non-native English speakers (including me!). In Chapter 6 there is a section on spelling written for native speakers

of English. The spelling of English words is difficult for several reasons:

1. One letter can be pronounced in different ways, depending on the word. This is different from languages such as Spanish, in which the letters do not vary much in sound. Note the variations for the letter "o" in the following words:
   - *o*nce
   - *o*nly
   - w*o*man
   - w*o*men (These last two words can be really confusing! The words are almost identical, but in the plural form the "o" sound changes to "i"!)

(If you are unsure of the differences in sound, ask a native speaker to read them aloud.)

2. Different combinations of letters can be pronounced in the same way, such as in l*ie* and rel*ie*ve. The letters "ough" have a variety of pronunciations, none of them including the letter g:
   - t*ough*—pronounced "tuhf"
   - thr*ough*—pronounced "throo"
   - d*ough*—pronounced "doe"
   - b*ough*t—pronounced "bawt"

3. Different spellings can be pronounced the same way. Consider the following examples with the sound "ee":
   - m*e*
   - m*ee*t
   - m*ea*t
   - ch*ie*f
   - p*eo*ple

Following are a few more with the sound "oo":
   - f*oo*d
   - r*u*de
   - cr*ew*
   - gr*ou*p
   - thr*ough*
   - bl*ue*
   - sh*oe*

4. In some words, not all the syllables are pronounced. For example, some words with three syllables have only two sounds when spoken, and some with three syllables have two sounds. See Table 4-4 for some examples.

These examples demonstrate why you simply have to memorize the spelling of many words. In fact, according to one source, to become a moderately competent speller of English, you have to memorize at least 3700 words that have unpredictable spellings.[9] This is almost four times the number of unpredictable spellings of any European language. You may wonder why English has such a variety of vocabulary and spellings. It is largely because English has a number of different of roots: Anglo-Saxon, Latin, and Greek.

TABLE 4–4	Examples of Words with Silent Syllables	
Word	**Syllables in Written Form**	**Syllables in Spoken Form**
aspirin	as-pi-rin	as-prin
different	dif-fer-ent	diff-rent
temperature	tem-per-a-ture	tem-pra-ture
comfortable	com-fort-a-ble	comf-table
vegetable	veg-e-ta-ble	veg-table

Other languages have contributed vocabulary to English, including Danish and Norman French. This is why we have so many different and overlapping spelling patterns. It also explains why English has such a large vocabulary: different words meaning the same thing were adopted from various languages.

There are some major spelling rules, and these are listed in Chapter 6 (more proof that even native English speakers need this help!). These rules can be helpful. However, as one author puts it, they are like weather reports. We can use them but cannot depend on them to be correct 100% of the time.[10]

Improving Your Grammar

Every language has its own set of rules for constructing sentences, using verbs, punctuating, and so on. When we are speaking our native languages, many of us never think too much about grammar. We just speak and write out of habit. When learning or improving our skills in another language, it can be helpful to learn grammar rules.

Rules help organize a language to make communication easier and increase understanding. Some points of English grammar present special problems for speakers of other languages. A number of these are explained, along with examples, in the following sections. You may find it helpful to study this material, along with Tables 6-3, 6-4, 6-5, and 6-6 in Chapter 6. The intention here is not to offer a complete coverage of English grammar, but to present a review of some common challenges. If you find something you don't understand or that has been a problem for you, I suggest that you seek more complete explanations and practice exercises.

Finally, a couple of comments: (1) There are some grammatical terms used in the following sections. The point is not to learn these terms. They are used only to have a term to discuss them in the explanation and examples. Using English, not describing it, is the goal. (2) The grammar checkers included in word-processing software often do not catch errors. Worse, their suggestions frequently suggest constructions that contain mistakes. This can be a problem for students who have limited experience with English. I suggest that you do not use them.

Note: Much of the material in the following sections is adapted from Hacker D: *A writer's reference,* ed 6, Boston, 2007, Bedford St Martin's Press.

Articles: Using *a, an,* and *the*

- Articles tell you that a noun is about to appear. They are used directly before nouns and before adjectives followed by nouns.
  a patient
  a sick patient
  the room
  the examining room
- "A" is used before words beginning with a **consonant.**
  a nurse
  a busy nurse
- "An" is used before words beginning with a vowel or vowel sound.
  an obstetrician
  an obstetric nurse
  an hour
- Other words, called **determiners**, can also be used before nouns.
  my book
  your notes
  this patient
  that examining room
  most students
  some therapists

If there is a determiner, it is usually not necessary to use an article.
  Incorrect: *this a patient*
  Correct: *this patient* or *a patient*
  Incorrect: *my the book*
  Correct: *my book* or *the book*
- Some exceptions:
  A few of the x-ray films were lost.
  The most accurate diagnostic test requires a specialist to interpret.
  All the physical therapists from the hospital were at the meeting.
- Use *a* or *an* with nouns that can be counted and whose specific identity is not known. Use *the* with nouns whose identity is known. For example:
  We need *a* surgical technologist. (Not a specific one; any surgical technologist.)
  We need *the* surgical technologist who was here this morning. (Now we have someone specific in mind.)
  Mr. Singh needs to go to the lab for *three* tests. (The kinds of tests are unknown or not specified for the listener or reader.)

Mr. Singh needs to go to the lab for *the three* tests. (The kinds of tests are known to the listener or reader.)

- Do not use *the* with plural nouns that mean "all" or "in general," as is done in some languages, such as Spanish.

  Incorrect: *The* physicians must study many years before they can practice medicine. (*The* is not needed because the statement refers to physicians in general.)

  Correct: Physicians must study many years before they can practice medicine.

  Incorrect: *The* blood tests are often used to diagnose diseases. (*The* is not needed because the sentence refers to blood tests in general, not specific tests.)

  Correct: Blood tests are often used to diagnose diseases.

Using Verbs Correctly

- Certain **helping verbs** called **modals** are used to add to the meaning of verbs. They are always used with the **base form of a verb** (the form without the word "to").

  Incorrect: I *can to study* in the library.

  Correct: I *can study* in the library.

  Incorrect: I *must to study* more for the test.

  Incorrect: I *must studied* more for the test.

  Correct: I *must study* more for the test.

- Using *do, does,* and *did*

These helping verbs are used with the base form of a verb to ask questions, express negatives, and positively emphasize the main verb. For example:

Do you *have* the patient's consent form?

Mrs. Caceres *does not need* any more physical therapy.

I really *did enjoy* the presentation you gave about preventing diabetes.

- Using *have, has,* and *had* with the **past participle**

Past participles are verbs that usually end in *-ed, -d, -en, -n,* or *-t.* For example: *operated, tested, sent, written.*

The surgeons *have operated* together before.

The lab technician *has sent* the reports to the physician.

The dentist *had written* the follow-up letter before it was requested.

- Irregular past participles

  Quite a few common past participles are irregular. For example:

Base Form	Past Participle
begin	begun
bring	brought
come	come
make	made
sting	stung
wear	worn

A comment about irregular verbs: They can be difficult and can seem to not make sense when we are learning a new language. However, they exist in many languages. We just don't notice them as much in our native language. If you grew up speaking Spanish, for example, you probably never think about verbs such as "ser" being highly irregular. But this is difficult for native speakers of English. Add to this the fact that in Spanish, both "ser" and "estar" are irregular—*and* they both mean the same thing in English! So deciding what is difficult just depends on our point of view.

- Using forms of "be" plus the **present participle**

  Present participles are verb forms that end in *-ing.* When used with forms of "be," they express continuous action. For example:

  Carla *is studying* to be a medical biller.

  Sara and Jaime *were taking* the anatomy exam when the fire alarm sounded.

  Note: Verbs that express a state of being or a mental state are not used in the progressive form.

  Incorrect: I *am wanting* to be a massage therapist.

  Correct: I *want to be* a massage therapist.

  Note that "be" must be preceded by a modal:

  Incorrect: I *be starting* school next week.

  Correct: I *will be starting* school next week. (In this sentence, "will" is the modal.)

- Forming the passive voice

In the passive voice, the subject receives the action instead of doing it. It is formed using a form of "be" plus the past participle.

  Active voice: Hahn *gave* the injection.

  Passive voice: The injective *was given* by Hahn.

  Active voice: Ms. James *teaches* the class.

  Passive voice: The class *is taught* by Ms. James.

- Present participles and past participles used as adjectives

Present participles are used for the person or thing causing an experience.

Past participles are used to describe the person or thing that is undergoing an experience.

  The procedure *was frightening.* (The procedure caused fright.)

  The patient *was frightened.* (The patient experienced fright.)

  The lecture *is boring.* (The lecture causes boredom.)

  The students *are bored.* (The students are experiencing boredom.)

- Using **gerunds** and **infinitives** after certain verbs

Gerunds are words that are derived from verbs but that function as nouns. They end in *-ing.* Examples: *observing, swimming.*

Infinitives are basic forms of verbs preceded by the word "to." Examples: to observe, to swim.

Some verbs can be followed by a gerund, but not an infinitive. Examples: *admit, appreciate, avoid, deny, discuss, enjoy, escape, finish, imagine, miss, postpone, practice, quit, recall, resist, risk, suggesting, tolerate.*

Incorrect: I *practice to give* injections during the lab sessions.

Correct: I *practice giving* injections during the lab sessions.

Incorrect: The instructor *discussed to handle* blood safely.

Correct: The instructor *discussed handling* blood safely.

Incorrect: Jaime *will finish to study* the chapter in about an hour.

Correct: Jaime *will finish studying* the chapter in about an hour.

Here are some common verbs that can be followed by an infinitive, but not a gerund: *agree, ask, bet, claim, decide, expect, have, hope, manage, mean, need, offer, plan, pretend, promise, refuse, wait, want, wish.*

Incorrect: I *need borrowing* a book from the library.

Correct: I *need to borrow* a book from the library.

Incorrect: Carolyn *is planning attending* this college next year.

Correct: Carolyn *is planning to attend* this college next year.

• Verbs that recommend or advise

When a speaker or writer uses certain verbs to tell someone to do something, a noun or pronoun must go between the verb and the infinitive. These verbs include *advise, allow, cause, command, convince, encourage, have, instruct, order, persuade, remind, require, tell, urge, warn.*

I *persuaded my father to see* the doctor about the pain in his arm.

The doctor *advised him to rest* the arm for the next two weeks.

My mother *reminded dad to take* his aspirin.

• **Phrasal verbs**

Many English verbs can be combined with prepositions to create idiomatic expressions in which the phrase has a meaning that is different from the meaning of the verb by itself. Following are some common examples:

call off—cancel

drop in—visit

drop off—deliver

get up—arise

look up—visit, find

run into—meet unexpectedly

The delivery service *dropped off* the medical supplies we ordered.

Jackie has to *get up* early because she works the morning shift at the hospital.

I *ran into* an old classmate at the workshop on protecting patient privacy.

Phrasal verbs can be confusing because looking up the individual words is not likely to give you the correct meaning. Because these are used frequently in English, it is suggested that you include them in your study of vocabulary. Lists are available from websites such as www.learn-english-today.com/phrasal-verbs/phrasal-verb-list.htm, or you can enter "phrasal verbs" into a search engine such as Google.

Conditional Sentences

In conditional sentences, the action in one **clause** in a sentence can take place only if something in the other clause takes place.

• With conditions that are always true, use the same tense in each clause:

When Dr. Harrison *sees* his patients, he always *remembers* their names.

• Predictive (If this, then that…)

If you *study* every day, you *will increase* your chances of earning good grades.

• Unlikely possibilities

If *Janet practiced* more, *she could speak* better Spanish.

If *I had* more money, *I would quit* my job while I'm in school.

• Events that did not happen in the past

If I had graduated last month, *I would have been hired* by the hospital.

• Conditions that are not real

If I were a doctor, I would want to be a pediatrician. (Note the use of "were" in this sentence. "I were" and "he [or she] were" are used only in the conditional, never in the past tense.)

Sentences Beginning with "Although" and "Because"

Mixed constructions, which are incorrect, occur when the following word pairs are used in one sentence:

although—but

although—however

because—therefore

Incorrect: *Although* the waiting room was full, *but* the office was running on schedule.

Correct: *Although* the waiting room was full, the office was running on schedule.

Correct: The waiting room was full, *but* the office was running on schedule.

Incorrect: *Because* this medication can cause drowsiness; *therefore,* you need to have someone drive you home. (Note that "therefore" is preceded by a semicolon and followed by a comma.)

Correct: *Because* this medication can cause drowsiness, you need to have someone drive you home.

Correct: This medication can cause drowsiness; *therefore,* you need to have someone drive you home.

Prepositions That Show Time and Place

English uses many prepositions. They are used to show relationships, such as direction, place, time, means, and cause, between other words in a sentence. Prepositions are placed before nouns and pronouns to modify (restrict or add to the sense of) and link them to the rest of the sentence.

Frequently used prepositions include *at, by, for, from, in, of, on, to, with.*

The medical assistant put the patient's chart *in* the file. (The preposition "in" shows the location of chart.)

The appointment was scheduled *at* 2 o'clock. (The preposition "at" indicates time.)

The patient was taken *by* ambulance *to* the nearest hospital. (The preposition "by" indicates means and "to" indicates direction.)

Choosing the correct preposition can sometimes be confusing, as shown in the following examples:

To get to the workshop, Carla will travel *by car.*

To get to the workshop, Carla will travel *on the bus.*

To get to the workshop, Carla will travel *on the train.*

 Go to page 115 to complete Prescription for Success 4-9

STUDENTS WITH LEARNING DISABILITIES

THE CHALLENGE OF LEARNING DISABILITIES

When people hear the term "learning disability," many of them picture a child struggling to learn to read or perhaps a youngster who can't sit still in the classroom. The fact is that there are a variety of conditions that interfere with learning, and many of these present problems for adults as well as children. There are no typical profiles of a "learning disabled student" of any age. Rather, there is a variety of learning disabilities, and some individuals may experience different combinations of challenges that interfere with their learning or even with carrying out their daily activities. (See Box 4-1 for examples of common challenges.)

You may have been diagnosed with a learning disability as a child or teenager. Or you may have simply wondered why you had, or are having, certain difficulties in school or even in learning on the job. Learning disabilities are not always obvious, even to the person who has them, and for this reason they

---

BOX 4-1   Challenges Associated with Learning Disabilities

- Rarely completing projects you start
- Rarely meeting deadlines
- Being unable to manage time realistically
- Constantly feeling the need to move around or fidget
- Being unable to handle sequential or serial information
- Being unable to stay focused for more than very short periods of time
- Getting distracted very easily
- Seeing letters and numbers in the wrong order
- Having letters go blurry or jumping around when you are reading
- Experiencing great difficulty remembering oral instructions
- Having trouble judging distance and determining direction, such as left and right
- Always feeling disorganized and out of control
- Being unable to write legibly or neatly, even when you try
- Easily forgetting material that is presented visually
- Experiencing great difficulty in communicating thoughts orally or in writing
- Constantly losing your possessions

---

are sometimes referred to as "hidden" or "invisible" disabilities. Actually, it doesn't really matter if you "have" a learning disability. What matters is that if you have noticed you have more difficulty than most people with certain tasks and this often gets in the way of your learning and living productively, there are positive actions you can take. As an adult, you have self-awareness and can monitor your own behavior and work to make changes.

First, however, there are some things you should know about learning disabilities:

- They are *not* related to intelligence. In fact, some research indicates that individuals with attention deficit disorder tend to have above-average IQs.
- They are based on biologic factors, mostly involved with certain specific brain functions. They are not a person's fault or caused by a person's unwillingness to try to do better.
- They are not always obvious and can result in puzzling contradictions. (See Box 4-2 for examples.)
- They do not prevent people from having successful and high-level careers.
- Some people with learning disabilities are creative and able to come up with innovative ideas.
- Being learning disabled has *nothing* to do with a lack of effort or laziness.

- Having a learning disability does *not* mean you can't learn. It simply means you learn in different ways from the crowd.
- There are many strategies you can use to overcome the challenges of learning disabilities.

You are encouraged to try the strategies presented in this chapter. They are organized by academic and life skills, such as reading and time management, and presented in Tables 4-5 through 4-15. Select strategies that correspond to difficulties you are having and that look appropriate for you. Not all of them will work for every student. For example, let's look at the following suggestion: "Take notes as you read your textbook to increase your concentration." Now, if one of your problems is difficulty with your handwriting, this might not be good advice. In that case, you could place your book next to your computer and take notes on your word processing program. But if you are very slow at keyboarding or very easily distracted, this might not work for you. So perhaps underlining key words in your text and making short notes in the margins might work best. Repeating the important points out loud may also work. Consider your own situation to determine what might work best for you.

If the suggestions don't work and you find yourself struggling with your studies, speak with your instructors and perhaps an administrator at your college. Don't wait until you experience feelings of desperation or panic. There is no need to miss achieving your academic and career goals when help is available.

GENERAL SUGGESTIONS

This section contains suggestions for individuals with all types of learning disabilities. The first involves your physical health and fitness. Because learning disabilities are biologically based, it makes sense that maintaining good health habits is important. Physical exercise, which has been found to help prevent diseases of all kinds, is also helpful in relieving some of the problems that accompany learning disabilities. Some students report that they are more able to concentrate and learn if they engage in just a little exercise each day.

On the other hand, it is important to get adequate rest. This may seem like a contradiction for a busy adult student, but if you have a learning disability, it is quite important. This is because it takes effort to concentrate and learn, especially when

---

BOX 4-2   Contradictions in Performance

- You can think logically but cannot write your thoughts in a paragraph.
- You are alert and skilled but have trouble following directions.
- You understand mathematical theories but get confused performing calculations.
- You practice for hours, but your handwriting is illegible.
- You have creative ideas but cannot explain them clearly to others.
- You write beautiful stories and essays, but your spelling is very poor.

TABLE 4–5	Communication
Difficulties	**Suggested Strategies**
You find it difficult to follow what people are saying.	Keep your eyes on the speaker to avoid getting distracted. Ask the speaker to speak more slowly or to repeat things, when necessary. If the person is the instructor, request a meeting outside of class. Ask if lecture outlines are available to help you follow along. Develop active listening skills (see Chapter 5).
You think you know what you want to say, but it doesn't come out right.	Practice speaking alone in front of a mirror. Use notes when engaging in an important conversation. Before speaking, take a few moments to think and be clear in your own mind about what you want or need to say.
You tend to ramble on and get lost in details when you are speaking.	Think about the purpose of your conversation: what do you want to get across? Practice being self-aware and observing your own behavior. When you catch yourself, use humor and say: "Oops, I'm rambling on again. The important thing is…." If appropriate, explain to your listener(s) that communication is difficult for you and that you may experience some problems.
You miss nonverbal signals that people give you during conversations.	Read about nonverbal communication. Practice observing others. Work with a friend who is willing to observe you and help you identify nonverbal language.

TABLE 4–6	Focusing
Difficulties	**Suggested Strategies**
You are easily distracted by extraneous noise.	When studying, wear headphone or earplugs or use a white noise machine. Sit close to the instructor during lectures (if seats are assigned, request permission to sit up front). Avoid sitting near students who talk during class. Choose quiet places to study, such as the library. Turn off your phone when you are studying.
You are easily distracted by visual stimuli.	Choose a seat where there are minimal distractions, such as away from a window or an interesting wall display. Work in an uncluttered area. Minimize the number of items on your desk that might draw your attention.
You are distracted by your own ideas that come up but are not needed at the moment. You are just bombarded with competing thoughts and ideas.	Keep a brainstorming log to note the ideas for consideration later. (I have 27 pages of writing ideas that popped into my head while I was working on something else.) Try doing meditation, a practice that has been shown to increase focus and attention (Box 4-3).
It is very difficult to stay with a task for any length of time—even a few minutes.	Try doing meditation, a practice that has been shown to increase focus and attention (see Box 4-3). Train yourself to keep on task by deciding how many minutes you will focus, even if it is just 5 or 10 to start. Write down the time, and keep bringing yourself back to your task until the stop time. Try focusing on what you will gain by completing the task at hand.
You find it difficult to both start and complete projects.	Think about your goal. Why is this project important to you? Build in rewards to encourage yourself to get things done. Break projects into small chunks with interim deadlines. Trying to do too much can be overwhelming and result in doing nothing.

BOX 4-3	Meditation, Yoga, and Guided Imagery

Purposeful relaxation and practices that clear the mind promote calmness and can increase our ability to focus and concentrate.

- *Meditation:* a process for quieting the mind. Meditation actually affects brain activity and has been shown to decrease blood pressure and offer other health benefits. It involves sitting quietly and clearing the mind of thought. This is not as easy as it sounds, especially for someone with ADD or ADHD. Ways to benefit from meditation include choosing a quiet area; eliminating distractions and interruptions; and using a focusing technique such as repeating a word, counting, or focusing on your breathing in and out.
- *Yoga:* an ancient practice of assuming certain body postures and focusing on breathing. There are many types of yoga, and the postures range from easy to advanced.
- *Guided imagery:* a method of visualization that involves focusing mentally on peaceful, pleasant scenes. Some individuals imagine a brilliant white light entering the top of their head and flowing through their body, spreading positive feelings of peacefulness and calm.

TABLE 4–7	Hyperactivity
Difficulties	**Suggested Strategies**
You cannot sit still or refrain from fidgeting for any length of time.	Engage in regular physical exercise. Choose something you enjoy doing. When appropriate, move around when you study. Try relaxation exercises, **yoga**, or **guided imagery** to help you relax and slow yourself down (see Chapter 3 for a relaxation exercise). When you are attending gatherings where you must sit for extended periods of time, engage your hands in an activity such as taking notes.
You have trouble settling down at night and sleeping.	Thirty minutes before bedtime, turn off the television and computer to reduce the sensory stimulation. Instead, engage in a quiet, relaxing activity. Develop a "going to bed" ritual that signals your body to slow down.

TABLE 4–8	Memory
Difficulties	**Suggested Strategies**
You cannot remember information given to you orally, especially things like multi-step instructions.	Ask the speaker to speak slowly, if necessary. Take notes. Ask if the instructions are available in written form. Ask the speaker to repeat anything you do not understand (it is very difficult for anyone to remember something they don't understand). Check your understanding of what people have said: "Let me make sure I've got this right…," then repeat what you heard or read from your notes. See the suggestions for improving your memory in Chapter 3.
You cannot remember what you have read or studied in class.	See the suggestions for reading in Chapter 5. Take notes of the main points as you read to increase your concentration. Writing also helps reinforce memory traces in the brain. Try the following to reinforce the material. Suppose you are studying diabetes. • *Visualize* how you might use what you are learning, such as in patient education. • *Associate* it with anyone you know who has diabetes. • *Think* about the causes and the increase in cases in the United States. • *Create* a mental picture of the pancreas. • *Discuss* what you are learning with others. • *Explain* what you are learning to others, such as the effects of untreated diabetes. • *Read* other sources, such as information on the Web or brochures about diabetes. • *Review* the material periodically.
You cannot remember new vocabulary.	Create a word list that you review daily. Use some of the techniques above to visualize, associate, and so on to "plant" the word in your memory. Try creating mnemonics such as the following: • Create a silly or interesting mental picture. Example: picture a *crane* lifting a large skull to remember *cranium,* the medical term for skull. • Link the new word to one with a similar sound and meaning. Example: *-stasis* is the medical word element for stoppage. It sounds like *stay.* If something stops, it stays in place.

TABLE 4–9	Note-Taking
Difficulties	**Suggested Strategies**
You cannot listen and write at the same time.	Request permission in advance to record class lectures. (Take care, however, to listen in class.) It is best if you use a recorder that has variable speed control so you can speed up or slow down the speech as needed. Request permission to copy notes from another student. Ask your instructors if they can give you outlines of their lectures. Try to copy down any information written on the board or screen.
You can listen and take notes, but what you write down doesn't make much sense.	See the sections on note-taking in Chapter 5.

you are overcoming learning difficulties. If you become overly tired, your learning efforts become counterproductive. The brain simply cannot function as it should when it is deprived of sleep and rest breaks. It is recommended that students break up their studying into chunks of 20 minutes or so, taking short breaks between sessions. The emphasis here is on "short" because you may need only a few minutes to rest your eyes and your mind. Because you may have to spend more time studying than students without learning disabilities, good time management and teaching yourself not to waste

time are especially important skills. For example, if you leave things until the last minute, you will find yourself rushed. This creates anxiety, even feelings of panic, and these feelings can prevent you from getting anything done at all.

There is a variety of groups and services you might find helpful. These include the following:

• Services for learning disabled students that may be available at your college or in your community

• Support groups that consist of students with learning disabilities, in which they share their experiences and ideas for overcoming challenges

TABLE 4–10	Numbers
Difficulties	**Suggested Strategies**
You have trouble copying strings of numbers in the correct order.	Break strings of numbers into groups of two or three digits. Write each small group, and check as you proceed. Cover part of the number as you read, especially if there are series of zeroes. When copying two numbers, cover the one that you are not copying.
You find it difficult to read tables that contain lots of numbers.	Draw an extra thick line under every third row. Highlight the sections in different colors.
You have difficulty performing math calculations.	Go over the review material in Chapter 7. Read the section on math anxiety in Chapter 7. Request permission to use a calculator when doing your work. If you have trouble reading numbers and following your calculations, try a talking calculator. It may be easier for you to catch errors if you hear them.
It is hard for you to measure accurately.	Take a deep breath and work calmly and slowly. Write down measurements as you go along so you don't forget them. Double check your work. If in doubt, have someone else check your work.

TABLE 4–11	Organization
Difficulties	**Suggested Strategies**
You lose things all the time.	Designate a place for everything, especially items such as keys and eyeglasses. Figure 4-4 shows an example of an organized workspace. Store items close to where you use them. Set up specific places for important items such as bills to be paid and assignments you are working on. Keep your desk and work areas as free of clutter as possible so important items don't get buried. Keep items such as your cell phone attached to your purse or belt so they can't get away from you.
Your desk is covered with piles of papers, folders, and notes, with many of their contents a mystery to you.	Work on clearing a small area at a time. Discard papers you no longer need. Create a simple filing system. Use colored file folders for different projects. (If you have trouble sequencing letters, and keeping files in order, make an alphabet arc. This is a semicircle with the letters of the alphabet written from left to right along the curved portion. Alternate idea: purchase a home filing system that comes with files, labels, and instructions for organizing papers and forms. Set up two accordion files: one with a section for each day of the week, and the other with a section for each month of the year. Place items that need attention in the corresponding file section. Be sure to check these files regularly. Alternate method: set up three trays labeled "This Week," "This Month," "This Term (or Semester)." Sort tasks accordingly; check the file labeled "This Week" daily and the other two weekly.
You frequently miss deadlines or appointments.	Keep a calendar or planner, either paper or electronic. Today's PDAs (**personal digital assistants**) include everything from calendars to wireless phones. Be disciplined about recording everything you need to do and checking your calendar frequently. Maintain a daily and weekly to-do list, either on paper or electronically. If on paper, use a small notebook, not little slips of paper that are easily lost.
You often find you don't have what you need for class, work, or household duties such as paying bills.	Create a list of things you must have each day and post it where you will see it, perhaps next to the front door. Each evening, set out what you will need for the next day. Do the same for your children to prevent the morning rush.
You feel so overwhelmed by everything that needs to be done that you often become "paralyzed" and don't do anything.	Get an "organization buddy" who can help you get things into perspective, make a plan, and keep you motivated. Your buddy can be a family member, a friend, or even an organization professional. It just needs to be someone who is organized, patient, and sympathetic to your situation. Work on gradually clearing clutter that can cause an overload of stimuli, visual stress, and distraction. Think about what really needs to be done and what can be put off until later. Consider the consequences of your choices. Divide large projects that seem impossible to complete into small pieces; estimate the time needed to complete each; designate deadlines for each piece and for the final project.

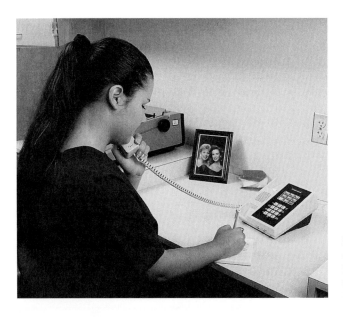

Figure 4–4 Working in an uncluttered area helps prevent distractions for individuals with attention deficit disorder. Set up your home office and desk in an organized manner, as the medical reception area shown in this photo has been organized. (*From Gerdin J:* Health careers today, *ed 4, St. Louis, Mosby, 2007.*)

TABLE 4–12	Reading
Difficulties	**Suggested Strategies**
You can't seem to remember anything you read.	Study the section on reading in Chapter 5 and try the methods suggested. The previewing and reviewing steps are especially helpful for students with retention problems. Use the following strategies, which are also listed in Table 4-8 (Memory). This time, let's suppose you are studying the process of digestion: • *Visualize* the path of a donut as it goes through the digestion system, naming each part of the anatomy it passes through. • *Associate* the digestive process with the energy you use going about your day. • *Think* about the functions of the various digestive organs. • *Create* a mental picture of the digestive organs. Imagine each one in a bright color. • *Discuss* what you are learning, such as the causes of indigestion, with others. • *Read* other sources, such as illustrated material on the Web. • *Review* the material periodically.
You have trouble keeping your place when reading.	Move your finger along text as you read. Place a ruler or piece of paper under the line. Use an **eye-level reading ruler**, a special ruler made of opaque and transparent plastic in a variety of colors. Its serves to underline and highlight text in a colored tint, thus helping with both tracking and reducing the glare. Use a reading window, a slotted piece of plastic that shows one line at a time to reduce distraction from surrounding text.
You have problems distinguishing letters and their order: 1. See letters in the wrong order 2. Confuse reversible letters, such as *b* and *d, m* and *w* 3. Confuse words that look similar, such as *were* and *where* 4. Mis-sequence letters in long words, such as *conversation* and *conservation*	Pay attention to the context and meaning of sentences. If a word doesn't fit, examine it carefully to see if you have misread it. Practice seeing words as separate groups of letters (syllables) instead of as long strings of letters. Examples: presentation = pre-sen-ta-tion, terminology = ter-mi-nol-o-gy Learn common **prefixes** and **suffixes.** A prefix is a letter or a group of letters attached to the beginning of a word that partly indicates its meaning. Examples: • *anti-* means against: anti viral → antiviral • *mis-* means wrong or bad: mis diagnose → misdiagnose • *trans-* means across: trans plant → transplant A suffix is a letter or a group of letters attached to the end of a word to form a new word or to alter the grammatical function of the original word. Examples: • *-less* means without: pain less → painless • *-ment* means action or process: treat ment → treatment • *-ed* indicates past tense: inject → injected
You have difficulty reading print on white backgrounds because it seems to glare. Letters are blurred and jump around on the page.	Copy written materials, such as class handouts, onto light colored paper (investigate to see which color works best for you). Use a colored overlay on your computer monitor screen, or change the background color on your screen, if possible. Investigate the use of colored overlays for placing on text or colored eyeglasses.

TABLE 4–13	Taking Tests
Difficulties	**Suggested Strategies**
You misunderstand instructions and what the questions are asking.	Ask the instructor to privately explain the questions. State what you think a question is asking and ask for feedback to let you know if you understood it correctly. *Note:* If you believe you will need this extra help, advise the instructor *before* the day of the test.
You read and write so slowly that you don't have enough time to finish all the questions.	Request extra time to complete tests. *Note:* If you believe you will need this accommodation, submit your request *before* the day of the test.
You are too distracted by noises in the environment to focus on the test.	Request permission to take the text in a quiet environment *Note:* If you believe you will need this accommodation, submit your request *before* the day of the test.

Note: See also the section on test anxiety and test-taking strategies in Chapter 6.

TABLE 4–14	Time Management
Difficulties	**Suggested Strategies**
You never come close to estimating the amount of time it will take to complete any given project or activity.	Keep a time diary for a couple of weeks. Write down start and stop times for your daily activities. Then analyze to see how long things really take. You may be astonished to discover that something you thought takes 15 minutes actually takes closer to an hour. Estimate how long it will take to complete an activity, then start by adding 50% to the time. You can adjust over time as you learn to set realistic goals.
You try to do too much during the time available and often end up feeling exhausted or burned out.	See the suggestion above for keeping a time diary. Try planning fewer activities than you normally would, and see how much you actually accomplish. Prioritize your tasks, and always do the most important ones first. Pace yourself. When doing something that requires concentration, work in blocks of 20 to 30 minutes at a time. Use a planner or calendar to mark final deadlines. Set interim deadlines for completing parts of the project, studying for a test, and so on.
You easily lose track of time. A 10-minute break becomes a 2-hour session of lost time.	Set timers or alarms when you go on a break, answer the phone, or look at your e-mail. Vibrating timers are available if more appropriate. Practice being aware of where you are, what you are doing, and the time.
You are rarely on time for appointments, classes, or social occasions.	Start recording how much time it actually takes you to get to places you commonly visit, such as school. Then try adding 5 minutes to your travel time. Resist doing "one last little thing" as you head for the door.

See also the section on time management in Chapter 3.

- Study groups with a variety of students
- Learning centers and tutors who help with specific academic skills and subjects

Lastly, what may be the most important advice of all: seek help from your instructors. Students with learning disabilities report that their greatest mistake was not getting help before they were struggling and feeling desperate. Your instructors want you to succeed. Give them the opportunity to help make that happen.

Tables 4-5 through 4-15 outline different learning challenges and offer strategies on how a student can work with these challenges.

 Go to page 116 to complete Prescription for Success 4-10

ACCOMMODATIONS

Knowing yourself and your needs is the first step toward **self-advocacy**, which means seeking solutions to your learning difficulties, trying alternate ways of learning, and asking for appropriate and necessary help. You may need to explain the nature of learning disabilities to people who don't understand them.

TABLE 4–15	Writing
Difficulties	**Suggested Strategies**
You have serious problems with spelling.	Review the spelling rules and strategies presented in Chapter 6. Use the spell-check feature on your word processor. Carry a handheld spell-checker. Consider purchasing a medical terminology spell-checker. Investigate **abbreviation-expander** software. You can enter codes for often-used words so you don't have to continually reenter—and possible misspell—them. Check into proofreading software to supplement what came with your word processing program. This is available in medical report versions.
You make mistakes copying written material.	Work slowly and carefully. Copy onto colored, nonglare paper. Use paper with a slot cut into it or a reading window to cover the lines you are not copying.
You have difficulty organizing your thoughts and presenting them logically on paper.	Use a computer to do writing assignments so you can easily correct mistakes and move text around. When students aren't worried about the mechanics of writing, they can focus on the content and meaning. Ask your instructor to review your first draft to help you get on the right track. Have someone critique and proofread your written work. See also the suggestions about writing in Chapter 6. Request extra time to complete long writing assignments. *Note:* If you believe you will need this accommodation, submit your request *before* the assignment is due.
You find that the white paper you are writing on seems to glare.	Request permission in advance to submit your work on colored paper (experiment with colors to see which works best for you).

Accommodations are often available for students whose learning challenges prevent them from learning in traditional ways and who cannot demonstrate what they actually know through typical testing methods. The laws that protect individuals with disabilities apply to some people who have learning disabilities, depending on the nature and severity of the condition. These laws are *not* intended to excuse students from having to fulfill the requirements of their certificate or degree programs. Their purpose is to help students find ways to acquire needed knowledge and skills and demonstrate that they have mastered them.

It is important that if you do seek extra help or time to complete a test, you do so only when absolutely necessary. Taking advantage of the situation is unethical and unfair to other students. You must also consider carefully the possible effects of your learning disability on your work in health care. Using this time during your training to find solutions you can apply to your working conditions will help ensure your future success.

LEARNING DISABILITIES DURING THE JOB SEARCH

Personal organization and good oral and written presentation are important aspects of a successful job search. You may want to seek assistance from qualified helpers to work with you as you look for a job. These might include the following:

- Career services personnel at your school
- Your organization buddy
- Your instructors
- Your mentor, if you have one (see Chapter 3)

If writing is a problem, have someone proofread your resume and any letters you send out. See if potential employers have applications you can fill out online; if not, ask if you can take the application home to fill out so you can check it over carefully. If you are called for an interview and communicating orally is difficult for you, ask for help from your school's career services personnel or an instructor. Perhaps they can spend some extra time helping you prepare.

A question many students have is if they should disclose their learning disability to a potential employer. The opinion of experts is that if your disability does not affect your job performance, then it is not necessary to mention it. If, however, you plan to request accommodations, you must disclose it to be eligible. (Do note that if you are not legally defined as "disabled," you may not be entitled to accommodations.)

Once on the job, there are things you can do to work more effectively, as follows:

- Ask your supervisor to help you prioritize tasks.
- Ask that oral directions be repeated or given to you in written form.

- Apply the strategies you used in school. For example, if you used an eye-level ruler to help with reading, keep one with you at work.
- Request permission to take notes at employee orientations, workshops, or important meetings.
- Copy material you must read onto colored paper.
- Keep a timer at your desk or work area—or a small one in your pocket—to limit phone calls and conversations with co-workers.

As discussed previously, the important thing is to identify your own weaknesses and work to find ways to overcome them. People with learning disabilities have successful careers and productive lives. Sometimes, it just takes a bit of extra effort.

⇨ SUMMARY OF KEY IDEAS

1. Adult students have different challenges and advantages than traditional students.
2. The challenges that adult students face can be handled.
3. English can be challenging to learn, but with study and practice, it can be mastered.
4. There is a variety of learning disabilities, but most can be overcome by using specific strategies.

Positive Self-Talk for This Chapter

Adult Students

1. I have many experiences that will help me become a successful student.
2. I face up to my fears and concerns and seek help when necessary.
3. By attending school, I am making a better life for myself and my family.

English-as-a-Second-Language Students

1. I have the advantage of knowing more than one language.
2. I am improving my English every day.

Students with Learning Disabilities

1. I am learning what I need to know about health care.
2. I am successfully using strategies to accomplish what I need to do.
3. I know my strengths and weaknesses and am a good self-advocate.

To Learn More

Adult Students

Adult Student Center

adultstudentcenter.com

Explore this website for inspiring stories about adults who return to school. Also contains links to dozen of Web resources providing help with specific subjects, locating references, and acquiring study skills.

Doolin M: *The success manual for adult college students,* ed 3, 2006, Booklocker.com.

Hardin CJ: *100 Things every adult college student ought to know,* Williamsville, NY, 2000, Cambridge Stratford Study Skills Institute.

Siebert A, Karr MK: *The adult learner's guide to survival and success,* ed 6, Portland, Ore, 2008, Practical Psychology Press.

www.adultstudent.com

The Internet companion to the book provides help with study skills and includes success stories and suggestions from other students.

Simon L: *New beginnings: a reference guide for adult learners,* ed 3, Upper Saddle River, NJ, 2006, Pearson Prentice Hall.

Walstrom C, Williams BK, Dansby CK: *The practical student,* Clifton Park, NY, 1999, Wadsworth Cengage Learning.

English-as-a-Second-Language Students

Activities for ESL Students

http://a4esl.org

The activities include grammar explanations, quizzes, and vocabulary practice.

Dave's ESL Café

www.eslcafe.com

The "café" contains links to many ESL sites, including grammar lessons and lists of idioms.

e Learn English Language

www.elearnenglishlanguage.com

This site contains short lessons, which include good examples, on dozens of topics.

English Club

www.EnglishClub.com

English Club provides grammar explanations with examples. Also included are quizzes with immediate access to correct answers. The site originates in England, so a few words, such as "favourite," have British rather American spelling. The grammar, however, is the same.

English Page

www.englishpage.com

Explore the online tutorials that teach English grammar and vocabulary. There are good practice exercises and links to dozens of other useful sites.

Flores K: *What every ESL student should know: a guide to college and university academic success,* Ann Arbor, 2008, University of Michigan Press.

Flores shares tips for learning English gathered from her years of teaching English to college students from around the world who come to the United States to study.

Hacker D: *A writer's reference,* ed 6, Boston, 2007, Bedford/ St. Martin's.

This is an excellent, easy-to-use book that includes explanations and examples of grammar, sentence structure, punctuation, and organization of content. One entire section is devoted to special help for ESL students.

Hospital English

www.hospitalenglish.com

Vocabulary is grouped into families of health care words such as diseases, patient-interaction vocabulary, and body systems. The site includes audio for pronunciation help and quizzes to check understanding.

Learn English Today

www.learn-english-today.com

This site has lessons on all aspects of English, including a good list of phrasal verbs.

Resources for English as a Second Language

www.UsingEnglish.com

This is a comprehensive site with lists of idioms, phrasal verbs, irregular verbs, grammar, and more. There are quizzes on all aspects of English, plus links to other useful websites.

Vocabulary University

www.vocabulary.com

This site contains links to groups of basic vocabulary, including one for health terms.

Purdue University Online Writing Lab

http://owl.english.purdue.edu/owl/resource/678/01/

A section of this excellent Writing Lab is designed for ESL students.

Students with Learning Disabilities

ADDitude Magazine

www.additudemag.com

The emphasis of this website is "living well with ADD and learning disabilities." It contains useful articles for adults with ADD, such as how to focus at a job interview.

Children and Adults with Attention Deficit Disorder (CHADD)

8181 Professional Place, Suite 201

Landover, MD 20785

800-233-5050

www.chadd.org

This organization provides helpful information and support as well as publishing *Attention!* magazine. The website contains questions to help adults identify the signs of ADHD.

Crossbow Education

www.crossboweducation.com/Eye_Level_Reading_Ruler.htm

Although this is a British website, it has good visual presentations of useful products to assist with dyslexia and reading problems, such as eye-level rulers and reading windows.

Dolber R: *College and career success for students with learning disabilities,* Chicago, 1992, VGM Career Horizons.

This book provides specific strategies for college students, including study techniques and personal organization tips.

Great Schools

www.greatschools.net/cgi-bin/showarticle/2479

This Web page contains an article on evaluating assistive devices.

www.greatschools.net/cgi-bin/showarticle/3080

This Web page provides information about abbreviation expanders and lists various types available.

International Dyslexia Association

www.interdys.org

This website contains fact sheets and other resources.

Learning Disabilities Association of America

www.ldanatl.org

Find comprehensive information that includes help for adults with learning disabilities in postsecondary education and in the workplace.

Learning Disabilities Research and Training Center

The University of Georgia

Roosevelt Warm Springs for Rehabilitation

http://people.rit.edu/easi/easisem/ldnoelbw.htm

This website contains many links to resources for learning disabled teens and adults.

Moody S: *Dyslexia: surviving and succeeding at college,* New York, 2007, Routledge.

This book provides practical information to help students succeed.

National Attention Disorder Association

1788 Second Street, Suite 200

Highland Park, IL 60035

847-432-5874

mail@add.org (e-mail address)

www.add.org

This organization is specifically for adults with attention deficit disorder. It prints newsletters and brochures, holds conferences, and maintains a helpful website.

National Center for Learning Disabilities

www.ncld.org

This organization provides useful information for adults as well as children with learning disabilities.

National Resource Center on AD/HD

www.help4adhd.org

Information and resources for all ages.

National Resource Center on AD/HD: *Succeeding in the Workplace,* 2003.

www.help4adhd.org/en/living/workplace/WWK16

This article discusses dealing with ADD in the workplace.

Sarkis SM: *10 Simple solutions to adult ADD: how to overcome chronic distraction and accomplish your goals,* Oakland, Calif, 2005, New Harbinger Publications.

This book provides tips for personal organization to help adults cope with attention deficit disorder.

Technology Matrix

www.techmatrix.org

This is a Web tool for finding and comparing products that address special learning needs.

REFERENCES

1. Siebert A, Karr MK: *The adult learner's guide to survival and success,* ed 6, Portland, Ore, 2008, Practical Psychology Press.

2. Ellis D: *Becoming a master student,* updated 8th ed., Boston, 1998, Houghton Mifflin.

3. Berkman LF, Leo-Summers S, Hoewitz RI: Emotional support and survival after myocardial infarction: a prospective, population-based study on the elderly, *Ann Intern Med* 117:1003-1009, 1992.

4. Williams RB, Barefoot JC, Califf RM, et al: Prognostic importance of social and economic resources among medically treated patients with angiographically documented coronary artery disease. *JAMA* 267:520-524, 1992.

5. Seeman T: Social support and social conflict. John D. and Catherine T. MacArthur Research Network on Socioeconomic Status and Health, 1998. Available at: www.macses.ucsf.edu/Research/Psychosocial/notebook/socsupp.html. Accessed January 12, 2009.

6. Special Analysis 2002: http://nces.ed.gov/programs/coe/2002/analyses/nontraditional/sa04.asp. Accessed 1/12/09.

7. Flores K: *What every ESL student should know: a guide to college and university academic success,* Ann Arbor, 2008, University of Michigan Press.

8. *Reading strategies.* John's ESL Community. Available at: www.johnsesl.com/templates/reading/strategies.php. Accessed 1/24/09.

9. Bell M: *Problems in learning to read and write.* Available at: www.englishspellingproblems.co.uk. Accessed 1/24/09.

10. Norquist R: *Top 4 spelling rules.* Available at: http://grammar.about.com/od/words/tp/spellrules.htm. Accessed 1/24/09.

INTERNET ACTIVITIES

Identify a problem you want to work on related to the topics in this chapter. Then choose three websites from the "To Learn More Section" to explore. Try suggestions you believe might be helpful and report on the results.

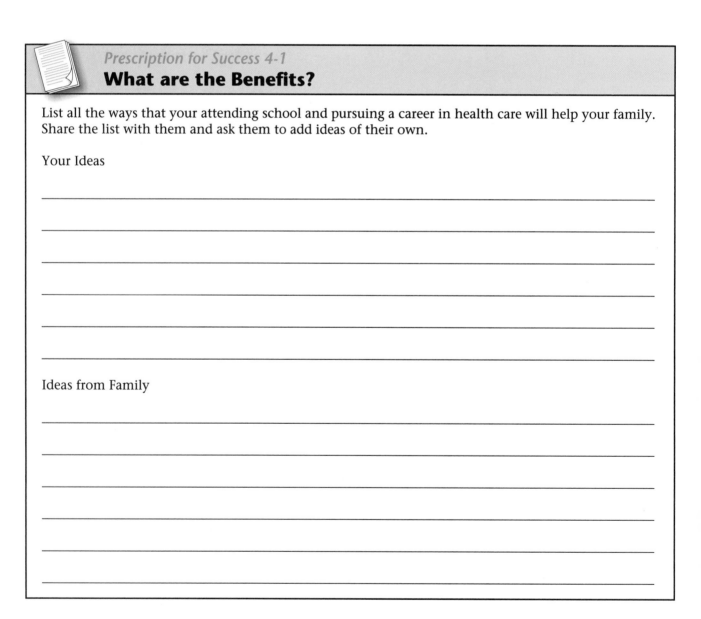

Prescription for Success 4-1
What are the Benefits?

List all the ways that your attending school and pursuing a career in health care will help your family. Share the list with them and ask them to add ideas of their own.

Your Ideas

_____

_____

_____

_____

_____

_____

Ideas from Family

_____

_____

_____

_____

_____

Prescription for Success 4-2
My Support Team

List the names of everyone you know who supports your decision to go to school.

_____

_____

_____

_____

_____

_____

From these names, who can you rely on when you need help?

_____

_____

_____

_____

_____

_____

Prescription for Success 4-3
What are my Challenges?

Look over the classes you will be taking and read any available descriptions. On the basis of these, list academic challenges that concern you.

_____

_____

_____

_____

_____

Continued

Prescription for Success 4-3 (Continued)

What can you do now to improve your skills? Create a plan with resources and timelines.

_____

_____

_____

_____

_____

Prescription for Success 4-4
Breaking It Up

Handling your various roles won't seem so overwhelming if you break what you need to do into bite-sized pieces. Choose a project or task you are currently working to achieve. Break it into a series of independent steps.

What is the task?

_____

_____

_____

Step 1:

_____

_____

_____

Step 2:

_____

_____

_____

Prescription for Success 4-4 (Continued)

Step 3:

_____

_____

_____

Step 4:

_____

_____

_____

Step 5:

_____

_____

_____

Prescription for Success 4-5
My Problems With English

Write a short description of up to five problems you have with English.

1. _____

_____

_____

_____

2. _____

_____

_____

_____

Continued

Prescription for Success 4-5 (Continued)

3. _____

_____

_____

_____

4. _____

_____

_____

_____

5. _____

_____

_____

_____

Prescription for Success 4-6
Create Your Own Dictionary

Start a vocabulary list of your own. It can be a paper list in your binder or an electronic list on your computer or PDA. When you see or hear a new word, add it to your list. Include pronunciation hints, the definition, and a sentence using the word.

Prescription for Success 4-7
Interesting Idioms

Idioms are commonly used in English. Learning them will add to both your comprehension and your speaking skills. Add them to your vocabulary list and practice using them each day.

Prescription for Success 4-8
Conversation Buddy

Make a list of native English speakers with whom you can practice each day.

_____

_____

_____

_____

_____

_____

_____

Choose someone on your list to be a "conversation buddy." Ask that person if he or she would be willing to talk with you regularly and be willing to help you with your pronunciation and vocabulary, when necessary. This will work best if you have scheduled times to meet. Write them here and on your calendar.

Meeting times: _____

Hint: If this person is also in your classes, you can talk about what you are learning and make even better use of your time.

Prescription for Success 4-9
For More Information

Many websites contain good explanations and examples of the grammar topics presented in this chapter. Choose topics for which you'd like more information, and use a search engine or the websites listed under "To Learn More" on pages 108 and 109. List sites you find useful for future reference.

1. Site name _____

   Site address _____ _____

   Contents _____

2. Site name _____

   Site address _____

   Contents _____

3. Site name _____

   Site address _____

   Contents _____

Continued

Prescription for Success 4-9 (Continued)

4. Site name _____

Site address _____

Contents _____

5. Site name _____

Site address _____

Contents _____

Prescription for Success 4-10
Helping Yourself

1. List up to five difficulties listed in the tables you believe to be obstacles to your academic and/or personal success.
2. From your list, choose one you want to work on.
3. Choose at least one strategy to try for 1 week.
4. Evaluate the strategy: how did it work for you?
Difficulties:

1. _____

2. _____

3. _____

4. _____

5. _____

Choose one: _____

Choose a strategy and describe how you will use it: _____

_____

_____

_____

Describe if the strategy worked for you. Why or why not was it helpful? _____

_____

_____

_____

Developing Your Paper Skills I: Intake of Information

CHAPTER 5

OBJECTIVES

The information and activities in this chapter can help you:

- Understand the importance of developing good note-taking skills.
- Use effective listening techniques to take advantage of learning opportunities.
- Develop a note-taking format and techniques that work for you in class and on the job.
- Convert your class notes into powerful learning tools.
- Use previewing and reviewing to learn as much as possible from your reading.
- Locate reliable sources of information to use in school and on the job.

KEY TERMS AND CONCEPTS

Active Listener: One who listens purposefully and attentively, focuses on what the speaker is saying, and asks questions when necessary for clarification.

Appendices: Sections at the end of a book that contain supplementary information. (Singular form is *appendix*.)

Concept: A general idea or reference to a unit of knowledge.

Cornell System: A method for taking notes in which space is left on each page for writing follow-up notes, questions, and summaries.

Edit: To correct, organize, and add to written materials.

Glossary: An alphabetical list of words with their definitions, usually located at the end of a book.

Internet: A system that connects millions of computers, providing access to all kinds of resources and services.

Key Terms: In note-taking, words that identify the most important concepts and ideas in a lecture.

Logical: In an order that makes sense, following some sort of pattern and showing relationships.

Objective: Statement of what students should know or be able to do as a result of a given learning activity.

Preface: An introduction for the reader, placed at the beginning of a book.

Preview: To look over a written selection, noting new vocabulary and content headings, before reading it carefully.

Rationale: An explanation or reason for something.

Research: To gather information from many sources.

Websites: The specific "places" you see on the computer screen when you are connected to the Internet.

NOTE-TAKING FOR SCHOOL SUCCESS

Taking good notes combines the art of listening and the act of selective writing. Many students report having trouble taking good notes, but it is a skill that can be mastered. Be optimistic about developing your ability to learn to take good notes. You actually have a big advantage because you can take in words much faster than your instructors can speak!

The most common teaching methods for health care courses are lectures, instructor demonstrations, and hands-on activities in the lab or at the clinical site. The first two require students to take notes they can use as study aids. You will have many opportunities to practice this important skill, and note-taking will serve you now and later on the job.

Some students wonder why they should even bother taking notes. Why not just look in the textbook later and find the information? There are a number of important reasons for taking notes in class in addition to learning to take good notes because it is an important health care skill:

1. Taking notes forces you to attend class, pay attention, process the material mentally, and selectively write down what you hear. It converts you from a passive to an **active listener.** Increasing the number of ways you interact with new material greatly increases your chances of understanding and remembering it, so hearing and writing it down in class give you a head start in learning.

2. Your instructors are likely to present more information than what appears in your textbook. They may have examples and additional techniques from their work experiences or new information from a seminar they just attended.

3. Some of the information in your textbook may be outdated. Although publishers do their best to ensure that textbooks contain the very latest information, it usually takes over a year from the time a book is written to get it ready for distribution to students. In a fast-changing field like health care, there is a continuous flow of new developments, and your instructors can provide you with the latest updates.

4. There may be information in your textbooks that does not apply to your geographic area. The scope of practice of professionals varies across the country. For example, some states allow medical assistants to take an active role in taking x-ray films. Therefore many medical assisting textbooks include information about positioning patients when taking x-rays. In some states, however, only graduates of approved x-ray programs who have also passed a state exam are allowed to perform these

procedures. Classroom instructors give you the rules and regulations of the area in which your school is located.

5. Your instructors can help you understand difficult sections of the textbook, presenting the material in a way you better understand. They may break it down into manageable chunks, provide examples, or explain it in different words. You can ask instructors questions, a definite advantage over textbooks.

6. Health care programs cover vast amounts of information. Your instructors' lectures can help you identify the most important points and give you clues about what will be included on tests.

7. You boost your personal efficiency. Taking notes saves you the time of looking up the information discussed in class that does not appear in your regular textbook and would require you to go to other sources.

8. Notes serve as powerful tools for studying and mastering important information needed for school and job success. In this chapter you will learn techniques for converting your notes into study aids.

Active Listening: Prerequisite for Good Note-Taking

Good note-taking requires good listening habits. You can't record what you don't hear. It is sometimes difficult to pay attention in class when you're tired, there are distractions, the instructor speaks too quickly or not clearly, or you don't find the subject matter interesting. However, listening is one of the most essential skills for the successful health care professional. In fact, poor listening skills can doom your professional life to failure. Patient surveys report that the failure of the health care professional to listen is a major cause of dissatisfaction.[1] The classroom provides the perfect opportunity to learn information and an essential life skill at the same time.

Success Tips to Develop Good Listening Skills

☐ Develop a positive attitude toward listening. Listening well increases your chances for success in life. Review your goals and think about how being a good listener will help you achieve them.

☐ Leave your mental baggage at the classroom or health care facility door. Try to go in with a clean slate for listening and learning. If you are having a bad day or your mind is distracted, look at class as an opportunity to focus, learn, and have a productive experience.

☐ Sit where you can both see and hear the instructor. Avoid sitting near people who talk or continually ask you questions during class. The distraction will disrupt your attention and can make you tense. (And don't you be the talker!)

☐ Concentrate on the content of the lecture, not the way it is delivered. It's easy to let the appearance, mannerisms, and voice of the instructor distract you from what is being said. Learning to focus on content is an important health care skill because patients will come to you with all kinds of physical and emotional conditions, and each merits your full attention.

☐ Reel in your wandering mind. Do your best to stay with the instructor mentally. If you think of something important, jot a quick note to yourself so you can take care of it later. This frees your mind to be in the moment and focus on the class.

☐ Keep your mind open and suspend judgment. It is common to stop listening when we disagree with something we hear. A better strategy is to write down the point of disagreement. After listening to the remainder of the presentation, ask the instructor to clarify the point. There may be several "right answers" or ways to perform a technique. Perhaps you heard or interpreted the information incorrectly. If the instructor did make a mistake, show respect. Enjoying "being right" in front of the class is unacceptable classroom conduct. On the job, it could be perceived as insubordination with a supervisor, and this behavior is generally not tolerated.

Learning Styles and Listening

Obviously, auditory learners have the edge when it comes to lectures. They can, however, get caught up in the listening and find it difficult to take adequate notes. This can be a problem because even good listeners won't remember every important point presented.

Visual learners may have more difficulty paying sustained attention and comprehending long lectures. If you are a visual learner, here are some techniques to help you get the most from lectures:

☐ Complete any reading and assignments related to the lecture before going to class. Knowing something about the topic, rather than starting out cold, provides a framework to guide your listening.

☐ Avoid sitting near visual distractions, such as a window with an interesting view or pictures and displays not related to the topic being discussed.

☐ Watch the instructor. Note movements, gestures, and facial expressions and see how they reinforce the material being presented.

☐ Pay attention to anything shown on the board or through other visual aids to help you better visualize and understand the material.

☐ Ask the instructor to write down any words or phrases you cannot understand orally.

☐ During lectures, refer to the sections of your textbook or handouts that relate to the material.

If you are a kinesthetic (hands-on) learner, you can benefit from the physical activity of writing when you take notes. Additional suggestions to improve your listening include the following:

☐ Think of applications for ideas you hear during lectures. (But be careful not to get too carried away and miss the next thing the instructor says!)

☐ Imagine yourself interacting physically with the topic: performing procedures, touching things, or operating a machine.

☐ Make slight movements that do not disrupt others: count off steps on your fingers, stretch your legs slightly, take occasional deep breaths, or move your hand down the page of your text or handout as the material is being explained.

☐ Take enough notes to keep busy, but not so many that you miss the important points as the instructor moves on.

 Go to page 140 to complete Prescription for Success 5-1

Advance Preparation for Taking Good Notes

Preparing for classes is an important part of listening and taking good notes. Advance preparation, according to many instructors, is the key to benefiting from class sessions. If you forget about class between meetings and just show up each time as the instructor begins to speak, you will lose out on a good part of your educational investment. To obtain maximum benefit from your in-class experiences, try the following suggestions:

☐ Complete any assigned reading and other homework. There is nothing more frustrating than trying to follow a lecture in which the instructor assumes you know something about the subject—and you know nothing! Give yourself every advantage by anticipating what the lecture might cover.

☐ Review your notes from the previous lecture. This gives you an opportunity to set the stage for a continuation of the subject and to recall questions or points you want to have clarified.

☐ Arrive at class a few minutes early. This gives you a chance to choose an appropriate seat, quickly look over your notes from the last class, and prepare yourself to take notes.

☐ Set your attitude for learning. Make the decision to get as much benefit as possible from every class. Be positive and expect to acquire useful information.

☐ Take all necessary supplies to class: a binder with extra paper, pencil or pen, textbook, and handouts. (Make sure they're in the "big bag" discussed in Chapter 3. If books and binders get heavy, consider using a flight bag on wheels to prevent stress on your shoulders.)

PERSONAL REFLECTION

1. Are you satisfied with your note-taking skills?

   _____

   _____

2. Does your note-taking system need improvement?

   _____

   _____

Note-Taking Materials

There are a variety of ways to take and organize notes, and these will be discussed in the following sections. When choosing the best one for you, consider your learning styles and personal preferences, your instructors' lecture styles, and the number and type of handouts distributed in your classes.

Taking notes in class is the first step in creating a personalized learning tool. Your notes are not completed when the instructor finishes the lecture. You still need to **edit** them to increase their value as a learning tool and then review them regularly.

Notes are useless, however, if you cannot find or identify them, so good organization is essential. Loose-leaf binders receive the highest marks from instructors for keeping notes together because they are the most flexible and easiest to organize and keep in order. You can add new information in any order you wish, something you can't do with spiral notebooks. Binders allow you to insert class notes, revisions of your notes, handouts, assignments, reference sheets, and skill check-off sheets. Binders also offer the best protection against weather and keep papers flat and neat. Portfolios and other types of folders with pockets tend to tear and get messy.

You can purchase several binders with thin vinyl covers and use one for each class. Or you can divide a large binder with indexed dividers. Each class can also be subdivided for class notes, handouts, reading notes, and assignments. Periodically review and tidy up your binder as needed.

Regardless of how you organize your binder, the important thing is to keep your notes for each class together and in order. Label the outside cover with the name of the class or classes. If you are using more than one binder, color-code or mark them in such a way that you never arrive at anatomy class only to discover you have your pharmacology notes! Label the individual pages with the name of the class and the date.

The Cornell System

The **Cornell system** is a method for laying out, editing, and studying from your notes to get the most benefit from them. It was devised by Professor Walter Pauk, who wanted to help his students improve their study habits. A key feature of the system is leaving enough blank space on the page to add specific kinds of information when you review and edit your notes. To do this, set up each page on which you will take notes by drawing a line about 2½ inches in from the left side. Then draw a line about 2 inches from the bottom. Figure 5-1 shows this page layout.

The large space in the center is for recording notes during class. The left side is used after class to write key words, headings, questions, and other notes. The bottom space is reserved for writing short summaries of the contents of the page. We will discuss how to use these spaces later in this chapter.

Deciding What to Record

Instructors can say a lot during a lecture, and sometimes it's difficult to decide what to write down. If this happens to you, you're not alone. Students report this to be the hardest part of note-taking. This is especially true when a subject is new and you don't have the background to help sift the must-know from the interesting-to-know. You need to write down enough to understand your notes later. But if you try to record every word, you're likely to miss half of what the instructor says. There are a number of things you can do to get the most important content from class lectures.

As mentioned before, and it is worth repeating, do the reading and assignments before going to class—even if it is not required. This will give you an

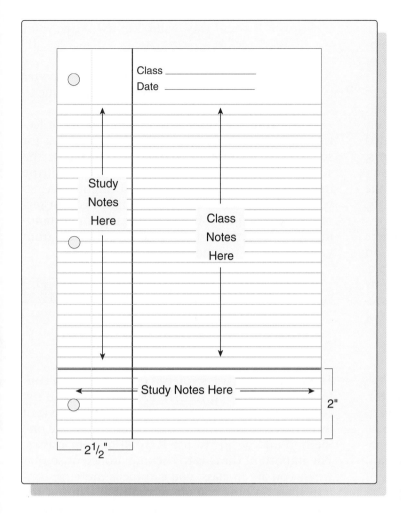

Figure 5–1 Example of setting up a page when using the Cornell note-taking system. After class, write additions and revisions on the reverse sides of the pages.

overview of the topic. Your textbook has headings and other ways of emphasizing the major points of a subject. Use these to develop a mental outline. If you find the subject especially difficult and have the time, prepare a written outline of the chapters before the lecture.

In class, listen for the main ideas. Your prereading is an excellent way to help you identify what these might be. Listen carefully to your instructors. They may list important points, introduce them and provide details and examples, and/or tell you what is most important. As you become familiar with the material and health care topics in general and take quizzes and tests, you will find it easier to identify the major points.

Organizational Patterns in Lectures

Most lectures follow an organizational pattern. Recognizing some of the ways that instructors present information can help you improve your note-taking.

1. **Clusters of information:** Topics are divided into chunks of related material, and the instructor covers one chunk before moving on to the next. Examples: the human body parts and functions are usually grouped by systems—skeletal, digestive, and reproductive. The topic of scheduling appointments for the medical office is usually organized by the different methods used to set them.

2. **Procedures:** These are often explained in a step-by-step sequence. Examples: how to measure an infant; how to perform one-person, adult cardiopulmonary resuscitation (CPR).

3. **Concepts** *or procedures with* **rationale:** Material is first introduced, and then important reasons are given to explain and support it. Examples: legal reasons for maintaining patient confidentiality; why standard precautions must be followed.

4. **Definitions:** In addition to medical terminology, each area of health care has its own vocabulary. Lectures may be organized around explanations of new terms. Example: discussion of terms related to medical insurance billing.

5. **How things work:** Descriptions and explanations are given. Examples: parts and operation of the microscope; safe use of the autoclave.

6. **Lists:** descriptions and/or explanations of a number of items of equal importance. Examples: purpose and interpretation of a series of lab tests; different medications and their use.

7. **Patterns:** These are created by instructors to present material in a specific order. Example: anatomy and physiology course in which information about body systems is always presented in the same order, such as (1) names of parts, (2) purpose and function of each part, (3) common disorders of the system, (4) causes of the disorders, (5) diagnostic tests, (6) treatments, and (7) prevention.

8. **Verbal signals:** Certain words tell you where the lecture is going. Examples: "Let's go on to…" signals the transition to a new topic. "Therefore" and "In conclusion" let you know a summary statement is coming. "First," "second," and so on tell you there will be a list of items of equal importance.

Clues from Instructors

Listen and watch for clues from the instructor. Instructors plan their lectures to help students learn the subjects they are teaching. They want you to succeed, so many of them provide clues, both consciously and unconsciously, about what is important in their classes. Here are some common instructor behaviors that say, "Write this down!"

☐ Saying, "This is important" or "You must know or be able to do this when you are working in the field" or "Write this down" or "This will be on the test." (They really do say these things. This is what you might miss if you are absent from class or daydreaming when you *are* there.)

☐ Emphasizing certain words or concepts by saying them loudly, writing them on the board or overhead, or repeating them. (It is a good idea to copy everything the instructor writes down.)

☐ Expressing extra interest or enthusiasm. This may indicate an area the instructor believes to be especially important.

☐ Illustrating points with stories and anecdotes.

☐ Asking questions of students during the lecture. These are usually points the instructor considers to be important.

A technique to keep yourself on track is to mentally ask yourself questions, based on the topic, and then listen for the answers during the lectures. Here are some sample questions:

☐ Why is thi s important?

☐ How does it work?

☐ What are the main parts?

☐ Why is it done this way?

☐ How is it done? How will I do this? When will I do this?

☐ How will I apply this in my work?

☐ How will this knowledge help me be a better health care professional? How will it help me to help patients?

If you continually miss the major points of lectures, see your instructor outside of class. Ask for suggestions to improve your listening, follow the style of lecturing, and take better notes. Ask if the instructor has lecture outlines you might have, so you can follow along in class. If English is your second language and you have difficulty understanding spoken and/or written English, seek help from your instructor or school advisor.

 Go to page 141 to complete Prescription for Success 5-2

Deciding How to Record Your Notes

There are several ways you can organize lecture content as you record it. When choosing formats to try, consider your learning style, the instructor's style of lecturing, and the subject matter. You may like one method and decide to use it in all of your classes. The important thing is to become proficient so that when you are in class, you can focus more on content than on how you are recording it. Four of the most common methods for taking notes, described in the following sections, are:

1. Informal outline
2. Paragraphs
3. Key words
4. Write it all

The description for each method is written in the format being presented to show what the methods look like.

Informal Outlines

How to use
   Create indentations to organize ideas
   Write phrases
   Don't use numbers or letters
When to use
   Student is linear thinker
   Lecture is easy to follow
Advantages
   Helps you organize thoughts
   Keeps materials in logical order
Disadvantages
   Difficult if lecture is disorganized, rambling
   May distract from lecture content
      Trying to make neat outline
   Holistic thinkers need time to formulate outline

Paragraphs

Writing in paragraphs helps when lecture hard to follow. Use phrases. Create paragraph for each main idea. Mark important points during lecture. Organize later by creating outline.

Difficult for some. Must write quickly and neatly. Must decide what to write. Advantage for kinesthetic learners—involves activity. Lots of writing.

Key Words

Main ideas only
Relationships
Supporting facts
Auditory learners
Reminders
Fill in later
Difficult material—may miss facts
Easy to forget!

Write it All

A few students are successful with writing everything down. They are more comfortable knowing they haven't missed anything the instructor says. Must use shortened sentences, phrases, and abbreviations, but they try to record all that instructor says. Might work well for kinesthetic learner, who needs activity, or for students who have trouble concentrating and find that this method helps them concentrate. Method not recommended for most students because if you don't write fast you can get behind and get very frustrated. Usually unnecessary to write everything down. Lose important ideas in details.

Examples of Note-Taking

Figures 5-2, 5-3, and 5-4 contain examples of notes taken in the various styles, based on the lecture segment from *Today's Medical Assistant* by Bonewit-West, Hunt, and Applegate[2] (Box 5-1) as if it were presented as a lecture.

 Go to page 142 to complete Prescription for Success 5-3

Note-Taking Guides

Some instructors distribute preprinted outlines to help their students focus on the important points of their lectures. These can be very helpful but

---

BOX 5-1   Lecture Segment on Anxiety

Anxiety is a response to a perceived threat. A person who is moderately to severely anxious is not able to converse coherently and will not pick up on nonverbal cues that he or she would normally notice. When working with a patient who is anxious, the medical assistant must first get the person's attention, slow down the conversation, and then help the person to focus on the conversation. It is important to validate the patient's concern, which reduces his or her anxiety level. This allows the patient's energy to be channeled in a more productive way. When patients are anxious, they may not remember what they are told. The medical assistant can help the patient by creating memory aids. For example, the medical assistant can prompt the patient to record a follow-up appointment in his or her appointment calendar. It is also a good idea to write the instructions down or provide the patient with a preprinted instruction sheet.

Severe anxiety can be medically problematic. Physical symptoms occur with a full-blown anxiety attack, often termed a *panic attack*. An overly anxious person hyperventilates, has an extremely rapid heart rate, and becomes unresponsive. Some people experience numbness in their fingers and toes; others feel a sensation of fluid in their ears. Some people become intensely fearful and have an overpowering sense of dread.

An anxiety attack must be dealt with as a medical issue first. Helping the patient acknowledge the anxiety is important. Acknowledging the anxiety helps a person gain control. In addition, having strong emotions accepted by another person decreases the sense of fear that many people have about their emotions.

If the patient is breathing rapidly, the medical assistant should encourage the patient to take slow, deep breaths. Experts no longer recommend having a patient breathe into a brown paper bag because this may cause blood oxygen levels to fall dangerously low.

If possible, the medical assistant should encourage the patient to validate that anxiety is present without minimizing its significance. If the patient has not experienced severe anxiety before, he or she may not realize the effects it can cause. The medical assistant can explain that any physical symptoms are the result of anxiety and stay with the patient until the symptoms begin to subside. With most patients, the symptoms begin to diminish after 1 or 2 minutes. After the person has returned to a level of relative calm, it may be possible to discuss how the person handles anxiety. The physician may also refer the patient to a counselor to work on strategies to manage it.

From Bonewit-West K, Hunt S, Applegate E: *Today's medical assistant: clinical and administrative procedures*, St Louis, 2009, Elsevier, p 68.

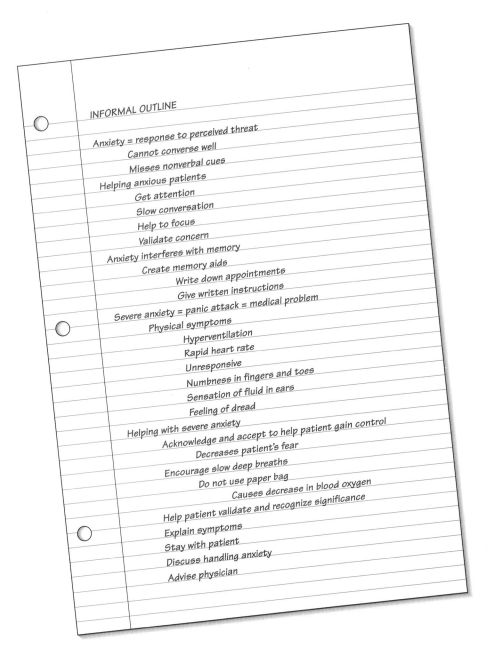

INFORMAL OUTLINE

Anxiety = response to perceived threat
    Cannot converse well
    Misses nonverbal cues
Helping anxious patients
    Get attention
    Slow conversation
    Help to focus
    Validate concern
Anxiety interferes with memory
    Create memory aids
        Write down appointments
        Give written instructions
Severe anxiety = panic attack = medical problem
    Physical symptoms
        Hyperventilation
        Rapid heart rate
        Unresponsive
        Numbness in fingers and toes
        Sensation of fluid in ears
        Feeling of dread
Helping with severe anxiety
    Acknowledge and accept to help patient gain control
        Decreases patient's fear
    Encourage slow deep breaths
        Do not use paper bag
            Causes decrease in blood oxygen
    Help patient validate and recognize significance
    Explain symptoms
    Stay with patient
    Discuss handling anxiety
    Advise physician

Figure 5–2 Example of notes using an informal outline. This is probably the most commonly used method. (*Data from Bonewit-West K, Hunt S, Applegate E:* Today's medical assistant: clinical and administrative procedures, *St. Louis, 2009, Elsevier.*)

should be used with caution. It can be tempting to go on "automatic pilot" during lectures and listen only for the points listed on the guide. Another habit students sometimes fall into is copying down exactly what the teacher says. This is appropriate for recording definitions, formulas, and rules. However, you increase your chances of learning the material when you use your own words to take notes.

To Record or Not to Record

There are conflicting opinions about the value of taping lectures. Some educators believe that students who record their lectures pay less attention in class. And recordings don't include important nonverbal language and visual aids. Also, listening to recordings later is time-consuming. On the other hand, recording can be useful if listening is an effective way for you to review. It can also help students who have trouble understanding English. If you decide recording is a good idea for you, be sure to obtain your instructor's permission. Some schools and/or individual instructors don't allow lectures to be recorded. They believe students must develop good listening skills in class as part of their career training. And they have a good point!

Shortcuts with Symbols and Abbreviations

Creating your own symbols and abbreviations can help you take notes more quickly and can make them more useful. Here are some ideas for symbols:

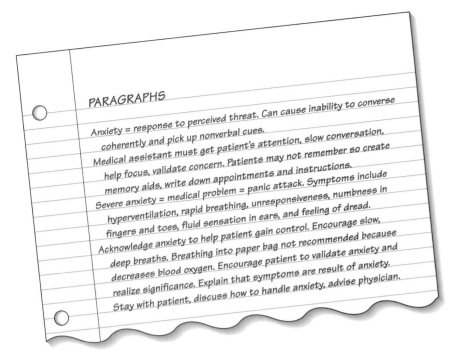

Figure 5–3 Example of writing notes in paragraph form. (*Data from Bonewit-West K, Hunt S, Applegate E:* Today's medical assistant: clinical and administrative procedures, *St. Louis, 2009, Elsevier.*)

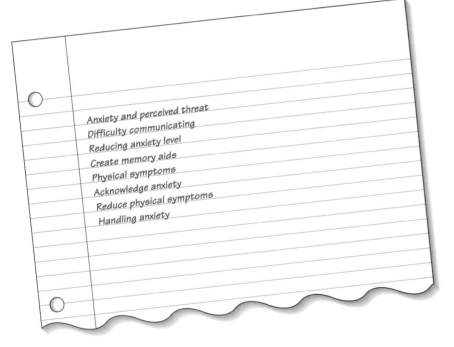

Figure 5–4 Example of using key words to take notes. (*Data from Bonewit-West K, Hunt S, Applegate E:* Today's medical assistant: clinical and administrative procedures, *St. Louis, 2009, Elsevier.*)

T= test item (instructor announced or hinted).

?? = got lost and need to fill in later.

P= personal thoughts: your own ideas about the topic. You can also bracket ()your own thoughts to distinguish them from what the instructor says.

J= important for job success, something employers look for.

Creating abbreviations can help increase your note-taking speed. Try standard abbreviations or invent your own—or use a combination. See Table 5-1 for a list of suggestions you might find useful.

If you create your own set of abbreviations, it's a good idea to put together a directory to keep with your notes in case you forget your coding system. Because you can't anticipate all the words you might shorten during a lecture, write out potentially confusing abbreviations as soon as possible after class. Figure 5-5 shows how the informal outline notes, from Figure 5-2, might look if symbols and abbreviations were used. (Note, however, that using original abbreviations when charting or creating notes for others is unacceptable on the job because of the chance for confusion.)

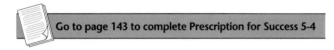

Go to page 143 to complete Prescription for Success 5-4

Success Tips for Taking Great Notes

☐ Be there! Do your best to be present for both the beginning and end of class. Introductions and conclusions often contain valuable information about what the instructor considers to be most important. Conclusions may clarify points that seemed fuzzy or unrelated earlier in the lecture.

☐ Leave some blank space on your pages between the major ideas or clusters of related information so you can make additions when you edit and review. If you get lost and have gaps in your notes, leave extra space to fill in later.

☐ Write out examples, definitions, formulas, and calculations.

☐ Write on only one side of the paper so you can lay the pages out and see all your notes at once. Some students use the blank facing pages to create

TABLE 5–1 Symbols and Abbreviations for Note-Taking

STANDARD ABBREVIATIONS

Word	Standard Abbreviation
and	&
and so forth	etc
equals, same as, means	=
for example	eg
less than	<
greater than	>
negative	–
not the same as, does not equal	≠
number	#
of, per	/
positive	+
regarding	re

STANDARD ABBREVIATIONS—(Continued)

Word	Standard Abbreviation
therefore	∴
times	×
to, toward, leads to, goes to	→
versus	vs
with	w/ or c̄
without	w/o or s̄

SPELL WORDS AS THEY SOUND, LEAVING OUT SILENT LETTERS

Examples	Phonetic Spelling
although	altho
through	thru

SHORTEN WORDS BY LEAVING OUT THE VOWELS

Word	Shortened Form
blood	bld
book	bk
homework	hmwrk
learn	lrn
patient	pt

MAKE UP YOUR OWN SHORT FORMS OF COMMON WORDS

Word	Shortened Form
anatomy	anat
appointment	appt
because	bec
determine	det
important	imp
information	info
introduction	intro
necessary	nec
procedure	proc
psychology	psych
venipuncture	venip

LEARN COMMON MEDICAL ABBREVIATIONS

Word	Abbreviation
cardiopulmonary resuscitation	CPR
electrocardiography	ECG
medical assistant	MA
occupational therapy	OT

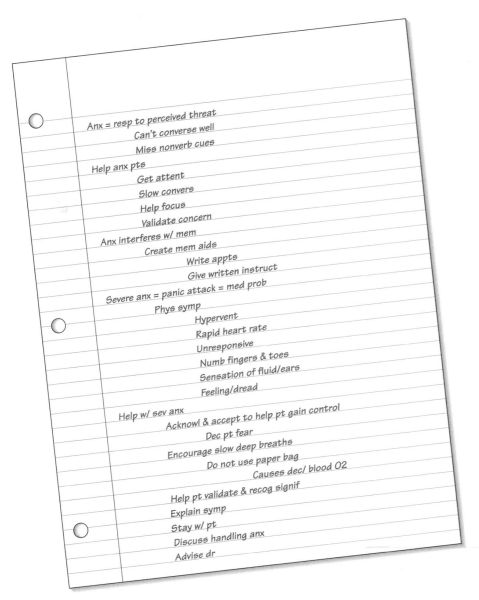

Anx = resp to perceived threat
Can't converse well
Miss nonverb cues
Help anx pts
Get attent
Slow convers
Help focus
Validate concern
Anx interferes w/ mem
Create mem aids
Write appts
Give written instruct
Severe anx = panic attack = med prob
Phys symp
Hypervent
Rapid heart rate
Unresponsive
Numb fingers & toes
Sensation of fluid/ears
Feeling/dread
Help w/ sev anx
Acknowl & accept to help pt gain control
Dec pt fear
Encourage slow deep breaths
Do not use paper bag
Causes decl blood O2
Help pt validate & recog signif
Explain symp
Stay w/ pt
Discuss handling anx
Advise dr

Figure 5–5 Example of how abbreviations and symbols can be used to take notes efficiently. (*Data from Bonewit-West K, Hunt S, Applegate E:* Today's medical assistant: clinical and administrative procedures, *St. Louis, 2009, Elsevier.*)

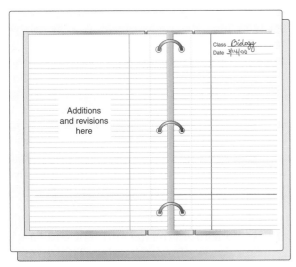

Figure 5–6 Use the reverse side of previous pages for adding to and revising your notes.

additional study notes. Figure 5-6 illustrates how this works.

☐ Do your best to write down words you don't know. Guess at the spelling and circle the words so you can look up their meanings or ask the instructor.

☐ Write as neatly as possible. If necessary, practice improving your handwriting or try printing if it doesn't slow you down too much. Aim for a balance between speed and legibility. Recopying notes to make them neater takes time you could use more productively. There are, however, a few circumstances in which rewriting, typing, or word processing notes is recommended. If you have strong keyboarding skills, you may find that this process serves as a good review of the lecture. If you are a kinesthetic learner, you may benefit from the activity of keyboarding or rewriting. Finally, on those occasions when your notes are a total disaster, it may be worth your time to clean them up.

☐ Erasable pens are good for taking notes, although regular pens can be used if you make corrections neatly. Pencils can break or need sharpening, and the writing tends to fade and smudge over time.

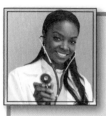

USING ABBREVIATIONS ON THE JOB

Abbreviations are used in health care work, so learning to apply them is an important skill. The following is an example of notes on a patient history form.[3]

Chief complaint: Ⓛ shoulder pain p̄ playing basketball this AM.

Present illness: Soreness and immobility Ⓛ shoulder ×8 hours; strained on collision w/another player

Important note: Abbreviations used on medical records *must be standardized* (the same for everyone who adds information), so be sure to use only those that are approved by the facility in which you work. Also, some abbreviations are no longer allowed because they lead to confusion and medical errors. The Joint Commission and the Institute for Safe Medication Practices have both published lists of abbreviations that should not be used on the job.

Make Your Notes Work for You

It takes work to take good notes in class. Now let them work for you. Start by reviewing them as soon as possible after class. Try not to wait more than 24 hours because the average person forgets more than half of what was said during a typical class lecture within that time. Even a quick review will help create memory pathways for the new information.

Begin your review by reading over your notes and filling in any missing words or abbreviations with meanings you might forget. Next, fill in ideas or reorganize your notes, as needed. If there are gaps where your mind wandered or you did not understand well enough to take clear notes, look in your textbook, ask a classmate, or make a note to ask the instructor for help.

Consider rewriting your notes if they are extremely disorganized or if you think a different format might help you better learn from them.

For example, if the topic emphasizes relationships and you wrote paragraphs, create a mind map. If the lecture was organized by classifications, put together a chart that lays out the various categories.

Use a highlighter or colored pen to mark key words and phrases. You can also personalize your notes with drawings, arrows to show relationships, pictures from magazines, or anything else that helps you focus on and better understand the material. Auditory learners might record their edited notes for reviewing. See Figure 5-7 to see how Emily personalized and added to the notes she took in her Interpersonal Relations class.

Using the Cornell System

Figure 5-1 illustrated a page layout for taking notes. The space in the left column on each page is for writing key words or phrases (Figure 5-8) or your own quiz questions (Figure 5-9). The space at the bottom of the page is for writing summaries, in your own words, of the material on the page. (If you have trouble writing a summary, this is a good indication you may not fully understand the material.) If you don't have enough room on the page containing your notes, use the back of the previous page, as discussed earlier in Figure 5-6.

Reviewing Productively

The most important thing you can do with your notes is to review them often, at least twice a week. If your classes last for less than 1 month, review your notes even more often. As we discussed in Chapter 3, the key to long-term memory is repetition over time. Your review sessions don't have to be long, but make them a regular part of your study schedule. Keep in mind you are not simply learning to pass a test but are accumulating knowledge to apply when you are working as a health care professional.

Engage your mind actively when you review. Passively reading and rereading your notes will not store them in your mind. Use the review column to the left of your notes to prompt recall of the information. Cover the notes you took in class, and explain the key words or answer the questions you wrote. This is the most effective part of the review because it forces you to think and helps transfer the content of your notes into your long-term memory.

Think about your own past experiences and how what you are learning relates to them and to what you already know about the topic. This gives you reference points and makes new information more meaningful.

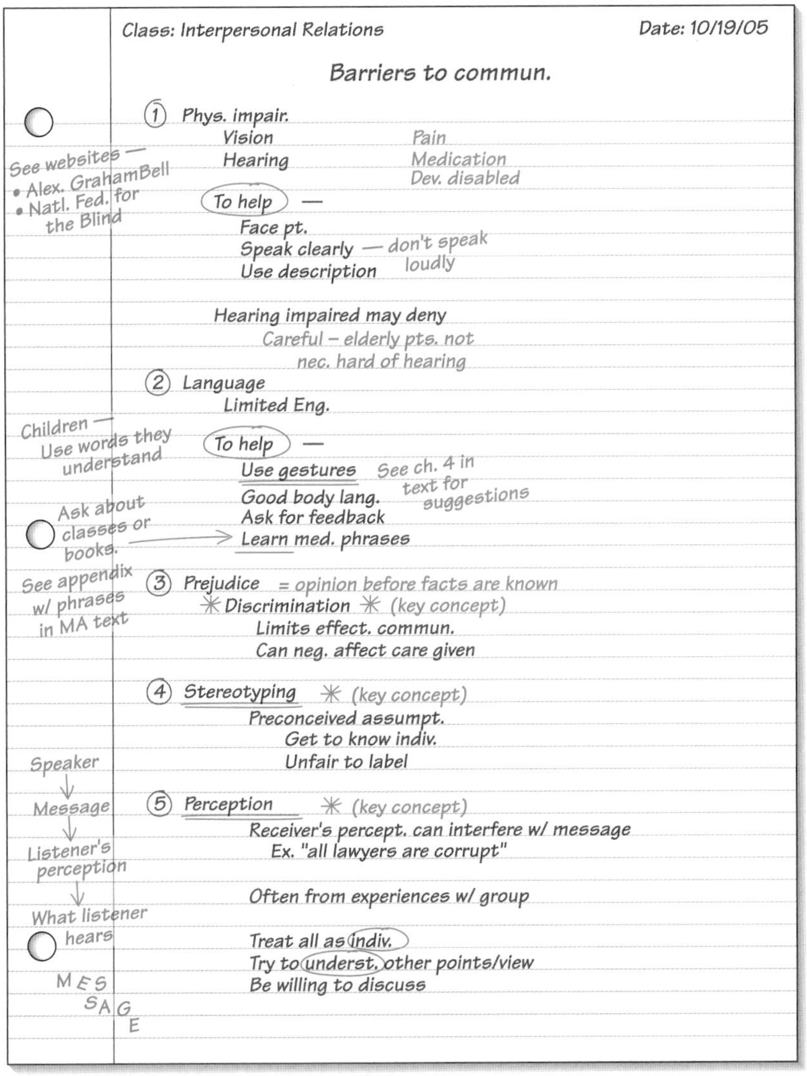

Class: Interpersonal Relations   Date: 10/19/05

Barriers to commun.

① Phys. impair.
    Vision   Pain
    Hearing   Medication
                Dev. disabled

See websites —
• Alex. GrahamBell
• Natl. Fed. for the Blind

(To help) —
    Face pt.
    Speak clearly — don't speak loudly
    Use description

Hearing impaired may deny
    Careful – elderly pts. not
        nec. hard of hearing

② Language
    Limited Eng.

Children —
Use words they understand

(To help) —
    Use gestures See ch. 4 in text for suggestions
    Good body lang.
    Ask for feedback
    Learn med. phrases

Ask about classes or books.

See appendix w/ phrases in MA text

③ Prejudice = opinion before facts are known
    ✳ Discrimination ✳ (key concept)
        Limits effect. commun.
        Can neg. affect care given

④ Stereotyping ✳ (key concept)
    Preconceived assumpt.
    Get to know indiv.
    Unfair to label

Speaker
↓
Message

⑤ Perception ✳ (key concept)
    Receiver's percept. can interfere w/ message
        Ex. "all lawyers are corrupt"

Listener's perception
↓
What listener hears

    Often from experiences w/ group

    Treat all as indiv.
    Try to underst. other points/view
    Be willing to discuss

M E S
S A G E

Figure 5–7 Emily personalized her notes by adding details, writing questions, noting sources for more information, and marking key concepts.

Use what you know about your learning styles when studying from your notes. Here are a few ways to do this:

□ **Visual:** Picture the words and concepts in your mind as you review; label drawings from memory; draw sketches. Rough ones are fine—no one is grading the art!

□ **Auditory:** Review out loud, even if you must speak in a soft voice. Have someone read your key words and questions and check your answers as you give them out loud. Listen to recordings of your notes.

□ **Kinesthetic:** Stand up, move around, re-create the lecture. Or teach someone else by explaining one on one. Use movement and gestures to emphasize important points. If the content concerns a procedure or something that involves movement, act it out or actually perform it as much as possible.

□ **Interactive:** Exchange notes with a study partner or group. Discuss and quiz.

□ **Global:** Write out concepts, then create a list of supporting related details.

□ **Linear:** Look for **logical** patterns in the material.

Finally, create practice tests based on your notes. You can write your questions to the left of your notes or on a separate page. You can also record them. Don't take your "test" for at least 3 days. Here are some suggestions for questions:

1. What is the definition of _____?
2. What is the meaning of _____?
3. What are the steps in performing a _____?
4. What is important to remember about ____?
5. Why must you _____?
6. What are the principal parts of _____?
7. How does _____ function?
8. What is the purpose of _____?

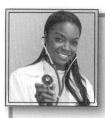

NOTE-TAKING ON THE JOB

Note-taking is a skill that health care professionals use on many occasions. Figure 5-10 shows some common examples. The medical assistant may be called on to take notes as the physician examines a patient. And when patients themselves explain their health background, symptoms, and reasons for seeking care, the information must be recorded correctly. Patient records serve as the basis for giving appropriate and consistent care; therefore it is critical that they be both accurate and legible. In addition, they serve as legal documents and are used in court cases to defend the actions of health care providers.

Good handwriting is important on the job because the quality of patient care depends on the ability of other health care professionals to read your written documentation. In spite of jokes about doctors' chicken scratches, there is nothing funny about illegible medical records.

READING TO LEARN

"To read without reflecting is like eating without digesting."

—Edmund Burke

Reading, along with listening and taking notes, is one of the most important ways you will acquire information as a student. Like effective listening, reading to learn requires you to pay attention and participate actively. It should be approached purposefully because you must work at understanding, remembering, and applying new material. If you were reading instructions about how to perform a medical procedure, you would ask yourself, "Do I understand this? What, exactly, am I supposed to do?" and then you would read carefully to make sure you got it right. The goal when reading your textbooks is also to comprehend and think about what to do with your new knowledge. You will spend a great deal of time reading textbooks, so it makes sense to learn how to gain the most benefit from your efforts.

Earlier in this chapter, we discussed why you should take notes. You might wonder why you have to read and take notes. There are several reasons, as follows:

1. The more ways you take in information, the more likely you are to remember it. Paths are worn over time by many walkers. If no one uses them, they disappear. Your memory paths are also created and maintained by repeated use. Even if a subject is discussed in class, reading gives you one more encounter with it.
2. As we suggested in the section on taking notes, reading will give you background information for class lectures. It also reinforces what you hear in class.
3. Textbooks provide a permanent means of saving information. You can refer back to them over and over as needed.
4. Books usually contain more supporting details, examples, graphics, and organizational aids than lectures.

Getting Ready to Read

There are several prereading activities you can do to make your reading easier and more beneficial. The first is to clear your mind of clutter. Reading requires concentration, and this is difficult when you have unfinished business on your mind. If something is bothering you that can be handled quickly, take care of it before you start studying. (But try not to let "urgencies" be an excuse to put off getting together with your books indefinitely.) If it will take more than a few minutes of your attention, write it down (your planner would be a good place) so you can deal with it later.

Next is to find a place that encourages reading rather than sleeping or daydreaming. Many people find that a straight-backed chair at a desk works best (you will be doing some writing as you read). Give your back good support, and make sure the lighting is adequate. An uncomfortable environment can tire you and cut your reading time short.

You need more than just your textbook to read actively, so gather your tools: notebook, pen or pencil, highlighter or colored pen, and dictionary. Develop the habit of gathering needed supplies before you start studying. This is an important health care practice, too. You would not want to interrupt a patient procedure because you forgot to bring something from the supply room. Your study time is valuable, too, and should not be interrupted while you look for the dictionary.

Previewing

"Advice worth repeating: Work smarter, not harder."

KEYWORDS	LECTURE NOTES

Anxiety
  Resulting
  behaviors
	Anxiety = response to perceived threat
	Cannot converse well
	Misses nonverbal cues

Helping pts.	Helping anxious patients
	  Get attention
	  Slow conversation
	  Help to focus
	  Validate concern

Effect on memory	Anxiety interferes with memory
	  Create memory aids
	    Write down appointments
	    Give written instructions

Panic attacks
  Symptoms
	Severe anxiety = panic attack = medical problem
	Physical symptoms
	  Hyperventilation
	  Rapid heart rate
	  Unresponsive
	  Numbness in fingers and toes
	  Sensation of fluid in ears
	  Feeling of dread

Helping with severe
attack
	Helping with severe anxiety
	Acknowledge and accept to help patient gain control
	  Decreases patient's fear
	  Encourage slow deep breaths
	    Do not use paper bag
	      Causes decrease in blood oxygen
	  Help patient validate and recognize significance
	  Explain symptoms
	  Stay with patient
	  Discuss handling anxiety
	  Advise physician

Figure 5–8 Write key words in the left margin of your notes. To use these as prompts when studying, cover the main section and recall what you learned in class. (*Data from Bonewit-West K, Hunt S, Applegate E:* Today's medical assistant: clinical and administrative procedures, *St. Louis, 2009, Elsevier.*)

Many methods have been developed to help students gain maximum benefit from their reading assignments. Some methods have many steps and others just a few, but they all recommend that you **preview** before you start reading. Using our medical procedure example, you would never perform a treatment on a patient without taking a few preliminary steps: (1) identify the patient, (2) introduce yourself, (3) verify the procedure, (4) gather the necessary supplies, and (5) put on gloves. Previewing in reading means that you look over the entire selection, learn any new vocabulary, pay attention to the headings, and use clues in the text to anticipate and think about the content. Fortunately, most textbooks are set up to help you and contain many features to guide your previewing and reading.

Anatomy of a Textbook

When you get a new textbook, take a few minutes to look it over carefully. Don't wait until the end of the course to discover something that could have made your life easier. Every textbook contains at least a few of the following useful features:

1. **Preface:** An introductory section at the beginning of the book. It typically contains a statement of the author's purpose and an overview of the book's content and structure. Some prefaces include information of special value to students, such as how to use the different features, study tips, and career ideas.

2. **Table of contents:** Some books supplement the usual list of chapter titles with a complete listing of chapter sections. This detailed format gives you a good overall view of the topics covered.

3. **Appendices:** Extra materials placed at the back of the book. Their contents are based on the book's subject and vary widely. Look these over when you first begin using the book, because you may discover valuable resources to help you understand both the textbook and the subject. There may also be sources of career information and reference guides. Examples

YOUR QUIZ QUESTIONS	LECTURE NOTES
What is the definition of anxiety?	Anxiety = response to perceived threat
How can anxiety affect patient patient behavior?	Cannot converse well Misses nonverbal cues

What are ways the health care professional can help anxious patients?	Helping anxious patients
	Get attention
	    Slow conversation
	    Help to focus
	    Validate concern

What can the health care professional do to help anxious patients remember important information?	Anxiety interferes with memory
	    Create memory aids
	Write down appointments
	    Give written instructions

What is a panic attack?
What are the physical symptoms associated with severe anxiety?
	Severe anxiety = panic attack =
	                medical problem
	Physical symptoms
	Hyperventilation
	Rapid heart rate
	    Unresponsive
	    Numbness in fingers and toes
	    Sensation of fluid in ears
	    Feeling of dread

What actions can the health care professional take to help patients who are experiencing severe anxiety?	Helping with severe anxiety
	    Stay with patient
	    Acknowledge and accept patient's
	      feelings
	    Help patient validate and recognize
	      significance of anxiety
	    Explain symptoms
	    Discuss ways of handling anxiety
	    Advise physician

Why is breathing into a paper bag no longer recommended for patients who are hyperventilating?	Do not have patient's breathe into paper bag Causes decrease in blood oxygen

Figure 5–9 Make up questions based on your notes and write them in the left margin. Cover the main section and review by answering your "quiz" questions. This is reported to be *the* most effective way to learn from reading. (*Data from Bonewit-West K, Hunt S, Applegate E:* Today's medical assistant: clinical and administrative procedures, *St. Louis, 2009, Elsevier.*)

from recent editions of health care textbooks include guidelines for infection control, important abbreviations, a metric conversion chart, Spanish translations of common health care phrases, laboratory test values, and a Celsius-Fahrenheit conversion scale.

4. **Index:** An alphabetical listing of all the topics in the book and the page numbers on which they appear. The items included are much more specific than those listed in the table of contents. The index is located at the back of a book and is very useful when you need specific information or are reviewing.

5. **Bibliography and/or references:** A list of source materials used by the author and/or recommended readings for students who want to learn more about the subject. Each chapter may have its own bibliography, or there may be one list at the end of the book. Bibliographies can be excellent resources for expanding your knowledge of specific areas in which you are interested.

6. **Glossary:** An alphabetical list of words with their definitions, usually located at the back of the book.

7. **Vocabulary or key terms:** Lists of new words, often placed at the beginning of each chapter. Because reading is based on understanding words, learning new vocabulary before you begin to read is essential for comprehension. Take a few minutes to study the terms listed before you read the chapter, marking any words you find difficult. Word lists may also contain clues about what the author considers to be most important.

8. **Objectives:** These are statements telling you what you should learn or be able to do as a result of studying and applying the information in the chapter. Knowing the chapter objectives gives structure and purpose to your reading. Objectives are also useful to check

PATIENT HISTORY   Soc Sec Number _203-46-7809_

Patient Name _Sean D. Austin_   DOB _03/03/83_
Address _1234 Crown Ave._   City _Dayton_   State _Ohio_   ZIP _24354_
Home Phone _(937) 123-4567_   Work Phone _____   Emergency Phone _(937) 545-4415_
Status   M Ⓢ W D   Spouse's name _____   Referring Physician _____
Occupation _student_   Employer _____   Phone _____
Primary Insurance _Anthem BC/BS_   Policy Holder _John Austin_   Policy No. _AN232435545_

Chief Complaint Ⓛ shoulder pain p̄ playing basketball
              this AM.
Present Illness _soreness and immobility_ Ⓛ _shoulder x 8_
hours; strained upon collision w/ another player

HT	_62"_	Sc Fever	—
Weight	_112#_	Rheum Fev	—
Past yr + –	_8#_	Measles	+
Temp	_98.4°F_	Mumps	—
Pulse	_72_	Rubella	—
Resp	_12_	Chicken Pox	+
BP	_108/64_	Asthma	—
LMP	_NA_		

FAMILY HISTORY

Heart	Father	Mother	Brother	Brother	Sister	Sister	MGM	MGF
Heart	—	+	—	—			+	
Bld Pressure	—	—	—	—			—	
Diabetes	—	—	—	—			—	
Bld Diabetes	—	—	—	—			—	
Asthma	—	+	—	—			—	
Epilepsy	—	—	—	—			—	
Stroke	—	—	—	—			—	

SURGICAL HISTORY

	Surgery	Year	Physician	Surgery	Year	Physician	Surgery
	Adenoidectomy	1986	Smith				
	BTTI	1986	Smith				

WHILE YOU WERE OUT

FOR: _Pt Billing_   DATE: _05/04/00_   TIME: _10:20 am_

FROM: _Bonita Henderson_

OF: _(Dr. Arewells Pt)_

PHONE NUMBER: (_771_)- _423-6740_

FAX: (   )-

RX REFILL: PHARMACY: RX#:

REMARKS: ☒ telephoned   ☐ needs to talk to you
          ☐ will call back   ☐ will call again
          ☐ stopped by   ☐ needs to see you
          ☒ please return call   ☐ urgent

MESSAGE:
Questions about her April bill and insurance

taken by: _G. Chester, CMA_

REVIEW OF SYSTEMS

HEENT

Head	Acne	—					
Eyes	Vision	—	Glasses	—	Pain	—	
Ears	Hearing	—	Pain	—	Discharge	—	Tinn
Nose	Obstruction	—	Discharge	—	Epistaxis	—	Sinu
Throat	Teeth	—	Tongue	—	Gums	—	Thro
NECK	Swelling	—	Stiffness	—	Hoarseness	—	
BACK	Pain	—					
LUNGS	Cough	—	Hemoptysis	—	Sputum	—	Pain
HEART	Chills	—	Fever	—	Nightsweats	—	Whe
GI	Pain	—	Dyspnea	—	Edema	—	Palp
	Appetite	good	Diet	"normal"	Nausea	—	Vomit	—
	Diarrhea	—	Constipation	—	Jaundice	—	flatulence	—
GU	Belching	—					
	Frequency	—	Dysuria	—	Burning	—	Nocturia	—
MENSES	Incontinence	—	Hematuria	—	Discharge	—	Vaginal irritation	—
PREG HX	Menarche	—	Regularity	NA	Duration	NA	LMP	NA
LIBIDO	Cramping	—	Menorrhagia	NA	Metrorrhagia	NA	
EXTREM	#Pregnancies	—	Miscarriages	NA	Abortions	NA	Live births	NA
ENDO	Frequency	—	Satisfaction	NA			
SKIN	Joint pain	—	Weakness	—	Varicose veins	—	Swelling
NEURO	Hair	—	Nails	—	Sensitivity to temp	—	
HABITS	Dryness	—	Perspiration	—	Itching	—	Eruption	—
STRESS	Paralysis	—	Tingling	—	Numbness	—	Tremor	—
	Faint	—	Dizziness	—	Memory loss	—	Convulsion	—
	Sleep	8hr/night	Caffeine	16oz/day(pop)	Smoking	—	Alcohol	—
	Home	some	Work	—	Finances	—	General disposition	—
							"easy going"

CHARTING NOTES   _02/10/97_ | _9am   c/o sore throat. T—99⁴F, P—72, R—18, BP—120/68,_
Throat culture obtained. Amoxicillin 500 mg P.O. given to pt.
P. Dunham, CMA

Figure 5-10   Note-taking and record-keeping are important health care skills.

your understanding after reading the material. Here are some examples of objectives:

☐ Describe the steps in the communication process.[2]

☐ Identify key differences between law and ethics.[2]

☐ List and describe the three stages of a fever.[2]

☐ Explain the advantages of outpatient intravenous (IV) therapy.[2]

9. **Chapter introductions:** In addition to giving an overview of chapter content, these often contain explanations of why the material is important and how it relates to your career.

10. **Section headings:** Words or phrases that divide and identify sections of text. Headings give you an idea of the content that follows. An important part of previewing is going through the assigned reading page by page and reading

the headings. You will see they are organized like an outline, often with several levels of sub-headings. Some books distinguish the levels with different colors and lettering styles. The following example of headings comes from a chapter entitled "Interacting with Patients" in *Today's Medical Assistant*[2]:

Communicating with Patients

Verbal and Nonverbal Communication

Interference with Communication

Listening Skills

Nonverbal Measures to Facilitate Communication

Interviewing Techniques

    Closed Questions

    Open Questions

    Keeping the Conversation Going

    Drawing Out Patients

    Avoiding Responses That Inhibit Communication

Headings provide a logical structure to guide your reading. In the example, you learn three things before even reading the chapter: (1) interviewing techniques are used when communicating with patients; (2) there are at least two kinds of questions; and (3) some types of responses interfere with good communication.

One effective way to increase learning is to relate new information to what you already know. After reading the headings, but before reading the material, take a few moments to think about what you know about the topics.

You may be thinking that previewing is a waste of time and that it would be better to just jump into the reading and get it done. Not true! You are not "just reading." You are engaging in a learning activity, and previewing increases your ability to comprehend and remember the information presented in your textbooks. Previewing is actually an excellent investment of your time.

 Go to page 143 to complete Prescription for Success 5-5

Getting the Most from Your Reading

Two activities to help you interact with your textbooks are asking and answering questions and marking or highlighting. These actions focus your attention and serve as comprehension checks as you proceed through the text.

To use the question-answer method, change each section heading into a question and look for the answer as you read. When you find it, stop and answer the question aloud or quietly to yourself. This technique was developed almost 60 years ago when methods to increase the speed of learning were researched for World War II soldiers.[3] To this day, it has proven to be one of the most effective ways to master written material. See Table 5-2 for examples of study questions based on a few of the headings from "Communicating with Patients."

To benefit from questions, it's usually not necessary to write out the answers, although you may find

TABLE 5-2	Examples Using the Question-Answer Study Method
Section Headings	**Study Questions**
Verbal and Nonverbal Communication	What is the difference between verbal and nonverbal communication? How are the two types of communication used by health care professionals when working with patients?
Interference with Communication	Give examples of factors that can interfere with effective communication.
Listening Skills	How can good listening skills be developed? Why are good listening skills important when working with patients?
Nonverbal Measures to Facilitate Communication	What is meant by "nonverbal measures"? When should the health care professional employ nonverbal measures?
Interviewing Techniques	When do health care professionals use interviewing techniques when communicating with patients?
Closed Question	What is an example of a closed question? When should closed questions be used when one is interviewing a patient?
Drawing out Patients	What are two ways to draw out patients during the communication process?
Avoiding Responses that Inhibit Communication	Explain what is meant by "responses that inhibit communication." What are responses that the health care professional should avoid when communicating with patients?

it helpful with difficult material. (You must, however, say the answers, either silently or out loud.)

 Go to page 144 to complete Prescription for Success 5-6

The second interactive reading activity is marking your book by highlighting or underlining the most important information. Do this after you finish reading each section. If you highlight as you read, you may end up marking just about everything in the book. This defeats the purpose of highlighting. Try highlighting only key words and phrases, rather than whole sentences. This will draw your attention to the important points when it's time to study for an exam.

In addition to highlighting, you can further increase your learning by writing in your book. This can take the form of key words, short summaries, questions, or responses. Use logical and easy-to-remember symbols, like the ones suggested earlier in the chapter for taking notes:

T means the instructor has indicated you will be tested on this material

?? means "I don't understand this and need to ask about it"

* means this information is important

** means this information is very important

circled word means this is a new word and I need to learn it

Many students like to use colored highlighters to mark their books. If this is your preference, avoid very bright colors because they can cause eye strain. You might want to use a pen or pencil to underline and make notes. A tool that combines the features of the highlighter and pen is a colored pen. When it is used to underline, the color draws your attention for easy review. Use the same pen to write in your book. This saves time because you don't have to switch back and forth between a highlighter and a pen.

Success Tips for Reading

☐ Look up unfamiliar words as you come to them by using the book's glossary, a general dictionary, or a medical dictionary. You can write the definition in your book, in your own glossary you keep in your notebook, and/or on flash cards. (An exception to this for English-as-a-Second-Language [ESL] students is explained in Chapter 4.)

☐ Take advantage of illustrations, charts, lists, and boxed text. These are designed to give you examples and additional opportunities to master the material. Boxes often provide summaries of text content and serve as handy review aids.

☐ Read through procedures carefully, paying special attention to the rationales. It is important for health care professionals to understand the reasons behind their actions because nothing in health care is routine. You must think through every action and know why you are performing it.

☐ Read in short sessions. Depending on the difficulty of the material, you may find you are able to read and absorb for only 20 to 30 minutes without a short break. Experiment to see what works best for you. Just don't wander off too far or get involved with a 2-hour movie on TV!

☐ Don't worry about your reading speed. Health care textbooks contain lots of technical and detailed information. Your goal is not speed; it is comprehension. Read at a rate that keeps your attention and also allows you to understand the material. One way to prevent getting bogged down is to avoid saying each word, even if you are only doing this mentally. Try to read in phrases. When you drive a car, you see and act on many things at once. The same is true for reading, and with practice, you can see and process several words at a time.

Reviewing

As we discussed in the section on note-taking, reviewing regularly soon after your first exposure to new material is the key to ensuring its storage in long-term memory. Effective review techniques for material you have read are similar to those suggested for reviewing your notes. A good habit is to review within 24 hours. Start laying down memory paths before you forget most of the information. What a waste to spend an entire evening reading an assignment, only to forget most of it by bedtime the next night! Even a quick review is helpful.

Reading to learn requires more than simply reading passages over and over. You need to actively engage with the material. Quiz yourself on the material you have read without looking at the text. This forces you to think and checks your understanding. If you have difficulty remembering, review the section and try again. If you continue having trouble, this is a sign you don't understand the material.

As suggested for reviewing your notes, consider your learning styles when studying from your textbook:

☐ **Visual:** Use text illustrations to reinforce the material. Create stories about the illustrations to help anchor concepts in your mind. Attach significant concepts to people in a photograph. While looking at a picture of a piece of equipment, recall the name and function of each part, as well as how and for what purpose the equipment is used. Cover the labels on drawings and say or write down the names. Later you can call up the pictures in your mind as a trigger for remembering facts and concepts.

☐ **Auditory:** Do "out-loud" activities. Read the text aloud. Explain what you are reading in your own words. Create a dialogue to discuss the material. Have someone ask you questions. Record important points about the text or your questions and answers created from the headings.

☐ **Kinesthetic:** Stand up or move around while you review. Point to illustrations as you describe them. When appropriate, imagine how something feels. Health care texts typically describe processes and procedures. Go through them as realistically as possible in your mind or act them out. For example, open and close your hand as you read about how the heart pumps blood. Imagine yourself taking a file off the shelf, opening it to the correct section, and entering patient information.

☐ **Linear:** You may find outlines helpful because they form a logical structure for new material. Use the headings in the textbook as a guide. Charts that show relationships are also good. If the text does not include them, create your own.

☐ **Global:** Create mind maps or concept maps of the material.

☐ **Deductive:** To be sure you master the concepts along with the facts, try writing short summaries in which you state the principal ideas.

☐ **Inductive:** List the important facts that support the major ideas. Make flash cards with facts on one side and explanations or details on the other.

In addition to asking yourself questions as you read, make up written practice tests. Converting chapter objectives into questions is an excellent way to review. Table 5-3 contains a few examples. Another idea is to form a study group and have each member make up several quiz questions to exchange with the others.

TABLE 5–3	Converting Chapter Objectives into Quiz Questions
Chapter Objectives	**"Quiz Questions"**
List and describe the parts of the medical office.[2]	What are the various parts of the medical office? What is the purpose of each?
List and describe the seven parts of the health history.[2]	What are the seven parts of the health history? What is the content of each?
Explain the purpose of OSHA.[2]	What is the purpose of OSHA? How does OSHA affect the work of the health care professional?

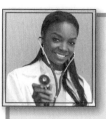

READING ON THE JOB

Reading is an important skill in your professional life. Directions for the proper use of medications and medical equipment, as well as instructions for performing procedures, come in written form. Your ability to understand and follow written directions has an impact on patient well-being.

Reading is also necessary for keeping up with the rapidly advancing field of health care. Discoveries about how the body works, such as in the field of genetics; the development of new medications and treatments; and the invention of new machines and devices, such as computerized robots that perform surgery, will make your current knowledge outdated in only a few years, if not months. Literally thousands of journals are devoted to medical and health care topics, and reading at least some of them will be an important way of staying up-to-date in your field.

Most health care certifications and licenses require continuing education credits for renewal, and this presents another need for reading and comprehending written material. Credits can often be earned through self-study, such as reading an article, and then answering questions or taking a test.

DOING RESEARCH TO LEARN

Research is not limited to finding information for a paper you have to write. We do research all the time, such as when we investigate which car to buy, how to find the best auto insurance, and how to change a tire. Research simply means finding sources of reliable information and obtaining what you need from those sources.

Library

Your school's library may be large and contain thousands of books and loads of other material, or it may be small and focused on the specialized materials needed to support the programs offered at the school. You should get to know both your school library and your local public library. If there are other schools of higher education nearby, inquire whether they allow the public to use their libraries. Some give checkout privileges for a yearly fee. Hospitals and clinics often have libraries for employees. It is possible you will have access to these during your clinical experience.

Today's libraries have many resources in addition to books and journals. Most offer Internet services, videos, DVDs, and other multimedia materials. Every library is different. Walk around and explore. Look for informational brochures and how-to guides, and ask the librarian for help.

 Go to page 144 to complete Prescription for Success 5-7

Internet

The **Internet**, a connection of many millions of computers throughout the world, is a valuable source for all kinds of information. Literally anyone or any organization can create a **website** on the Internet for everyone to access. Following are a few examples of what is available:

- Articles from newspapers and magazines
- Informative articles by researchers
- Directories
- Dictionaries
- Opportunities to communicate with experts
- Job postings and applications
- Information about diseases and injuries for both patients and health care professionals
- Career advice from professional organizations
- Photographs
- Video presentations
- "Stores" from which you can order almost any product or service imaginable

If you don't own or have access to a computer, check with your school to find out what is available. A complete discussion on how to search the Internet is outside the scope of this book. However, it is easy to use and doesn't require a significant amount of computer experience. If you don't have much experience searching the Internet, online tutorials are available and can be accessed by entering the key words "Internet tutorials" or "online search tutorials."

You can find information on the Internet in several ways. The first is by using a website address. All sites have one, just like houses. If you know the address, you simply type it in. If you do not know which sites have the information you are looking for, you can use a program called a *search engine*. You simply enter key words and the search is on! Here are the three general search engines recommended by the University of California (UC), Berkeley[4]:

- Google: www.google.com
- Yahoo!Search: www.search.yahoo.com
- Exalead: www.exalead.com/search

Some search engines are limited by subject area, such as the following:

- fealth! is limited to health: www.fealth.com
- Scirus is limited to science: www.scirus.com

General subject directories contain information categorized by topic, including health. The following two examples are recommended by UC Berkeley[4]:

- Infomine: www.infomine.ucr.edu
- About.com: www.about.com (for resources limited to health: www.about.com/health)

Evaluating Websites

A word of caution—the Internet is not controlled by any organization or agency that checks on content or keeps the connections up-to-date. For serious research, be sure to check the credibility of the information supplier. Here are some questions you should ask about a website:

1. Who is the sponsor? Universities, government agencies, professional organizations, research institutes, and established publishers are usually good sources. (This is not to say that commercial sites do not contain excellent information. Just note whether their purpose is to inform or advertise a product.) The endings of the web address indicate sponsorship:

   university: .edu
   government: .gov
   professional organization: .org
   commercial enterprise: .com

2. Who is the author? He or she should have education and/or experience in the subject matter. Can you contact the author?
3. What is the purpose of the website? Many sites are designed to sell products or persuade viewers to believe in a cause. The material provided may be biased and/or not well researched.
4. How are claims supported? Check for statistics and references to original sources of information.
5. How current is the information? Are dates given? Advances and changes in health care and its delivery occur continually.
6. What is the purpose of the document? To present facts? To give an opinion? To sell a product or service?

Examples of Health Care Sites

The Internet is a relatively new technology. Websites close down, merge with others, or change their addresses, and this can be a source of frustration. The following are examples of reliable sites that have a wealth of information about health topics:

- Agency for Healthcare Research and Quality www.ahrq.gov
- Centers for Disease Control and Prevention

http://cdc.gov
- Family Doctor
  http://familydoctor.org/
- Healthy People
  http://healthypeople.gov
- MedlinePlus, sponsored by the National Library of Medicine and the National Institutes of Health
  http://medlineplus.gov
- National Institutes of Health
  http://health.nih.gov
- University of Iowa Hospitals and Clinics
  www.uihealthcare.com/topics/catindex.html
- Web MD
  www.webmd.com

Health care professional organizations have websites. Appendix A contains a list of many organizations with their contact information.

Interviewing

The informational interview, described in Chapter 1, is a form of research. Many important studies are based on interviews, and interviews can help you find information not available from other sources. To interview effectively, you need to identify your purpose in advance and prepare good questions. You use note-taking skills to record all the key points given by the interviewee. Here are some examples of interviews that you might conduct as a student or health professional:

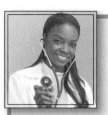

INTERVIEWING ON THE JOB
Providing good health care depends on the quality of information gathered from the patient. Asking good questions and listening carefully are used when collecting this important information. Nurses conduct assessments when developing care plans for their patients, and part of this assessment involves interviewing patients to learn about their health status. A common task of medical assistants is to interview patients and fill out the patient history (see Figure 5-10). And physical and occupational therapists gather the information needed to develop appropriate rehabilitation by interviewing their clients to determine their goals and needs. These are just a few examples of professionals who use interviewing skills to provide appropriate health care.

- Request career advice from a graduate of your school to learn how you can make the most of your education.
- Ask a medical specialist a series of questions about a health condition in which you have a special interest.
- Talk with personnel at community offices of organizations such as the American Heart Association and American Cancer Society to learn what information and services they have available.

 Go to page 145 to complete Prescription for Success 5-8

SUMMARY OF KEY IDEAS

1. Class notes can be powerful study aids.
2. Effective listening is one of the most valuable skills for academic and professional success.
3. Repetition is the key to storing new information in your long-term memory.
4. Reading to learn is an active process.
5. Research is an everyday activity.

Positive Self-Talk for This Chapter

1. I am an active listener.
2. I take good notes in class.
3. My notes are good study tools, and I review them regularly.
4. I use techniques I enjoy to help me learn.
5. I learn from my reading assignments.
6. I use a variety of sources to conduct research.

To Learn More

Dartmouth College Academic Skills Centers
www.dartmouth.edu/~acskills/videos/index.html
Although created for college students who live on campus, the videos on note-taking and reading contain useful information for all post-secondary students.

Pauk W, Owens R: *How to study in college,* ed 9, Clifton Park, NY, Cengage.
Professor Pauk developed some of the most successful study techniques, which are still being used by students today.

Study Guides and Strategies
www.studygs.net
This website has been a public service since 1996 and contains hundreds of helpful strategies categorized by topic.

Study Skills Help Page: Learning Strategies for Success
Middle Tennessee State University (MTSU)
http://frank.mtsu.edu/~studskl
Created for students at MTSU, this site contains dozens of helpful study tips.

REFERENCES

1. Anderson R, Barbara A, Feldman S: *What patients want: a content analysis of key qualities that influence patient satisfaction.* www.drscore.com/press/papers/whatpatientswant.pdf (Accessed 2/9/09)

2. Bonewit-West K, Hunt S, Applegate E: *Today's medical assistant: clinical and administrative procedures,* St Louis, 2009, Elsevier.

3. Wahlstrom C, Williams BK: *The commuter student: being your best at college and life,* Belmont, Calif, 1997, Wadsworth Publishing.

4. University of California, Berkeley: Teaching Library Internet Workshops. Available at: www.lib.berkeley.edu/TeachingLib/Guides/Internet/SearchEngines.html. (Accessed 2/14/09).

BUILDING YOUR RESUME

Review the Resume Building Block #5 form at the end of Chapter 2. Use the research skills described in this chapter to learn more about certifications and/or licenses, either voluntary or required, for your career.

INTERNET ACTIVITIES

For active links to the websites needed to complete these activities, visit **http://evolve.elsevier.com/Haroun/career/.**

1. Enter the key words "active listening," and find five suggestions for improving listening habits.
2. Use the key words "effective note-taking" and you will find sources sponsored by universities. Choose among these and look for three note-taking tips you believe might help you.
3. The Academic Resource Center at Utah State University developed a series of over 40 Idea Sheets to help students. Review the list and choose five to read. Prepare a report on what you learned.
4. Search for tips on evaluating Internet sources. By entering terms such as "Internet source evaluation" you can locate information published by university libraries. Develop a fact sheet of evaluation criteria.
5. Using one of the search engines or web addresses given in this chapter, conduct an Internet search for information about a health topic of your choice. Write a summary of what you find, including the source of your information and why you believe it is reliable.

Prescription for Success 5-1
My Listening Habits

You can start improving your listening skills by practicing awareness. One way is to listen to the news or other programming on the radio for several minutes at a time. Pay attention to when your mind wanders or you lose track of what is being said. (You can try the same technique in your classes if you don't have time to listen to the radio and only if it does not distract your attention further from the lecture.)

1. Think about your listening. Is there a pattern to the breaks in your concentration? (For example, you are distracted by something visual or your private thoughts, you don't understand every-thing being said, it is difficult to follow long periods of speech.)

_____

_____

_____

_____

_____

_____

_____

_____

2. How might you improve your listening habits?

_____

_____

_____

_____

_____

_____

_____

_____

_____

_____

Prescription for Success 5-2
Applying What You've Learned

1. Review the notes you have taken for this or another class. How effective are they in identifying the key points and helping you prepare for tests?

_____

_____

_____

2. Practice listening for organizational clues in your classes during the next week. Choose two lectures and take a couple of minutes afterward to record how they were organized.

_____

Class or Subject 1   *How Lecture was Organized*

                                                  _____ Clusters

                                                  _____ Procedures

                                                  _____ Concepts with rationale

                                                  _____ Definitions

                                                  _____ How things work

                                                  _____ Presentation patterns

                                                  _____ Other (explain) _____

Class or Subject 2   *How Lecture was Organized*

                                                  _____ Clusters

                                                  _____ Procedures

                                                  _____ Concepts with rationale

                                                  _____ Definitions

                                                  _____ How things work

                                                  _____ Presentation patterns

                                                  _____ Other (explain) _____

3. Do your instructors give clues about what they consider to be most important in their lectures? Choose two lectures (from different instructors, if possible), listen and observe carefully, and check any behaviors you notice.

Continued

Prescription for Success 5–2 (Continued)

Class or Subject 1	*Class or Subject 2*	*Behaviors or Clues*
		Tell you directly that something is important
		Emphasize words
		Say words louder
		Write on board or overhead
		Show enthusiasm
		Ask questions
		Other (explain)

Prescription for Success 5-3

What Works for You?

1. Choose or create a note-taking method you believe might work well for you.

   _____

2. Try it during the next few class lectures you attend, and report on how it works. For example, did it make it easier or harder for you to take notes?

   _____

   _____

   _____

   _____

3. If this method didn't work well for you, choose or create another one to try.

   _____

   _____

   _____

   _____

   _____

Prescription for Success 5-4
Create Your Own Abbreviations

Create 20 abbreviations to use in your note-taking.

1. _____ 11. _____

2. _____ 12. _____

3. _____ 13. _____

4. _____ 14. _____

5. _____ 15. _____

6. _____ 16. _____

7. _____ 17. _____

8. _____ 18. _____

9. _____ 19. _____

10. _____ 20. _____

Prescription for Success 5-5
Book Report

Look over your current textbooks. Which of the following features do they contain?

_____ Preface

_____ Detailed table of contents

_____ Appendices

_____ Index

_____ Bibliography

_____ Glossary

_____ Vocabulary or key terms

_____ Objectives

_____ Chapter introductions

_____ Headings

_____ Other

Prescription for Success 5-6
Increasing Your Learning with Questions

Using this or any other textbook, fill in the chart with a list of 10 chapter objectives or 10 section headings within a chapter. Then convert each into a study question.

Objective or Section Heading   *Study Question*

1. _____   1. _____
2. _____   2. _____
3. _____   3. _____
4. _____   4. _____
5. _____   5. _____
6. _____   6. _____
7. _____   7. _____
8. _____   8. _____
9. _____   9. _____
10. _____   10. _____

Prescription for Success 5-7
Check Out the Library

Visit your school and/or local public library to learn about and create a list of the services offered.

_____
_____
_____
_____
_____
_____

Prescription for Success 5-8
Go to the Source

Choose a topic in which you have an interest, and locate five different sources of reliable information. Briefly describe each source and state why you believe it to be reliable.

Topic:

Name of Source	*Description of Source*	*Why Source Is Reliable*
1. _____	_____	_____
	_____	_____
	_____	_____
	_____	_____
	_____	_____
2. _____	_____	_____
	_____	_____
	_____	_____
	_____	_____
	_____	_____
3. _____	_____	_____
	_____	_____
	_____	_____
	_____	_____
	_____	_____
4. _____	_____	_____
	_____	_____
	_____	_____
	_____	_____
	_____	_____
5. _____	_____	_____
	_____	_____
	_____	_____
	_____	_____
	_____	_____

Developing Your Paper Skills II: Output of Information

OBJECTIVES

The information and activities in this chapter can help you:

- Explain why it is important for health care professionals to have good writing skills.
- Evaluate your own writing skills and, if necessary, devise a plan to improve them.
- Plan and organize various types of writing projects.
- Locate and use writing tools and references to help you write more effectively.
- Describe how tests are part of the daily life of a health care professional.
- Use tests as incentives to learn rather than as instruments of torture.
- Apply effective techniques to maximize your performance on classroom tests.

KEY TERMS AND CONCEPTS

Audit: To check an organization to see if it is following required laws, regulations, and/or professional standards. This is also a noun meaning the process of checking.

Auditor: An individual who performs an audit.

Bibliography: A list of information sources, including books, journal articles, websites, movies, and interviews, for any type of writing assignment.

Consonant: All the letters in the alphabet *except* A, E, I, O, and U.

Criteria: Established standards used to measure performance.

Documentation: Written records. In health care, it refers to detailed recordings, either on paper or electronically, of facts about and observations of patients and their care.

Draft: The first version of a piece of writing.

Essay: A short piece of nonfiction (based on facts and reality) that is meant to inform, persuade, or entertain the reader.

Fraud: Dishonesty or trickery, especially in business.

Freewrite: To record ideas as they come to you without worrying about perfect organization, grammar, and spelling.

Grammar: A system of rules for putting words and sentences together.

Protocols: Established ways of performing procedures.

Reimbursement: Payments from a third party for services given.

Suffix: A syllable attached to the end of a word such as *-ing* or *-ly*.

Syllable: The shortest part of a word that can be pronounced as a unit. For example, immunization has five syllables: im-mu-ni-za-tion.

Text: Written material, as contrasted with illustrations, drawings, graphs, and so on.

Vowel: Any of the following letters: A, E, I, O, U, and sometimes Y.

YOUR WRITING ABILITY: A KEY TO PROFESSIONAL SUCCESS

Good written communication is critical for the delivery of high-quality health care. Notes on patient charts and entered onto computers, letters to insurance companies, and printed instructions for patients must be written clearly and accurately. Consistency of care, **reimbursement** for services, and good relations between health facilities and the public they serve depend on the quality of written documents. You may think you won't do much writing in your future work. Not true! Almost every job in health care today involves paperwork and some writing tasks.

Your writing is like a personal advertisement, representing who you are. It influences the opinions of other people about you and your work. Writing is a form of permanent communication. Unlike speaking, which can be revised and corrected so your listener understands what you are saying, you have only one opportunity to express yourself in writing. Readers must rely on what they see on the page and may question your competence if you make grammatical and spelling errors or organize information poorly. How well you write makes an impression on potential employers when you are applying for jobs. Once you are hired, it reflects on your employer and the health care facility where you work. In short, writing is an important skill to master. Written communications skills are included in the National Health Care Standards and Accountability Criteria:

- 2.31 Recognize elements of written and electronic communication (spelling, grammar, formatting, and confidentiality).
- 2.32 Describe techniques for planning and organizing written documents.[1]

Contrary to what you might think, the computer age has actually increased the importance of good writing skills. E-mail, in which you correspond electronically over the computer, is replacing a lot of the communication that until recently was conducted over the telephone. Although e-mail messages tend to be informal and often use phrases instead of complete sentences, they must be expressed clearly and in an organized fashion to be useful to the receiver. The growing use of electronic health records also requires the ability to record information clearly and accurately. Technology is actually increasing, rather than decreasing, the need for you to develop your writing skills.

Many students find writing difficult and dread assignments in which they have to write more than a few words. Maybe this applies to you. Perhaps you thought your previous English classes were boring or you were never required to do much writing. Or maybe English is not your first language. Whatever the reason, it is not too late to upgrade your skills. Although a complete writing course is beyond the scope of this book, this chapter contains information about the basics of good writing and includes suggestions to help you write more effectively. The main goal is to encourage you to care about your writing skills and motivate you to improve them, if necessary.

WRITE ON! DEVELOPING GOOD WRITING SKILLS

There are two components to good writing: content and form. Content refers to *what* you write: the information and ideas. Form is *how* you present it: grammar, spelling, and formatting. You must pay attention to both content and form in order for your reader to receive your intended message. Employers today rank this as an important job skill.

Content: Determine Your Purpose

The first step when starting to write is to think about what you want to accomplish. Your purpose determines what you say and how you say it, so it needs to be clear in your own mind. It will be based in part on who your audience is. (Identifying and addressing the needs of readers will be discussed later in this chapter.)

The following examples illustrate common writing goals of students and health care professionals.

1. **Demonstrate your knowledge and/or inform your readers.** This is one of the reasons why instructors ask you to write research papers (also called "term papers" or "reports") and answer essay test questions. They use these assignments to assess what you have learned about a subject. To do well on papers and tests, you must know about your subject, state information clearly, and provide accurate facts to support what you write. When your purpose is to show what you know, it is important not to pad your writing with repetition or statements that add nothing meaningful to the content. Although instructors often assign papers by numbers of words or pages, a common mistake of students is to use many words to make it look as if they've said a lot when they really have said very little.

2. **Persuade your readers.** A common class assignment is to write a paper about a controversial topic in which you must convince the reader to accept your point of view. Outside of class, you may have opportunities to write with the goal of influencing the reader to take certain actions. For example, you may write application letters to include with your resume when you are looking for employment. The purpose of these letters is to convince prospective employers to interview you. Persuasive writing can be used on the job to present your ideas about how the facility might run more smoothly or to request a promotion or a pay raise. Supervisors often ask that you submit these ideas and requests in writing, so it is important to know how to write convincingly.

There are various ways to persuade readers. One is to present facts that support your arguments. In the case of the letter to a prospective employer, you could list the ways you can be of benefit and can help provide great service to patients. Another method is to appeal to readers' emotions. For example, if you want to convince them to take action against cigarette advertising aimed at children, you could point out the need for adults to express their love for vulnerable children by protecting them from potential health hazards. It is generally most effective to use both facts and emotions so they support each other and strengthen your case. In the argument against cigarette advertising, you could cite the number and ages of children who start smoking each year, along with statistics about diseases and deaths caused by smoking.

3. **Make a request.** This is related to persuasive writing, but it is usually more direct and has the goal of initiating a definite response. Although writing a request is not a common school assignment, you might use this form for tasks at school outside of class. For example, some schools require you to submit a written request if you need a leave of absence. Or you may fill out an application for a scholarship or write a request for information about your student loan. During your job search, you may submit requests to health care facilities for information about their application procedures. Once on the job, you may submit requests to vendors for information about their products, compose letters to physicians asking them to send you patient records, or write to insurance companies requesting action on unpaid claims.

4. **Provide an explanation.** Some school assignments, such as exercises in workbooks, ask you to explain the steps in a procedure or explain why something is done a certain way. Test questions that require short answers are often requests for explanations. On the job, you may write instructions for patients or directions for co-workers. It is important that this type of writing be very clear and organized in a logical order. Including information about why something should be done or why it should be done in a specific way strengthens your writing because people tend to be more willing and able to follow instructions when they understand the reasons behind them.

5. **Narrate a story or event.** If you take an English or a writing class, writing an original story may be one of your assignments. Although stories are not commonly used in workplace writing, they can add interest and provide examples in persuasive or explanatory works. The main considerations in story writing are to use your imagination and to write good descriptions. An example of the use of creative writing in the workplace would be writing a story to help children overcome their fear of the dentist. A word of caution: stories used in the workplace should be directly related to the situation. And it is inappropriate, even dangerous, to share work stories based on real people and events outside the facility.

Many pieces of writing have more than one purpose, and these can be combined so they reinforce each other. For example, when preparing instruction sheets for patients, they can be more effective if you include persuasive language that encourages the patients to follow their special diet or perform their exercises every day.

 Go to page 175 to complete Prescription for Success 6-1

Content: Gather Information

Writing sometimes requires research and always requires thought. This may sound obvious, but many people simply start writing without any preparation or in-depth thinking. The result is a collection of words and sentences that don't say much. There are many sources of information, and the first one may surprise you—your own knowledge and experience. Start by writing down what you already know in whatever format you find most useful, such as lists of key ideas and facts, a mind map, or an outline.

After assessing what you know, identify what you need to find out. If the instructor has assigned a topic about which you know very little, consider developing a list of questions to help guide your research. For example, if you are to write about infectious diseases in the world today, your questions might include the following:

☐ What are the major infectious diseases?
☐ What are the symptoms?
☐ What causes these diseases?
☐ How are they spread?
☐ How are they treated?
☐ How widespread are these diseases? How many people are affected each year?
☐ What is the annual mortality rate?

If you know very little about the topic, start your research with resources that provide definitions and general information. Examples of these resources include encyclopedia and journal articles, textbooks, nontechnical books for the general reader, and websites for the general public. Once you have an overall view of the topic, you can narrow your research to specific areas of interest. Your instructors may require you to consult certain types and numbers of resources beyond your textbook. They may also have good suggestions for additional sources of information.

As you consult each resource, record the important facts and ideas. Some people like to use note cards. Try using a separate card for each topic or subtopic. If you need more than one card for each topic, number or mark them in some way to keep them organized. Another method is to take notes on sheets of paper (one side only), organizing by resource rather than topic. You may have several pages for each source. When it's time to organize, you can cut up the papers and sort the pieces by related information. Other methods are to leave the sheets whole and color-code the different topics or write key words in the margins to identify the various topics. You can then quickly scan the pages for needed information as you write. You can also take and organize your notes using the computer.

Whichever way you take your notes, you also need a system to keep track of your resources so you can create your **bibliography** or reference list. This includes all the books, journal and magazine articles, brochures, websites, and any other resources you have used. See Table 6-1 for examples of what information to record about each kind of source. There are several standard styles you can use for organizing your bibliography, so check with your instructor to find out which one you are to use. Table 6-2 contains examples of two popular formats, one from the Modern Language Association (MLA) and the other from the American Psychological Association (APA). Compare the examples and you will notice they contain almost the same information, just presented in a different order. Even if your project does not require a bibliography, it is a good idea to write down your sources so you can find them later if you need them. One way to keep

TABLE 6–1	Information Needed for Various Sources	
Source	**Facts You Need**
Book	Author(s) or editor Title of the book Publisher Location of publisher (city) Year published Edition
Journal or magazine article	Author(s) Name of the journal or magazine Title of the article Volume number of journal Issue number Page numbers of the article
Newspaper article	Author(s) Name of the newspaper Title of the article Date of the newspaper Page numbers of the article
Website	Author(s) or creator(s) of site, if available Title of the site or "home page" if no title Name of any organization associated with the site Date site was created or latest update Date you accessed the site Complete site address

track of your sources is to create a numbered list and then write the corresponding number on each card or page of notes.

Content: *Organize Your Information*

"Since it is not possible to think about everything all at once, most experienced writers handle a piece of writing in stages."

—Diana Hacker

When you are assigned a research paper or have a report to prepare for work, it can be difficult to decide how to get started and then how to organize what you want to say. Some instructors require students to prepare an outline as the first step in writing. If you find it difficult to think in outline form (you're just not linear) or you just don't know where to start, outlining can be as intimidating as writing the paper itself. Don't despair. There are some other ways to tackle the problem of getting things in order and getting started. Suppose you are assigned to write a paper about electronic health

TABLE 6–2	Examples of Bibliographic Styles
Style	**Book**
Modern Language Association (MLA)	Young, Alexandra P., and Deborah P. Kennedy. *Kinn's the Medical Assistant.* 10th ed. St Louis: Saunders, 2008.
American Psychological Association (APA)	Young, A. P., & Kennedy, D. P. (2007). *Kinn's the medical assistant* (10th ed.). St Louis: Saunders.
	Magazine
MLA	Mattick, John S. "The Hidden Genetic Program of Organisms." *Scientific American* Oct. 2004: 60+.
APA	Mattick, J. S. (2004, October). The hidden genetic complex organisms. *Scientific American, 291,* 60-67.
	Website
MLA	Hopkins, M. E. "Critical Condition." *NurseWeek* 12 March 2001, 3 Jan. 2002 <http://www.nurseweek.com/news/features/01-03/shortage.asp>;
APA	Hopkins, M. E. (2001, March 12). Critical Condition. *NurseWeek.* [On-line] Available: http://www.nurseweek.com/news/features/01-03/shortage.asp [2002, January 3].

records. Here are some ways you can gather and organize your information:

1. **Questions.** List questions you would like answered, such as the suggestions in Figure 6-1. Your information falls into place as you research and find the answer to each question.

2. **Idea sheets.** As you think of major ideas, write each one at the top of a separate sheet of paper. Then list all related and supporting ideas on the pages. To organize, lay the sheets out and move them around until you find the best way to order them. Figure 6-2 contains an example of an idea sheet.

3. **Note cards.** Dave Ellis, writer of popular student success books, recommends the use of note cards for generating creativity and promoting organization.[2] List all your ideas, both major and supporting, on 3 × 5 cards, one idea per card. Sort the cards by topics or categories, and then arrange them in logical order. You can lay them out on a flat surface or pin them to a wall or large bulletin board as illustrated in Figure 6-3.

4. **Mind maps.** Mind maps, illustrated in Figure 6-4 for our topic, are diagrams drawn freehand that link and arrange words and ideas around a central key word or idea. Mind maps can be helpful if you don't have a clear idea of the order you want for your material. Some people find mind maps useful when brainstorming because they don't require ideas to be organized in a linear way. The result is a "map" illustrating how ideas relate to and support one another. If you have several major ideas, you can make a series of maps.

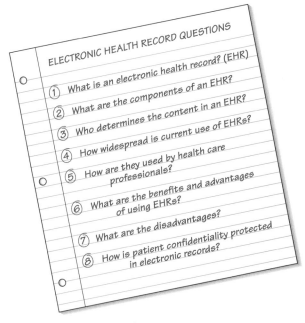

Figure 6–1   Organizing information using questions.

Who Are My Readers?

Effective writers consider the needs of their readers. This is especially important in health care, where safe and consistent care depends on how well health care professionals communicate with patients and with one another. Whenever you write, take into account the readers' ages, cultural backgrounds, knowledge of health issues, and purpose for reading the material. Remember that you will not usually be present to clarify information,

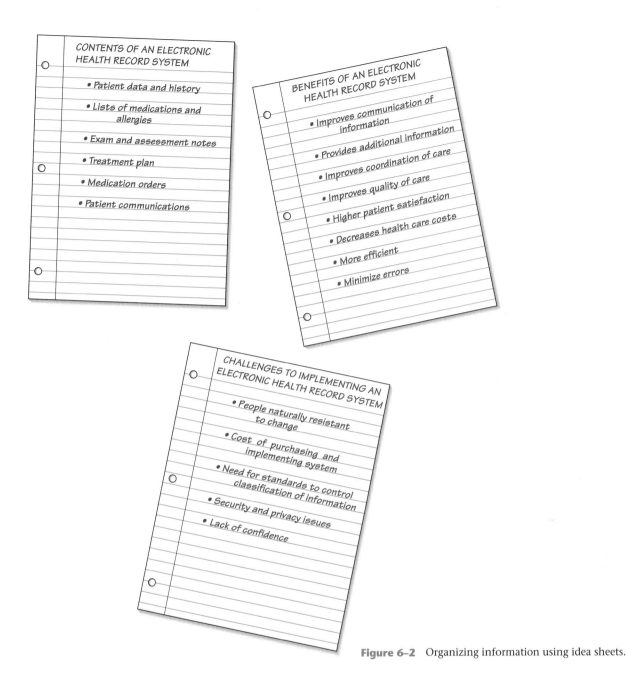

Figure 6–2 Organizing information using idea sheets.

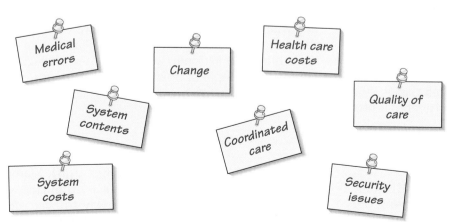

Figure 6-3 Organizing information using note cards.

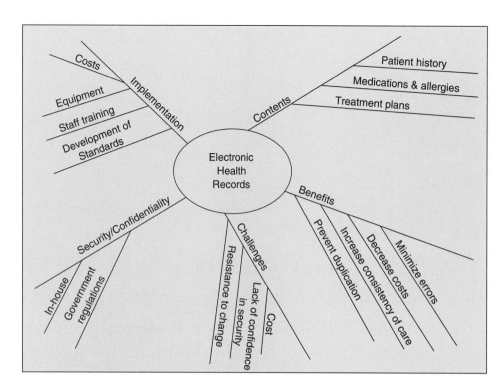

Figure 6–4 Organizing information using a mind map.

answer questions, or see from their facial expressions that they do not understand or agree with what you have written. This is why it is so important to write clearly and organize your **text** so readers can follow it easily. If you are addressing a mixed audience, plan your writing for the readers who are most likely to have difficulty understanding. When writing class assignments and tests, your instructor is the audience. He or she wants you to demonstrate what you know about a subject and how well you express yourself. There may also be specific requirements about the form of writing you are to use.

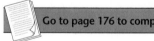
Go to page 176 to complete Prescription for Success 6-2

Organize Content for Your Readers

Everyone prefers to read material that is easy to follow. Good writers achieve this by organizing material logically, and you can do this too. How you organize your content is based on the type of document you are writing. Letters, research papers, and long essay answers are easier for the reader to follow if they are divided into sections:

1. **Introduction.** Present your major points. Tell what you are writing about. State your purpose.
2. **Middle or body.** Develop, support, and explain your ideas. You may have several sections, one for each topic or idea.

3. **Conclusion.** Show how everything you have written pulls together. Give your "final word" on the subject. Summarize your points. State what you have attempted to prove with your information. Tell the readers what action you hope they will take as a result of your writing. Figure 6-5 shows how a paper on electronic health records might be organized.

Short answers to test questions and brief letters and notes require tight organization to cover all necessary material in a small space:

1. Give your answer or state your purpose or main point in the first sentence.
2. Give supporting details in one or two paragraphs.
3. Limit your conclusion to one or two sentences.

Instructions and directions can be organized into lists of steps or activities in the order in which they should be performed or in order from most to least important. Rationale or purpose (reasons why something should be done) can be included just before or after the step or action to which it relates. See Figure 6-6 for an example of how written instructions can be organized.

Starting to Write

Don't aim for perfection on your first **draft.** Many people find a piece of blank paper very intimidating, even professional writers. A good way to beat the blank-paper monster is to just start writing. Begin

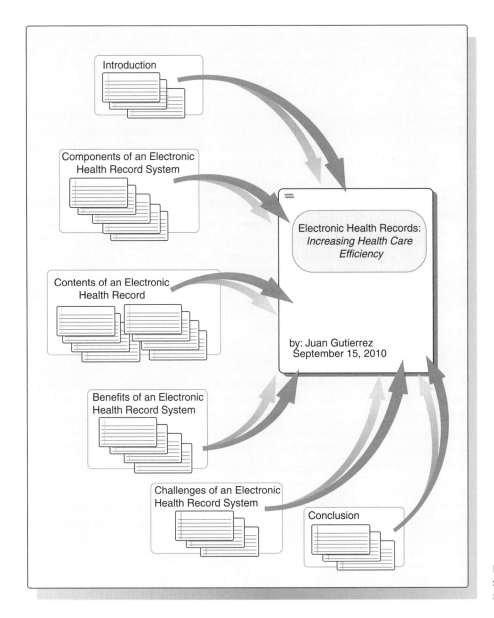

Introduction

Components of an Electronic
Health Record System

Contents of an Electronic
Health Record

Benefits of an Electronic
Health Record System

Challenges of an Electronic
Health Record System

Conclusion

Electronic Health Records:
*Increasing Health Care
Efficiency*

by: Juan Gutierrez
September 15, 2010

Figure 6–5 Organize your materials
so the information will be easy for
readers to follow and understand.

with a rough draft, and don't worry about how rough it is. Writing creatively and writing perfectly and correctly require different intellectual skills that can actually cancel each other out. Peter Elbow, a professor who wrote a very helpful book about how to write, says that trying to write perfectly the first time is "dangerous writing" because you can't generate good ideas and be critical of your work at the same time.[3] He recommends that you spend half of the time on a project **freewriting** the rough draft and the other half revising. (This is a good argument for starting your writing assignments well in advance of the due date!)

When freewriting, don't worry about starting with the introduction because this can put unnecessary pressure on you to start out "just right" with good opening sentences. You may not even know at this point how your piece is going to turn out because writers develop and come up

with new ideas throughout the writing process and you may add or delete topics. Go ahead and start with the middle section if that works for you. (An exception is when you are writing answers to essay questions on timed tests. State your answer at the beginning and spend the rest of the time supporting it.)

A technique called "brain dump" can work when you're really stuck getting started. It works like this: Get out some paper and just start writing, using the information you have gathered. This will be easier if you have used one of the techniques described earlier: outline, idea sheets, questions, and so on. Write quickly, and get as much down on paper as possible. Then go back and look for ideas and themes you can put in logical order. Although this is not always the fastest method for completing a paper or report, it can get you started when you find yourself with a bad case of writer's block. You may end up with

Preparing an Informed Consent for Treatment Form

GOAL: To adequately and completely inform the patient regarding the treatment or procedure that he or she is to receive, and provide legal protection for the facility and the provider.

EQUIPMENT AND SUPPLIES

- Pen
- Consent form

PROCEDURAL STEPS

1 After the physician provides the details of the procedure to be done, prepare the consent form. Be sure that the form addresses the following:

- The nature of the procedure or treatment.
- The risks and/or benefits of the procedure or treatment.
- Any reasonable alternatives to the procedure or treatment.
- The risks and/or benefits of each alternative.
- The risks and/or benefits of not performing the treatment.

Purpose: To make certain that the patient is fully informed about the procedure or treatment and the risks and/or benefits of having or not having it performed.

2 Personalize the form with the patient's name and any other demographic information that the form lists.

Purpose: To correctly identify the patient and the procedure.

3 Deliver the form to the physician for use as the patient is counseled about the procedure.

Purpose: To avoid charges of practicing medicine without a license. The physician should explain procedures, risks, benefits, alternatives, and answer all of the patient's questions.

4 Witness the signature of the patient on the form if necessary. The physician will usually sign the form as well

5 Provide a copy of the consent form to the patient.

Purpose: To make certain that the patient is fully informed regarding the procedure and has a copy of the information for his or her personal records.

6 Place the consent form in the patient's chart. The facility where the procedure is to be performed may require a copy.

Purpose: To maintain a permanent copy of the signed consent form.

7 Ask the patient if he or she has any questions about the procedure. Refer questions that the medical assistant cannot or should not answer to the physician. Be sure that all of the questions expressed by the patient are answered.

Purpose: To make certain that the patient is fully informed.

8 Provide information regarding the date and time for the procedure to the patient.

Figure 6–6   What features make these instructions effectively written? *(From Young AP, Proctor D: Kinn's the medical assistant: an applied learning approach, ed 10, St. Louis, 2007, Saunders.)*

a jumble of ideas that has to be unsnarled, but at least you have something on paper, and the chances are good you'll have something you can use. Many writers use brain dump to promote creativity and get ideas flowing.

Once you have completed your first draft, let it rest for a couple of days (or hours, if the due date is directly ahead). Then assume the role of your readers and try to imagine you are reading the piece for the first time. Read it aloud to hear how it sounds. Better yet, have someone else read it so you can listen for the following points[4]:

- Do you have an introduction?
- Is your purpose clear?
- Do your ideas flow smoothly, one to another?
- Have you supported your ideas?
- Is there enough information about each topic or idea?
- Have you included unnecessary details that should be left out?
- Do you repeat yourself unnecessarily?

- Does the conclusion summarize your information?
- Do you achieve your stated purpose?

Go to page 176 to complete Prescription for Success 6-3

Form: Attending to the Details of Writing

Your content may be important, interesting, and well organized, but poor **grammar** and spelling can cause your readers to misunderstand what you have written and even to question your competence. You may believe that worrying about grammatical details is unimportant. However, work in health care demands that you attend to details every day. Performing accurately and following exact procedures are valuable health care skills. In many types of written and electronic health care **documentation,** the contents are strictly controlled by federal and state laws as well as by nongovernmental regulatory

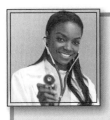

WRITING ON THE JOB

Getting a job involves several writing tasks: your resume, cover letters you send to prospective employers with your resume, and thank-you notes you send after interviews. These written pieces demonstrate some of your qualifications, including your ability to write. You can imagine how important it is to use good organization and correct grammar and spelling.

Once you are on the job, an increasingly important task of health care professionals is accurately recording information about patients. The quality of this information can affect the consistency and quality of care patients receive. It also has an effect on reimbursement—that is, how much money the physician, hospital, or other provider of services receives from insurance companies. And something you may not know is that medical records can be used as evidence in court. For example, if a doctor is sued for malpractice, the clarity and completeness of medical records can help—or hurt—the case.

agencies. For example, California law requires that reports prepared to document patient home care visits be written on the day of the visit, contain specific information, use certain abbreviations, show any corrections made in a specific way, and record the time of the visit using the 24-hour system.

Written documentation is often the only proof to show that patients have received appropriate care. It is recognized in court and by **auditors** who perform compliance reviews of medical institutions. A standard rule in health care is "If it was not documented, it was not done." We might add "If it's written poorly, it's not documented properly and may not have been done properly!" Most patients are covered by some type of insurance, and payment to the health care provider depends on clear and accurate claims submitted by health care facilities. Even if your job does not include preparing insurance claims, your notes may provide the information on which the claim is based. Writing correctly and paying attention to details are skills that today's employers require.

First Aid for Grammar

All languages are organized into systems with rules that determine how words are organized. These systems and rules help listeners and readers make sense of what they are hearing or reading because they know what to expect. Comparing the structure of different languages is one way to illustrate the role grammar plays. Let's look at word order. In English, we usually place describing words (adjectives) in front of the words they describe (nouns). If a friend said to you, "I live in the house blue with the trim white," it might take you a few moments to figure out what she was talking about. You are not accustomed to this word order. But in Spanish, this would be correct. Spanish speakers expect to first hear the noun before the adjective.

Another example is the methods used in language to let you know who the subject is; that is, who is doing the action. In English, we use pronouns such as "I," "we," and "they" to tell who this is: I swim, we studied, they will graduate. Again, using Spanish for our comparison, these words are not always necessary because the last letters of verbs change to indicate the subject: estudi*o* = I study; estudi*amos* = we study; estudi*an* = they study.

There are many differences among the thousands of languages spoken the world over. The point is that each has its own grammar, the purpose of which is to help people communicate effectively. Mastering the grammar of the language(s) you use improves your ability to communicate. Correct grammar is especially important in writing. Listeners may not notice the mistakes we make when we are speaking. If something is unclear, listeners can ask us to repeat or explain what we mean. Written material, however, must stand on its own. If it is unclear, the reader is not likely to have an opportunity to ask for clarification. Worse yet, readers may follow directions incorrectly, and this can result in costly mistakes when dealing with matters of health. In addition to helping ensure safety, proper grammar results in writing that reflects competence and professionalism.

Tables 6-3, 6-4, 6-5, and 6-6 contain grammatical rules you may have forgotten or perhaps never learned. They are not intended to be complete lists of "writing rules" for English. If you need to improve your writing skills, ask your instructors about other resources and find out whether your school offers English classes and/or has tutors. Many good books and websites with information about grammar and writing exist. (A few examples are listed at the end of this chapter.) The extra time you spend now will help you in valuable ways on the job.

A couple of notes about grammar references: First, many professional organizations have preferred styles for writing. For example, the American Association of Medical Assistants' book of style states that abbreviations for time should be written in lower case using periods: "a.m." for morning,

TABLE 6–3	Parts of Speech		
Part of Speech	**What It Is**	**Examples**	**Sentence Examples**
Noun	Name of a person, place, thing, idea, or process (such as a medical procedure)	Dr. Gutierrez, nurse, Texas hospital, microscope thought, urinalysis	**Mr. Samuels** is a **pharmacist** at the local **drugstore**. The **stethoscope** was lying on the **table**. The **technician** gave **Sarah** the **results** of the **test**.
Pronoun	Substitutes for a noun	I, he, she, it, we, they, me, him, her, it, us, them, this, that, these, those	**He** is the pharmacist at the local drugstore. **It** was lying on the table. **He** gave **her** the results of the test.
Verb	Expresses action or state of being	study, graduate, work, enjoy, am, is, are	Emily had to **work** hard to **finish** school, but after graduation she **got** a job she **enjoyed**. Now she **is** a medical assistant at a local clinic.
Adjective	Describes a noun or pronoun	kind, little, active, intelligent	The **kind** dental assistant gave the **little** girl a **comforting** hug. (*kind* describes the medical assistant; *little* describes the girl; *comforting* describes the hug)
Articles	Three small words that are used with nouns	the, a, an Note: Use "an" before words that start with vowels (a, e, i, o, u), the letter "h" when it is silent, and words that begin with a vowel sound, such as M&M.	**The** physical therapist worked with **a** patient for more than **an** hour. Johnny asked the nurse for **an** M&M as **a** reward for getting **an** injection.
Adverb	Describes a verb, adjective, or other adverb	Quickly, gently, very, really	The nurse **quickly** gave the injection. (*quickly* describes "gave") The veterinary assistant **very gently** picked up the kitten. (*very* describes *gently*; *gently* describes "picked up")
Preposition	Placed in front of a noun or pronoun to form a phrase (two or more words) that describes another word	as, at, between, of, on, out, since, than, to, with	The road **to** the clinic was really crowded today. The medical biller placed the files **on** the table.
Conjunction	Joins single words or groups of words Different kinds of conjunctions are used to indicate different types of relationships between the words they join	and, but, or, either…or, not only…but also, although, because, finally, however, meanwhile	She took classes **and** worked in the dental office. You need to take **either** medical terminology **or** anatomy this semester. Janet originally wanted to be a nurse; **however**, she decided to become a respiratory therapist.
Interjection	Expresses surprise or emotion	Oh! Hey! Wow!	**Oh!** I'm so sorry. I didn't see you coming this way. **Wow!** I can't believe I did so well on that test!

"p.m." for afternoon and evening). Other references suggest using uppercase to show time: A.M., P.M. Find out if there are style books or references for your profession.

Second, a word about grammar checkers on word-processing software. I am writing this book using a popular computer program. To my surprise, most of the suggested changes have been incorrect. In many cases, making the "corrections" would result in sentences that don't make sense. At the same time, many obvious errors are not caught. Although word-processing software has made writing and making corrections easier, the final judge is still the human writer.

TABLE 6-4	Common Sentence Ailments	
Ailment	**Example**	**Corrected**
No subject	Said that his tooth hurts.	He said that his tooth hurts.
Run-on (no punctuation or connecting word)	He needed an x-ray exam the radiologist was called.	He needed an x-ray exam, so the radiologist was called.
Pronoun does not agree with the noun it replaces	Each patient should take their prescription to the pharmacy.	Each patient should take his or her prescription to the pharmacy. *or* All patients should take their prescriptions to the pharmacy.
Subject and verb do not agree	Both the nurse and the physician sees the fracture on the x-ray film. The equipment you need to perform an ECG are in the other room.	Both the nurse and the physician see the fracture on the x-ray film. The equipment you need to perform an ECG is in the other room.
Split infinitive (unnecessarily separating "to" and the verb)	After this type of surgery, it is good for patients to frequently walk around to avoid stiffness.	After this type of surgery, it is good for patients to walk around frequently to avoid stiffness.
Dangling modifier (when a subject is not named for an action)	While giving the patient a bath, it got cold in the room. (In this example, "it" appears to be giving the patient a bath.)	While the nursing assistant was giving the patient a bath, it got cold in the room.
Incorrect pronoun	Jamie and me are working at the same dental office. Please give your urine sample to the nurse or to myself. The AARC has a special newsletter for we respiratory therapists.	Jamie and I are working at the same dental office. Please give your urine sample to the nurse or to me. The AARC has a special newsletter for us respiratory therapists.
Incorrect verb form	The patient already drunk the glass of water. Mr. Daley has broke the same leg twice.	The patient already drank the glass of water. Mr. Daley has broken the same leg twice.
Meaning is unclear because of the word order	When he hit his arm against the window, it broke. (Which broke—his arm or the window?)	When he hit his arm against the window, his arm broke. *or* He broke his arm when he hit it against the window.

 Go to page 177 to complete Prescription for Success 6-4

First Aid for Spelling

Many people, even good writers, have difficulty with spelling. English is a combination of many languages and contains silent letters, different ways of pronouncing the same letter, different ways of spelling the same sound, and other irregularities. There are a few rules, but the spelling of many words simply must be memorized. Developing a good learning system for spelling will be helpful when you are learning medical terminology. Spelling medical terms correctly is critical because errors can negatively affect patient care. Some medical words look alike and can be confused. Here are a few common examples:

- ilium—part of the hipbone
- ileum—part of the intestine
- alveoli—tiny air sacs in the lungs
- areola—brown pigmented area around the nipples

Begin now to practice good spelling habits by learning everyday English words. Tables 6-7 and 6-8 have spelling rules and a list of commonly misspelled words. Table 6-9 contains commonly confused words. You may have wondered about some of these yourself—words that are spelled the same with different pronunciations, and those that are spelled differently but have the same pronunciation!

You can use these tables, in addition to other spelling aids, as a study guide. Make them even more useful by adding your own problem words. If the sample suggestions given in Table 6-9 for learning commonly confused words don't make sense to you or seem silly, you might want to create your own hints for remembering them.

TABLE 6–5	Cures for Capitalization Problems
When to Use	**Examples**
First word of a sentence	The result of the test for strep throat was negative.
Proper nouns and adjectives: names of people, places, organizations, institutions, religions	Diane is working as a nurse in Kenya on a United Nations project in a Catholic hospital.
Professional titles when used with the person's name	I understand that Dr. Nguyen is a leading oncologist. (BUT: I understand that the doctor is a leading oncologist.) They are here to see Nurse Edmonds. (BUT: They are here to see the nurse.)
The major words in the titles of books, articles, movies, software programs, etc.	Career Development for Health Professionals is the title of this book. Steel Magnolias is a movie in which one of the main characters is a young woman living with diabetes.
The first word of a quotation	The physical therapist told the patient, "It is very important that you do these exercises every morning and evening."
Days, months, and holidays	I think Christmas was on a Friday last year.
Trade names of products and brand name drugs	The physician recommended Sudafed for the patient's nasal congestion. The lab technician used Acetest to confirm the presence of sugar in the patient's urine.
Abbreviations	AIDS (acquired immunodeficiency syndrome) CPR (cardiopulmonary resuscitation) ECG (electrocardiography) RDA (registered dental assistant)

 Go to page 177 to complete Prescription for Success 6-5

Success Tips for Spelling

☐ Try the memory techniques suggested in Chapter 3.
☐ If you have children in school, make spelling a family activity.
☐ Work on spelling in a study group: quiz one another, have contests, give small prizes, and make learning fun.
☐ Start your own dictionary and spelling list to keep in your notebook or on your computer.
☐ Make flash cards to quiz yourself.
☐ Put cards on the bathroom mirror and other places where you'll see them every day.
☐ Spell aloud.
☐ Create a "mental movie screen" on which you visualize the words spelled out in large colored letters.
☐ Create hints and associations.
☐ Write the words over and over. Try using colored pens and/or writing larger than you usually do.
☐ Record practice words to listen to at home or in the car.

TESTS: PART OF SCHOOL, PART OF LIFE

Taking tests is not limited to your life as a student. Much of what the health care professional does every day is a kind of test. Let's compare some typical classroom test questions with the performance of a procedure on a patient.

Test for A Class	Performance of A Procedure
Supply definitions	Know when to use the procedure
List items needed to perform the procedure	Gather equipment and supplies for the procedure
Recall information	Create mental checklist of steps
Write explanations	Provide patient with clear explanation and instructions
	Perform procedure correctly
Write short answers to questions	Record results accurately on patient chart

Using Tests to Your Advantage

Classroom tests and work on the job both involve interpreting sets of instructions (questions and job tasks), performing within time limits (class session and appointment schedules), following given standards (instructor **criteria** and facility **protocols**), and being measured by indicators of the level of

with a Health Care Professional Dolores Michaels

Dolores, a nurse in a large California medical clinic discusses the importance of good writing skills in the medical field.

Q Is being able to write well really that important for a health care professional?

A Absolutely! In fact, in our clinic written communication is central to everything. We have individuals who take phone messages from patients. These messages get passed on to doctors or to nurses like me who are responsible for reviewing them and getting back to patients. If we can't read or don't understand the message, we waste time checking back with whoever wrote it. In a fast-paced clinic, this can really create problems.

Q Do you have any examples of problems that resulted from unclear writing?

A Well, the other day I got a written message that said, "Patient has planteritis." This was a mystery because there's no such thing as "planteritis." I didn't want to call the patient without having some idea of the problem, so I had to take time to find the person who wrote this. Turns out the patient had "plantar fasciitis," which is inflammation of the tissue in the bottom of the foot. I have to say that good spelling is really critical. Another problem is with abbreviations. When we're in a hurry we tend to use them, but they can cause problems. The other day a nurse wrote on a chart, "Will call tom for a dressing change." The other staff then wasted time looking for someone named Tom who the patient was supposed to call. It turned out that "tom" was an abbreviation for "tomorrow." Totally different thing.

Q So abbreviations can really be a problem?

A Yes. You have to be really careful when using them. An interesting example is the shortcut for "shortness of breath." This is a common condition, but if

someone simply writes "patient is sob," the meaning is open to interpretation. If this were the only sentence on a chart with no context, it could be really inappropriate! So you really have to be careful.

The idea is to save time, but if abbreviations aren't clear, they can waste time. One day a doctor wrote "brbpr." I had no idea what this was and had to take time to find the doctor. It turns out it meant "bright red blood per rectum," but there was no way I was going to figure this out.

Even when everyone agrees on a facility abbreviation, it can be confusing to personnel who move from department or facility to another as fill-ins. Something like "mltcb" means "message left to call back." But lots of medical personnel work in various departments and facilities, and this can be confusing.

Q It sounds like we're not talking about the kinds of writing that students think of as assignments, like papers and reports.

A No, I'm referring to things like memos and electronic notes. These aren't long, but they're extremely important. They must be clear and accurate because we need the right information to give appropriate patient care. It's important to be precise and include all necessary details. If you're describing a wound, for example, you need to note the location, size, condition—all the things that the next person who sees the patient can use to see if the wound is healing or getting worse.

What students also need to understand is that these are legal records. If there's a malpractice suit, for example, they can be used in court as evidence.

performance (grades, patient satisfaction, evaluations, and raises). In reality, performing on the job is more serious in terms of requirements and consequences than any classroom quiz or final exam. Students can repeat a test—or a class, if necessary—but correcting a medical error, winning back an unhappy patient, or reversing the poor opinion of your supervisor is more difficult. At the extreme is the possible damage done by an incorrect procedure or inaccurate medication dosage.

The intention here is not to terrorize the future health care professional, but to put the subject of tests in the classroom in perspective. Tests are a fact of life, and if approached with the right attitude, classroom tests can provide you with opportunities to increase your learning. For example, tests

PERSONAL REFLECTION

What are some other similarities between classroom tests and working on the job as a health care professional?

_____

_____

_____

_____

_____

TABLE 6–6	**Punctuation Remedies**	
Mark	**When to Use**	**Examples**
Period .	To end sentences, unless you use a question mark (?) or an exclamation point (!)	There are five patients waiting in the reception area.
	After some abbreviations	Dr. A.M.
Comma ,	Connect two sentences (independent clauses) into one with a connecting word (and, but, or, nor, yet, for, so)	The surgeon performed the knee replacement surgery, and the physical therapist directed the patient's rehabilitation program. The patient was very nervous about the procedure, so the physician ordered a sedative.
	Separate items in a series	Encephalitis, epilepsy, meningitis, and multiple sclerosis are disorders of the nervous system.
	After introductory phrases	While the patient filled out the necessary forms, the dental hygienist gathered her supplies. When the EMT couldn't detect a pulse, he quickly began to perform CPR.
	Around optional information (nonrestrictive clause)	Mrs. Washington, who has been seeing Dr. Gonzalez for several years, is doing well on her new medication. She is doing well with her diet; however, she needs to walk at least a mile each day.
	After transitions (however, therefore, for example, in other words)	Alternative medicine is gaining popularity in the United States; for example, many patients have found pain relief with acupuncture. Sincerely, Very truly yours,
	After the closing in letters	The surgery is scheduled for August 12, 1999, at Grand General Hospital. Dr. Sally Halloway, M.D., will perform the surgery.
	With dates, addresses, titles, and numbers with more than four digits	There were 86,000 procedures performed in the United States last year.
Semicolon ;	To connect two sentences (independent clauses) that are not joined with a connecting word	Occupational therapists help patients regain as much normal function as possible after a serious injury; they also help patients adjust psychologically to their disabilities.
	To connect two independent clauses that are joined by a transitional expression (examples: however, also, therefore, furthermore, meanwhile, as a result, in conclusion)	I believe that medical care should be available to everyone in the United States; furthermore, it should be affordable.
Colon :	After an independent clause that is followed by a list	There are several habits that contribute to heart disease: smoking, a high-fat diet, lack of exercise, and psychological stress. Dear Dr. Chang:
	After the salutation in a formal business letter	
	With hours and minutes	Your appointment is at 4:15 P.M.
	With proportions	The ratio of medication to water should be 2:1.
Apostrophe '	To show possession	The patient's cast needs to be changed today. Please get John Bergen's file out for the dentist.
	To substitute for missing letters in contractions	Let's see if we can find better prices for these supplies. You're doing well with your therapy. It's a good method for sterilizing instruments.
Quotation marks " "	Around direct speech	"You should eat at least five servings of fruits and vegetables each day," said the dietitian.
	Around titles of articles, poems, short stories, songs, TV programs	"The Rising Costs of Health Care" article that appeared in today's paper was interesting.
	Note: Put periods and commas inside quotation marks. Put colons and semicolons outside quotation marks.	"Nova," a public television program, had a good review of current AIDS research.
Dash —	To give emphasis or more information	Diseases that were thought to be conquered—tuberculosis, measles, and hepatitis—have once again become public health concerns.
	To show a change of thought	Mrs. Crawford—who reminds me of my grandmother—comes in every Wednesday for chemotherapy treatment.

TABLE 6–7	Spelling Prescriptions		
Rules		**Examples**	**Exceptions**
I before E except after C or when the word sounds like AY, as in SAY		relieve receive neighbor weigh	either foreign height seizure
Drop final silent E when adding a **suffix** that begins with a **vowel** Keep final silent E when adding a suffix that begins with a **consonant**		achieve—achieving care—caring achieve—achievement care—careful	change—changeable argue—argument judge—judgment true—truly
When adding -ING to a word that ends in IE, replace the IE with Y		die—dying tie—tying	
Double the final consonant of a one-**syllable** word when adding a suffix that begins with a vowel *unless* there are two vowels or another consonant before the final consonant		trim—trimming look—looking test—testing	
PLURALS			
Add S to most words		disease—diseases wound—wounds	
Words that end in a consonant + Y: change the Y to an I and add ES		laboratory—laboratories pregnancy—pregnancies	
Words that end in S, SH, CH, and X: add ES		crutch—crutches cross—crosses	
Words that end in SIS: change to SES		diagnosis—diagnoses urinalysis—urinalyses	
Words that end in a vowel + O: add S		radio—radios	
Words that end in a consonant + O: add ES		echo—echoes	

encourage students to study. Most of us perform best when there is a consequence for our actions. In Chapter 3 we discussed how "good stress" can stimulate us physically and mentally to be alert and take appropriate actions. In the same way, you can harness the anxiety experienced when thinking about future tests to energize yourself and focus your efforts on learning. You can use tests to mark your progress toward achieving your long-term goal of becoming a competent health care professional—which is, after all, the real reason for learning.

Tests also teach you to work under pressure, which is a daily reality for health care professionals. You can never take your tasks for granted, and classroom tests provide practice for working calmly and efficiently when it counts. Planning and preparing ahead, thinking about what you are doing, and performing to the best of your ability are habits that apply to both test taking and work.

Finally, test results give you opportunities to improve and advance your learning. Answer sheets and scores are not for the exclusive use of your instructors. And contrary to what you might believe, assigning you a grade is not the only

purpose of tests. Take advantage of them to help you as a student. They identify what you know and don't know. Review your answers to discover which material you haven't mastered. What did you not understand? What do you need to ask the instructor? What should you review again? Fill the gaps in your knowledge now, while you are still in school. Don't brush off wrong answers and hope the knowledge all comes together on the job. Remember why you are in school: to learn the basics of your profession. Sometimes you will make mistakes, a fundamental student right. Learning from your mistakes is a fundamental student responsibility.

What Tests Are—and Are Not

"Think of a test as a challenge instead of a threat."
—*Walter Pauk*

Tests can turn otherwise sensible individuals into quivering masses of anxiety. For many students, the grades earned on tests influence their feeling of self-worth. You may be worried about appearing stupid

TABLE 6–8	**Commonly Misspelled Words**		
absence	disease	leisure	receipt
absorption	efficiency	license	receive
accessible	eighth	loneliness	recognize
accidentally	eligible	magazine	recommend
accommodate	eliminate	maintenance	reference
accumulate	embarrass	management	resuscitate
achievement	emphasize	maneuver	rhythm
acknowledge	encourage	marriage	safety
acquire	enthusiastic	miscellaneous	satisfactory
address	entirely	necessary	schedule
affiliated	environment	negligence,	scissors
aggravate	equipped	negligible	secretary
analyze	equivalent	neighbor	seize, seizure
appropriate	especially	noticeable	sensible
assistant	exaggerate	obstacle	separate
association	exercise	occasion,	several
athlete	exhausted	occasionally	severely
beginning	experience	occur, occurrence	significance
behavior	extremely	often	similar
belief	fascinate	original	sincerely
beneficial	fatigue	pamphlet	strategy
bureau	February	parallel	strictly
business, businesses	fluctuation	particular	substantial
cafeteria	foreign	patience	succeed
caffeine	forty	perform	success
calendar	fourth	persistent	surprise
cancel, canceled	fragile	physically	sympathy
column	friend	physician	technique
coming	government	pneumonia	temperature
commitment,	handkerchief	possession	thorough
committed	harass, harassment	practical	though
committee	height	precede	tongue
communicate	hygiene	preference	transferred
comparative	impatient	prejudice	typical
competition	indefinitely	privilege	until
cooperate	infinite	probably	urgent
correspond	intelligence	proceed	useful
criticism	interesting	prominent	usually
criticize	jewelry	psychiatry	vacuum
decision	judgment	psychology	vague
definitely	knowledge	qualified	vegetable
describe	knowledgeable	quantity	view
despair	label	questionnaire	Wednesday
develop	laboratory	quiet	weight
discipline	legitimate	quite	writing

Use the following space for your own spelling list

TABLE 6–9	**Commonly Confused Words**	
Words	**Meanings**	**Sample Hints for Learning**
accept	to take or receive	t<u>a</u>ke—<u>a</u>ccept
except	excluding, all but	<u>ex</u>clude—<u>ex</u>cept
access	way of entering	
excess	too much	<u>ex</u>tra—<u>ex</u>cess
adapt	adjust	<u>a</u>djust—<u>a</u>d<u>apt</u>
adopt	to take as one's own	<u>o</u>wn—ad<u>op</u>t
advice	helpful suggestions	
advise	to give advice	
affect	to influence	
effect	result; to bring about	
allowed	permitted	
aloud	capable of being heard	<u>loud</u> sound
already	before now, so soon	
all ready	completely prepared	It's <u>all</u> done.
capital	official seat of government; form of wealth	
capitol	building in which elected members of federal or state governments meet	
choose	to select	
chose	selected (past tense of "to select")	
coarse	rough	The dog has a rough <u>coat</u>.
course	class; path or track	<u>Our</u> class is on track.
conscience	part of the mind that determines right and wrong	
conscious	awake; aware	
council	governing body	
counsel	advice; to give advice	
defer	delay	d<u>e</u>lay
differ	to be different; to disagree	<u>differ</u>—<u>differ</u>ent
desert	dry land area	1 rain <u>s</u>hower in the desert.
dessert	eaten at the end of a meal	2 cups of <u>s</u>ugar in dessert
incompetent	unable to function properly and/or manage one's own affairs	
incontinent	unable to restrain the discharge of urine	
it's	contraction of "it is"	The apostrophe replaces the letter "i"
its	possessive form of "it"	
later	after the usual time	
latter	the second of two	2 Ts = 2nd of 2
lay	put or place something (past = laid)	
lie	rest on a surface (past = lay)	
	(Yes, these words are confusing!!)	
lead	type of metal; to guide; connecting wire	

TABLE 6–9	Commonly Confused Words—cont'd	
Words	**Meanings**	**Sample Hints for Learning**
led	guided (past tense of "lead")	
loose	not tight	Bigger word, like a shirt, is looser
lose	to be unable to find	I lost one O.
maybe	perhaps	
may be	possible, permissible	
miner	mine worker	
minor	younger than the legal age	
overdo	to do too much	
overdue	late or past due	
patience	quality of being uncomplaining, unhurried	
patients	people under medical care	
passed	went by, earned satisfactory grade	
past	before now, ended	
personal	private	
personnel	employees	
principal	head of a school, main or most important	The principal is your pal.
principle	general truth or rule	A principle is a rule.
stationary	not moving	Stay in one place
stationery	paper for writing letters	Letters are written on stationery
than	compared to	
then	at that time	
their	possessive of they	
there	in that place	
they're	contraction of "they are"	Apostrophe stands for the letter "a"
to	toward, for the purpose of	
too	also, very, more than enough	
two	2	
weather	climate conditions	Weather can be wet and windy
whether	introduces alternatives	
who's	contraction of "who is"	Apostrophe stands for the letter "i"
whose	possessive of "who"	
you're	contraction of "you are"	Apostrophe stands for the letter "a"
your	possessive of you	Our is possessive; so is your

and wonder if you have the ability to learn. Or you may feel insecure about your test-taking skills. In reality, your own personal experiences may be helpful in dealing with tests and other stressful situations. Although there is no denying that tests are used as indicators of progress by both instructors and students, understanding more about tests and their purpose can help you control them rather than letting them control you.

Good tests measure your knowledge and ability in specific areas. They can also measure how much you have packed into temporary memory as a result of last night's cram session, so they may or may not indicate the extent of true learning or your ability to perform effectively on the job. Tests, however, are never a measure of your value as a person. You can be an "A" in life even if you do not receive straight As in the classroom. See Box 6-1 for some other realities about tests.

 Go to page 178 to complete Prescription for Success 6-6

Preparing Effectively for Tests

The best way to prepare for tests is the same way you prepare yourself for career success: Start preparing early and study to learn because being prepared for tests means mastering the content of your courses. Let's review a few study techniques that lead to successful test taking:

- Manage your time so that studying is a priority.
- Identify and use study techniques that correspond with your preferred learning styles.
- Use learning techniques that help move information into your long-term memory.
- Take good notes in class and review them often.
- Read textbooks actively and review them regularly.
- Seek help early if you are having trouble.

In addition to practicing good study habits, there are specific steps you can take to prepare for important tests.

1. Find out as much as possible about the test. Gather your notes and handouts and ask the instructor for suggestions on how to best prepare. Suggested questions to ask your instructor: "What type of questions will be asked (such as multiple choice and true-false)?" "Will there be a time limit?" "Will it be given at the beginning or end of class?" "Will you review first?"

2. Quickly review your notes, textbook, handouts, and any other class materials to check your comprehension. Is there anything you don't understand or can't remember, even after reviewing? Write a list of questions about the subject to ask in class. (This is why you start your review early, not the night before the exam!)

3. Make a schedule, and divide what you have to review over the time you have available so you won't run out of time before you have a chance to review everything (another good reason to start reviewing a few days before the test).

4. Review your textbook and use any supporting materials that came with it such as a companion website or CD.

5. Use the study tools you developed when you reviewed throughout the class—or create some now! Here are a few ideas:

   ☐ Keywords or questions to prompt recall of notes and text.

BOX 6-1 **Realities about Tests**

- **Tests ask for only samples of what you are expected to know.** Many students express disappointment when everything they studied does not appear on a test. They believe they have wasted their time and should have had to study only what was going to be on the test. The truth is that health care professionals must know a great deal of information. If instructors included everything on tests that students should know, there would be time only for testing and none left for teaching! Samples are reliable indicators of overall knowledge. For example, if you are expected to learn 1000 medical terms, the instructor may randomly select 50 for a test. The percentage of those 50 that you know is a good indication of how many of the 1000 you know. Or if you must know the steps to follow in 12 procedures you will use on the job, you may be asked in a classroom test to give the steps for three of the procedures. Keep in mind that you are learning for the future: certification exams and job performance. Knowing more than what is on the test is a requirement for job success, not a waste of your time.
- **Classroom tests provide instructors with feedback about their teaching.** They are paid to educate you, not to fail you! Tests help them adjust their classroom strategies to ensure that their students have every opportunity to master the subject and skills. If many students do poorly on all or part of a test, it may be an indication the information was not presented effectively and needs to be repeated.
- **Poorly prepared tests do exist.** Test writing is a skill, and good test questions are not easy to create. Even instructors with good intentions may write some questions that are unclear and confusing. They may teach more than one class and forget exactly which material was—and was not—presented in each section. They may ask questions that are different from those they announced would be on the test. This does happen, and the best strategy is to ask the instructor politely to review the information. If the problem continues, meet with the instructor privately to discuss the situation.

   ☐ Outlines, charts, or mind maps to help you organize the material and make it meaningful for you.

   ☐ Flash cards to practice recall. Put aside the ones that you know well and concentrate on the ones you have the most difficulty remembering. Your goal is to move all cards into the "know-these" pile.

   ☐ Saying aloud or writing answers to your prompts and practice questions.

6. Identify and concentrate on the material you find most difficult and have the most trouble remembering. Don't keep restudying material

Go to page 179 to complete Prescription for Success 6-7

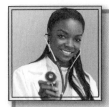

Test Taking On The Job

Many of the strategies that work for successful test taking have applications in health care work.

FOLLOW DIRECTIONS

This is a big one in health care. Your ability to follow directions can affect the safety of patients and the quality of your work. Examples include being willing and able to take direction from a supervisor, reading and understanding the instructions for a piece of equipment, following the steps to perform a laboratory test, and staying within legal guidelines for your occupation.

ASK FOR CLARIFICATION OF DIRECTIONS

You must be able to ask your supervisor questions about any aspect of your work that you don't understand.

KEEP YOUR COOL

Work in health care can be fast-paced. And you'll often be dealing with people who are frightened, in pain, and stressed out. Working calmly and carefully under all kinds of conditions is essential.

CHECK YOUR WORK FOR ACCURACY

Checking your work is another health care skill to ensure safety and accuracy. For example, it is essential to always check the identity of any patient you are working with. And a medication is never given to a patient until the label identifying it has been checked *at least three times*.

that you know. (Except when you are deliberately overlearning, as discussed in Chapter 3.)

7. Use the practice questions and quizzes you created from your class notes and from your reading. This may be the single best way to ensure you are prepared for classroom tests.

The Anxiety Monster

You have studied throughout the class, you have reviewed for the test, and you feel pretty secure about your knowledge of the material, but you are panic-stricken by the idea of your final exam. You just know you'll freeze up and won't be able to remember a thing. You may even feel physically ill when you enter the classroom on test days. There just doesn't seem to be any way around it—you just "can't take tests." This is a real problem for many students, and solving it is an important step toward achieving your professional goals. Following is a list of actions to help you manage test anxiety:

☐ Evaluate your study habits and test-review methods. Can you improve them? Are you really using your study time efficiently? For example, some students spend a lot of time reading notes over and over but never actually quizzing themselves without looking at the written information. They think they know it, but without their book or notes, they can't remember very much.

☐ Think about your actual test preparation. It may seem like you are spending a lot of time reviewing because you feel worn out by it. In reality, if you engage in a marathon review session the last 2 days before the test, you may feel as if you studied a lot but are too tired to remember much of the material.

☐ Be honest with yourself. Do you have trouble understanding in your classes but don't ask for help because you are embarrassed? Remember that instructors are there to help you, and asking for help is not nearly as embarrassing as failing a test or finding that you lack information needed to perform your job. Have you been an active participant in class? Do you lack the time after class to stay for extra help? Is there another reason? If you are serious about achieving your career goals, you must decide to make school a priority and organize your life so that you can study when and as much as needed.

☐ Don't let your classmates freak you out. If you worry about competing with them, such as finishing the test first or earning a higher grade, you can get distracted from focusing on your own performance. Your education is not a race with winners and losers; the goal of a health care program is for everyone to win by graduating as a competent professional. Although the awarding of grades tends to set up a competitive environment, modern health care is delivered by teams of individuals who must work cooperatively, not competitively. Some classmates are even more anxious about tests than you. These people often express their nervousness by talking a lot and predicting total gloom and doom. Be upbeat with them rather than letting their negative talk increase your own anxiety. Avoid participating in "ain't it awful" conversations around test time.

☐ Join forces with positive students. Organize a small group to review, share ideas, quiz one another, and cheer one another on. Have each person make up a few test questions and quiz the others. Seek out classmates who are dependable and will contribute to the group. Keep the number small (three to five) so that everyone can make a contribution. If the group is too large, it can be very difficult to plan meetings that accommodate everyone's schedule.

☐ Use visualizations and positive self-talk to promote learning and good test performance.

☐ Practice good health habits and the stress management techniques described in Chapter 3. Remember that physical exercise releases endorphins, the body's natural tranquilizers. Do your best to get enough sleep before major tests so that you're not exhausted and more subject to anxiety. Finally, the relaxation exercise described in Chapter 3 is effective just before taking a test. Take deep breaths to help quiet the mind. Help your body work for instead of against you.

If you review thoroughly and try the suggestions for relieving anxiety, but still find yourself freezing up during exams and feeling as if even dynamite couldn't blast facts out of your brain, you can try a technique called "desensitization." This is a treatment developed for people who have anxieties that interfere with their daily lives. It works by providing exposure to small doses of the source of the fear and then gradually increasing the size and number of exposures.[5] Develop a plan to increase your exposure to tests. Have a friend or family member make up and give you tests, starting with short quizzes. Make them as realistic as possible. For example, set and stay within a time limit. Ask your instructor to give you practice tests. Find out if you can take these in a classroom under conditions as close to those of a real test as possible. Many sponsors of professional exams have sample tests you can take. These techniques may seem like a lot of work and even a little embarrassing, but if test anxiety is running your future career off track, desensitization is worth trying.

Tripping Yourself Up

Some students procrastinate in preparing for tests (and starting other projects, such as term papers) because they are afraid of failing. Their fear causes a kind of paralysis that prevents them from taking positive steps to prepare. For other students, not studying creates an excuse for failure. After all, if they try their best and still fail an exam, this might mean they lack ability. Another problem is feeling overwhelmed. Students who feel there is just too much to learn may decide to give up without

really trying. If any of these behaviors sound familiar, make a deal with yourself to try something new. Study throughout the course, use the suggestions in this chapter on preparing for tests, ask for help, and work with a study group. The chances are very good you will experience success, and that can be habit-forming!

The Day of the Test

Okay, it's the day of the test and you feel reasonably prepared. You certainly don't want to perform poorly because you fail to follow some common sense test-taking guidelines. Here are some helpful hints you can apply to any test situation:

☐ You deserve a good start, so plan to arrive early. Don't stress yourself out by rushing in late, scrambling to find a seat, and missing the introductory instructions.

☐ Bring your supplies, including books, notes, and a calculator (if these are allowed). An erasable pen (blue or black ink) works well because you can make corrections neatly and your instructor will be able to read your answers.

☐ Read and/or listen to all instructions. Ask the instructor to explain anything you don't understand. This is not the time to be shy. You have a right to know exactly what is expected.

☐ Quickly review the *entire* test before starting. Read *all* directions on every page. If you have questions and the test has begun, go to the instructor and ask them quietly.

☐ If there are different types of questions, note which ones will take the most time to answer and/or are worth the most points. Then quickly plan how to divide your time among the different parts of the test.

☐ If the test is longer and/or more difficult than you expected, do *not* panic. Take a deep breath, follow the guidelines, answer the easiest questions first, and focus on doing your best.

☐ Give yourself a boost by answering the easiest questions first. When there are different types of questions, it is usually best to move from the shortest to the longest answers: true-false, multiple-choice, matching, fill-in, short essay, long essay. This is like giving yourself a warm-up. Also, the questions that have the answers provided for you to choose from may give you ideas for questions in which you must supply the answers from recall.

☐ Limit the time you spend on questions you find very difficult or don't know. Mark them and return later after you complete the rest.

☐ Proofread your answers before you turn in your test. Did you answer all the questions? Mark the correct boxes on the answer sheet? Follow all directions correctly? Check for spelling errors, words left out, and other careless errors.

☐ Use all the time allowed if you need it. You don't earn extra points by finishing early, and hurrying may cost you a few correct answers.

Specific Test-Taking Techniques

A message repeated throughout this book is the importance of mastering the knowledge and skills presented in your classes. The well-being of patients depends on what and how well health care professionals learn. The purpose of studying is to learn for the future, not just to pass tests. And the *best* way to prepare for tests is to know your material well.[6] That said, it is also true that learning about commonly used test formats can help you be more effective in showing what you know. Students who are unfamiliar with question formats can waste time and energy figuring them out.

It is important to keep in mind that some of the techniques suggested for answering test questions would be downright dangerous if applied to work in health care. For example, most study skills books recommend that if there is no penalty for incorrect answers, go ahead and guess. With true-false questions, you have a 50-50 chance; with most multiple-choice questions, the chance is 25%. But there is no room in health care for a 50-50 chance of correct performance. Some tasks, such as administering medications, must be 100% correct. There is no guesswork allowed here!

The suggestions given in the following sections are based on the experience of many students. However, they are only guidelines and do not substitute for knowledge.

True-False Questions

Purpose

Test your recognition of correct facts, statements, and cause-and-effect relationships, as well as your ability to distinguish fact from opinion.

Examples

Read each of the following statements. If the statement is true, circle the T. If it is false, circle the F.

T F **1.** Classroom tests are always good indicators of how well students understand a subject.

T F **2.** Test performance can be improved by cramming as much as possible the day before the test is given.

T F **3.** Reviewing material regularly throughout the course is the best way to do well on tests.

Suggested Techniques for Answering

☐ Be sure that every part of the answer is correct. If any part of it is false, the entire answer is false.

☐ Watch out for words like "always" and "never." Few things in life are that final, and statements with these words are often false. (There are exceptions, however. For example, there are safety rules in health care that must always be followed and legal rules, such as those concerning the release of patient records, that can never be violated.)

☐ Answers with middle-of-the-road words like "usually," "sometimes," and "often" tend to be true (except as previously noted).

☐ Do not spend a lot of time on true-false questions you really don't know, especially if they are at the beginning of a test that also contains more time-consuming questions

☐ Guess only as a last resort (and only if there is no penalty).

Multiple Choice Questions

Purpose

Test your knowledge of terminology, specific facts, principles, methods, and procedures.

Examples

Circle the letter to the left of the response that best answers each question.

1. Which is the best reason for learning to spell correctly?
   A. Patients are impressed by correct spelling.
   B. Patient care can be negatively affected if words are misspelled on medical documentation.
   C. Students who spell correctly get better grades in school.
   D. It increases the chances of receiving a promotion at work.

2. The Cornell note-taking system has proven helpful to students because it:
   A. prevents them from having to review notes after class.
   B. helps them record everything the instructor says.
   C. provides a format that encourages review.
   D. teaches specific active listening techniques.

Suggested Techniques for Answering

☐ Read the instructions and questions carefully. If the question asks you to identify the "best" answer, it is possible that more than one is correct. In the first sample question, all answers are good reasons for spelling correctly. So you need to think about which is the most important reason, and that is patient safety. Therefore B is the correct answer.

☐ If the direction states to select the correct answer (as opposed to the "best," "most complete," etc.), consider each statement separately and ask yourself if it is true or false. (Many professional exams, such as the Certified Medical Assistant exam, are multiple choice.)

☐ Read through all the answers before selecting one.

☐ Immediately eliminate answers that are obviously incorrect.

☐ If the answer requires a math calculation, do the problem yourself before you look at the answers.

☐ Match each answer to the question rather than comparing the answers to each other.

☐ If you are guessing, choose an answer that has information you recognize.

☐ You can sometimes eliminate choices by using logic. For example, if two answers say basically the same thing, they must both be incorrect. As with true-false answers, if any part of a statement is wrong, the entire answer must be wrong. If the answer is silly or farfetched (instructors sometimes like to have a little fun), eliminate it immediately.

☐ If you are allowed to write on the test, circle or underline key words in the question to focus your attention when you read the answers.

Matching Questions

Purpose

Recognize definitions of terms and identify correct facts based on simple associations.

Examples

On the line to the left of each number in Column A, write the letter from Column B that explains one of its uses.

COLUMN A	COLUMN B
_____ 1. Comma	A. Substitutes for letters that are dropped when contractions are formed
_____ 2. Semicolon	B. Indicates a change of thought within a sentence
_____ 3. Colon	C. Connects two sentences into one long sentence when a connective word is used
_____ 4. Apostrophe	D. Follows the greeting in a formal business letter
_____ 5. Dash	E. Connects two sentences into one long sentence without the use of a connective word
	F. Is placed at the end of a sentence

Suggested Techniques for Answering

☐ Read the instructions carefully. Note whether any item can be used more than once.

☐ Quickly count each column to see if both columns have the same number of items. Sometimes they do not. It is possible that an item may be used more than once.

☐ Read through both columns before you write in any answers.

☐ Do the ones you know first.

☐ Some students find it easier to read the longer answers first (usually placed in the right-hand column) and then look for the shorter match. See which method works best for you.

☐ Mark or cross out each item as you use it, if you are allowed to write on the test paper.

Fill-in-the-Blank Questions

Purpose

Test your ability to recall terminology, facts, and procedures and to interpret information.

Examples

Fill in each blank with a word or phrase that correctly completes the sentence.

1. The huge group of interconnecting computers located around the world is called the _____.

2. Learners who are both visual and global sometimes find that _____ is a useful note-taking technique to record information in a way that clearly shows relationships.

3. An explanation of why a procedure is performed in a certain way is called the _____.

Suggested Techniques for Answering

☐ Read the entire statement before attempting to fill in the blank(s).

☐ Write answers that fit the form and content of the words around them. For example, if the last word before the blank is "the," you know the answer is a noun.

☐ It sometimes helps to convert the phrase into a question in which the answer is the correct fill-in.

☐ The length of the space may be a clue to the answer, but there is a chance the person who typed the test didn't even know the answers and randomly chose the lengths. This is not a reliable way to select an answer.

Short-Answer Questions

Purpose

Recall facts and definitions or write explanations that demonstrate your understanding.

Examples

Write a short answer to each of the following questions using the spaces provided. Some questions have several parts. Your answers do not need to be complete sentences.

1. List three reasons why many educators recommend using a three-ring binder to keep your notes and class materials in order.
2. Explain why previewing is a critical part of the reading process.
3. Describe four ways of starting to write a paper when you are having trouble determining exactly what to write and/or how to organize it.

Suggested Techniques for Answering

☐ Read the instructions to find key words that tell you exactly what is expected in the answer. Are you asked to explain? Give two examples? List five reasons? Define? Give the steps?

☐ If you are asked to write several sentences, answer the question as directly and completely as possible without padding with unnecessary information.

☐ If you don't know the entire answer, write down as much as you do know. You may receive partial credit.

Essay Questions

Purpose

Demonstrate ability to select, organize, relate, evaluate, and present ideas. These questions provide an opportunity to show what you know about the topic.

Example

Write a well-organized essay at least one-page long explaining the meaning of this statement: "Study skills are career skills." Support your answer with examples and references to SCANS and the National Health Care Skill Standards. You will be graded on how well you demonstrate understanding of the concept, as well as on spelling and grammar.

Suggested Techniques for Answering

☐ As with the short-answer questions, read the instructions to find out what you are supposed to include in your answer. Provide evidence for your response? Give examples to illustrate? Give the sequence? Explain reasons and purposes? Defend your answer? Compare and contrast?

☐ Don't write answers that are too short. Even if the question does not specifically ask for examples or evidence, you should fully explain or defend your answer.

☐ Don't spend time with a lot of words that don't really mean anything, such as repeating the question or writing a long introduction. Answer questions directly.

☐ If you have trouble organizing an answer in your head, quickly jot down a few key ideas, an outline, or a mind map.

☐ Use the rule journalists use when they write a newspaper article: state the most important information first by answering the question as quickly as possible. Use the rest of the time to develop your answer, write examples, provide evidence, and so on. This way, if you run out of time, you know you have included the most important information.

☐ Include the principal ideas of the course, as appropriate, especially ones the instructor emphasized.

☐ Use the principles of good writing discussed in this chapter.

After the Test

Much as you'd like to forget about the test you just took, don't. Just like athletes who analyze each game to learn which plays worked and which didn't, you can use debriefing to your advantage. As soon as possible after finishing the test, review your notes and books to find the answers to the questions you were unsure about or just didn't know.

When the test is returned in class, try not to react emotionally. If you earned a top score, give yourself credit. Continue to review the material from time to time to reinforce and retain important facts and information. If you did poorly, don't lose heart. Instead, try the following:

- Listen to any review the instructor gives of the test.
- If you have to return it to the instructor, take notes on a separate sheet of paper.
- Pay special attention to the questions you missed and write down the correct answers.
- If the instructor explains information, be sure to take notes.
- Ask questions about anything you don't understand.
- If your instructor does not discuss the test with the class and you did poorly, make an appointment to discuss it privately.

At your earliest opportunity, review your notes and the marks you made in your books. Did you miss some of the major points? Study the wrong material? Not really understand it? What can you do to improve your performance next time? See Table 6-10 for suggestions on dealing with test problems commonly encountered by students.

TABLE 6-10	Common Test-Taking Problems
The Problem	**What to Do**
You didn't study at all or waited until the last minute and crammed.	You know what to do!
You studied but couldn't remember the information when you needed it for the test.	Check your understanding. Information you don't comprehend well can be very difficult to remember. Did you use prompts to study and review the material without looking at the answers? Or did you simply reread your notes and textbook? Passive review, simply looking at the material, is not an effective learning technique for most people.
You were extremely anxious during the test and froze.	Review the section in this chapter on anxiety and try using the techniques. If they don't work for you, seek additional help.
You made careless errors.	Allow time to proofread your test before turning it in.
You didn't understand what the questions meant.	When you are studying, be sure to look up any words you don't know. During the test, ask the instructor for clarification. If English is your second language, see your instructor for help.
The questions were not what you expected. For example, you memorized a list of facts and definitions, but the test asked you to apply information to new situations.	Review your notes or other information about the test to see if you misunderstood. Be sure to attend all classes so you will hear announcements about test content. If you believe the instructor was unclear about the format and/or content of the test, speak to him or her privately. Critical thinking and problem-solving skills, which involve applying information to new situations, such as test questions, are discussed in Chapter 7.

A WORD ABOUT PROFESSIONAL EXAMS

Many health care professions have exams you must pass to work in the field. The purpose of professional exams is to ensure high standards for practitioners by testing for knowledge and competence. These exams may be administered by a governmental agency or a professional organization. Passing them allows the professional to use one of several special designations such as "licensed," "certified," or "registered." Most exams require a fee. Your school may have included this cost in your tuition or fees. The school may also assist you in applying to take the exam. Some exams are given year round, others only on certain dates. Find out whether professional exams are required for your occupation. Learn as much as possible about the exam(s) while you are still in school.

Some professions do not require formal approval (certification, licensing, etc.) for graduates to work. At the same time, voluntary testing is available and recommended for many careers. For example, most states do not have licensing requirements for medical assistants. (States do regulate what procedures medical assistants can and cannot perform.) Many physicians, however, prefer to hire only certified or registered medical assistants, designations earned by passing professional exams administered by the American

Association of Medical Assistants and the American Medical Technologists, respectively. Some medical insurance companies require physicians to hire only credentialed professionals.

Success Tips for Passing Professional Exams

☐ Start preparing early (note the word is "prepare," not "worry"). This suggestion is not intended to add further stress to your already busy class and study schedule. It is a reminder that if you prepare over a period of time, you will learn more and experience less stress when the time comes to actually take the test.

☐ Keep your notes, handouts, and textbooks organized so you can find and use them for review before the exam.

☐ Pay attention to any information and advice your instructor gives you about the content of professional exams.

☐ Some textbooks refer to specific exams and requirements of professional organizations, and the authors of the textbooks design their content and review questions to help students prepare throughout their courses. Take advantage of these features!

☐ Find out if there are any review books available in your school library or for purchase or online materials to help you focus your studies on mastering the material likely to appear on the exam.

☐ Practice tests are available for many exams. Check with your professional organization.

☐ Find out whether review workshops are available in your area.

☐ Plan to take the exam as soon as possible after you become eligible. This is usually on graduation from your program, although some occupations also require work experience. You are less likely to forget information and lose your confidence if you do not wait too long.

☐ Think of the timed tests you take in school as opportunities to practice taking an important exam under pressure.

SOME HONEST TALK ABOUT CHEATING

Health care professionals must follow high ethical standards. High-quality patient care and safety depend on their actions, and there is no room for cheating in any form. Furthermore, governmental regulations have increased, and **audits** of health care facilities are common. The consequences for **fraud**, taking shortcuts, and even trying to just "get by" are severe, including costly fines and closures of health care facilities.

You may believe cheating on tests in school isn't as serious as cheating on the job, but this is not true. Health care graduates who cheat to pass their classes, instead of learning what they need to know on the job, may become dangerous practitioners. You are in the process of becoming a professional, and what you do now is setting the groundwork for your future actions. Integrity (honesty, sincerity) is an essential characteristic of the health care professional, and cheating undermines that integrity. Cheating is an unsatisfactory and potentially destructive way of approaching your education. It converts the opportunities offered by tests to develop effective study habits and to learn what you need to know into unacceptable behaviors.

Even if you do not cheat yourself, helping others to do so promotes incompetence in the health care system. Would you or one of your family members want to be treated by "professionals" who cheated to pass their classes? Do you want to carry the load at work for a co-worker who is used to taking the easy way out? Helping friends cheat allows them to avoid taking responsibility for themselves. This can lead to the habit of dependence and unsatisfactory performance on the job, resulting in negative consequences for everyone.

PERSONAL REFLECTION

What are some possible future effects on the job for students who passed their classes by cheating instead of studying?

_____

_____

_____

_____

_____

⇨ SUMMARY OF KEY IDEAS

1. Your competence is often judged by your writing ability.
2. Writing correctly takes effort and practice.
3. It is never too late to improve your spelling and grammar skills.
4. Tests are part of life.
5. Test anxiety can be conquered.
6. The best preparation for a test is to know the material.

Positive Self-Talk for This Chapter

1. I write clearly and effectively.
2. I spell and use grammar correctly.
3. I use the act of writing to help me learn new material.
4. I use tests to motivate me to do my best in school.
5. I prepare in advance for all my tests.
6. I manage test anxiety effectively.

To Learn More

Elbow P: *Writing with power: techniques for mastering the writing process*, New York, 1998, Oxford University Press.

This is one of the best books on writing I have found. It has many techniques to help you effectively put what you want to say on paper.

Hacker D: *A writer's reference*, ed 6, Boston, 2007, Bedford/St. Martin's.

This is an excellent, easy-to-use book that includes explanations and examples of grammar, sentence structure, punctuation, and organization of content.

Pauk W: *How to study in college,* ed 7, New York, 2005, Houghton Mifflin.

Professor Pauk developed many original and practical ideas to help students study more effectively.

Purdue University's Online Writing Lab.

http://owl.english.purdue.edu

Purdue offers information on dozens of topics related to writing of all types in its award-winning writing lab.

REFERENCES

1. National Consortium on Health Science and Technology Education: *National Healthcare Foundation Standards and Accountability Criteria.* Available at: www.nchste.org/cms/wp-content/uploads/2008/03/foundation_standards_ac_rev_01_08. (Accessed 2/13/09)

2. Ellis D, Toft D, Mancina D, McMurray E: *Becoming a master student,* ed 12, Boston, 2009, Houghton Mifflin.

3. Elbow P: *Writing with power: techniques for mastering the writing process,* New York, 1998, Oxford University Press.

4. Palau SM, Meltzer M: *Learning strategies for allied health students,* St Louis, 2007, Elsevier.

5. Fry R: *How to study,* ed 6, Franklin Lakes, Clifton Park, NY, 2004, Delmar Cengage.

6. Pauk W: *How to study in college,* ed 7, New York, 2005, Houghton Mifflin.

BUILDING YOUR RESUME

1. Review the Resume Building Block #5 form at the end of Chapter 2. Learn more about any exams needed to become licensed or certified in your career. Are there strategies in the test-taking sections of this chapter you can apply to start preparing for these exams?

2. Consider how developing your writing skills will help you put together a well-worded resume.

INTERNET ACTIVITIES

For active links to the websites needed to complete these activities, visit **http://evolve.elsevier.com/Haroun/career/**.

1. Purdue University has an excellent online writing lab that includes information sheets and quizzes. Explore areas you find interesting or with which you have problems and write a short summary of what you learn.

2. The *Merriam-Webster Dictionary* website includes definitions, pronunciation, and word games. Choose 10 unfamiliar words from this book or any of your other textbooks. Find the definitions and write a sentence using each word.

3. Study Guides and Strategies has an extensive list of topics in its resources. Read about at least two of the topics listed under "Preparing for Tests" to find techniques you can use.

4. Western Washington University has a good online tutorial center. Look for their hints on studying for exams, including a useful checklist. Try using this checklist when you are preparing for your next big exam.

Prescription for Success 6-1
What's the Purpose?

What do you think would be the major purpose of each of the following writing projects?

1. A three-page report about a skin disease that includes the causes, methods of diagnosis, and treatment.

   _____

2. An instruction sheet explaining how patients with leg casts can take a shower without getting the cast wet.

   _____

3. An **essay** in which you explain why quitting smoking can improve the quality of and increase the length of a person's life.

   _____

4. A letter asking for a transfer to a job at your facility that requires more experience than you currently have but for which you feel you are qualified.

   _____

5. A letter of recommendation for a co-worker who is moving to another state.

   _____

6. A letter to your local newspaper in which you express your ideas about the lack of affordable medical care for the poor.

   _____

7. Directions for using the office copy and facsimile (fax) machines.

   _____

Prescription for Success 6-2
Addressing Your Readers

Explain how instructions you write for a co-worker would differ from those you write for a patient.

_____

_____

_____

_____

Explain in what ways a letter asking for a job interview would differ from a letter you write to a friend.

_____

_____

_____

_____

Prescription for Success 6-3
What Works for You?

1. Which of the organizational techniques presented do you think best fits your learning style?

_____

2. Explain why.

_____

_____

3. Describe any other organizational or writing techniques that have worked for you.

_____

_____

_____

Prescription for Success 6-4
How's Your Grammar?

1. How would you rate your knowledge of English grammar?

   _____ Excellent _____ Very Good _____ Good _____ Fair _____ Poor

2. If you scored yourself "Fair" or "Poor," what can you do to improve?

   _____ Take classes at school

   _____ Use special services at school, such as a computer lab or tutoring program

   _____ Study on my own

   _____ Workbooks

   _____ Software

   _____ Videos

   _____ Other

Prescription for Success 6-5
How's Your Spelling?

1. Quiz yourself by having someone read the words in Tables 6-8 and 6-9 for you to spell.
2. After correcting your quiz, separate out any words that you missed. (Didn't miss any? Congratulations! Skip the rest of the assignment and consider volunteering to help classmates who have difficulty with spelling.)
3. For those of you who missed a few words, make a commitment to learn them in the next few weeks. Devise your own study plan, and reward yourself when you reach your learning goals.

Prescription for Success 6-6
Make Tests Work for You

Describe five ways you can use tests to your advantage as you prepare for a career in health care.

1. _____

_____

_____

_____

_____

2. _____

_____

_____

_____

_____

3. _____

_____

_____

_____

_____

4. _____

_____

_____

_____

_____

5. _____

_____

_____

_____

_____

Prescription for Success 6-7
Studying for a Test

1. Choose at least three study techniques to use when you prepare for your next test. List the ideas here.

   Technique 1: _____

   Technique 2: _____

   Technique 3: _____

2. Create a plan for using these ideas, including the actions you will take and a study schedule.

   _____

   _____

   _____

   _____

   _____

   _____

   _____

   _____

3. After you have taken the test, write a paragraph describing how the techniques worked for you.

   _____

   _____

   _____

   _____

   _____

   _____

   _____

   _____

   _____

   _____

CHAPTER 7

Developing Your Practical Skills

OBJECTIVES

The information and activities in this chapter can help you:

- Apply strategies to help you get the most benefit from laboratory sessions and master hands-on skills.
- Explain the importance of knowing how to apply math skills in health care.
- Approach the learning of math with a positive attitude and, if necessary, apply techniques to overcome math anxiety.
- Evaluate your own math skills and, if needed, devise a plan to improve them.
- List the purposes and benefits of the educational clinical experience.
- Describe how to maximize learning and gain the most benefits from clinical experience.
- Develop skill in using a problem-solving process to make good decisions in both your personal and your professional lives.
- Plan and start putting together a personal reference guide to help you in school, during your job search, and on the job.

KEY TERMS AND CONCEPTS

Aptitude: The ability to learn and apply new knowledge and skills.

Brainstorming: A problem-solving technique in which you generate as many ideas as possible without judging them for quality or practicality.

Contaminate: To make impure or infect by introducing organisms, such as bacteria, that can cause disease.

Critical thinking: A process of thinking purposefully in which you apply knowledge and use logic and reasoning to guide your actions, make decisions, and select the best choice among alternatives.

Dosage: The amount of medication to be administered.

Evaluate: To judge or determine the worth or condition of something.

Math anxiety: The fear of math. People with math anxiety don't believe they have the ability to learn math.

Metric system: A system of measurement used throughout the world that is based on meters (length), grams (weight), and liters (volume).

Nursing process: An orderly approach to patient care that nurses use to identify and resolve patients' health problems.

Protective equipment: Special clothing and accessories worn by health care workers to protect themselves against body fluids that may be infectious. Also referred to as personal protective equipment (PPE).

Role play: A way of practicing interpersonal exchanges in which students play the parts of health care professionals, patients, supervisors, and co-workers.

Standard or universal precautions: Practices for preventing the transmission of infection via body fluids.

Theory: Ideas and knowledge as seen in the mind. Also refers to systematic statements of principles.

LEARNING PRACTICAL SKILLS

Most jobs in health care involve a lot of hands-on activity, and the level of your performance is critical to your success on the job. Future health care professionals must master a variety of skills. Depending on your specific occupation, these skills range from filling out forms accurately to performing a urinalysis to taking an x-ray film. Learning to apply the theory you learn in class to practical situations is one of the most important components of your education.

It is important that students take learning practical skills as seriously as studying for their **theory** courses. This is because hands-on practice builds a bridge between school and the world of work, as illustrated in Figure 7-1. There is a big difference between knowing about a procedure and being able to actually do it well. Actually performing a blood draw, for example, is much different from hearing about it. Practice sessions provide you with opportunities to take risks in a safe, monitored environment where you can learn from your experience—and from your mistakes.

At the same time, it is important to learn the theory and background information that support the procedures you will practice in the lab. For example, giving injections requires an understanding of the principles of infection control. Insurance coding requires knowledge of basic human anatomy terminology and medical diagnoses.

LEARNING IN THE LAB

Depending on your program of study, practice may include performing procedures, engaging in **role play**, working on the computer, and completing pencil-and-paper activities. You may solve problems, work with "patients," conduct tests, or do calculations.

Being Prepared for Lab Sessions

Advance preparation will help you benefit fully from lab sessions. Lab time is often limited, and the instructor will expect you to get started on the assigned activities without delay. The first step in being prepared is to read your textbook. Don't depend on your instructor's explanations or on being able to "figure it out." Reading gives you time to think through the steps and, as we discussed in Chapter 5, gives you a framework for lectures and demonstrations. Many health care textbooks present procedures in recipe or how-to format. Read through each step. Note all hints and cautions that contain important safety information for you and the patient.

In addition to reading your textbook, study the illustrations. Are the health care professionals wearing gloves? How are they positioned in relation to the patients and equipment? What do the equipment and instruments look like? How are they held? In which direction should movements be made? For example, in disinfecting a surgical site on the skin, it is important that cleansing be done in a circular motion, moving from the center toward the outside edges, to not **contaminate** areas already cleaned. The effectiveness of a procedure is often based on details such as these.

If your instructor demonstrates a procedure in class, focus on the steps or actions involved. Take notes only if doing so doesn't prevent you from watching and listening. If action is involved, mirror

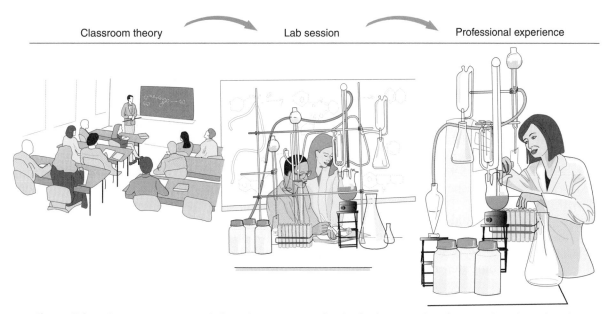

Classroom theory   Lab session   Professional experience

Figure 7-1   Laboratory sessions and clinical practice provide a bridge between class theory and work on the job.

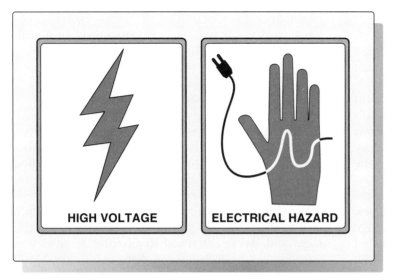

HIGH VOLTAGE   **ELECTRICAL HAZARD**

Figure 7-2   Pay special attention to all warnings and safety rules when working in the lab. In addition to maintaining a safe learning environment, this is good practice for when you are on the job and responsible for the safety of others. (*From Stepp CA:* Woods' laboratory procedures for medical office personnel, *Philadelphia, 1998, Saunders.*)

the instructor as closely as possible. For example, when watching a demonstration of the proper way to hold a syringe, use your highlighter or pen to copy the motion. Developing the ability to observe carefully is, in itself, a valuable health care skill.

Don't hesitate to ask questions about any point you don't understand. Get as complete an understanding as possible before going to the lab, to minimize mistakes and avoid wasting practice time.

Last—but very important!—pay special attention to learning safety rules. Many textbooks, as well as labs, use warning diagrams like the ones shown in Figure 7-2. Your future job may require you to operate expensive and potentially dangerous equipment and to handle chemical and biological hazards. The human immunodeficiency virus (HIV) and the hepatitis B virus can be spread by mishandling blood and certain body fluids. Laws regulate the proper disposal of contaminated items. All health care professionals must learn and follow the **standard or universal precautions** developed by the U.S. Centers for Disease Control and Prevention. The time to start applying these precautions is in your lab classes.

Success Tips for Learning in the Lab

☐ Take along any study materials, reference books, supplies, or **protective equipment** needed to participate in the scheduled activities. Set them out the evening before if you have an early start the day of the lab.

☐ Work with "real patients." Treat the students you work with in lab as you would if you were on the job. Demonstrate courtesy and concern. (Remember, "Your career starts now.") If you are entering patient data on the computer or practicing patient scheduling, work as if the exercises involved real people who are depending on your ability to maintain accurate and efficient records and schedules.

☐ Aim for accuracy. All health care tasks depend on accuracy to ensure safe, high-level patient care. You will also be expected to follow various laws and regulations, both in the lab and on the job. In many procedures, "almost correct" is not good enough. Only perfection is acceptable. For example, a sterile field is a germ-free area prepared to prevent infection during procedures such as minor surgeries. It is either sterile or it is not. Brushing an ungloved hand against an object in the sterile field may seem like a small error, but the field is no longer sterile. Work carefully in the lab. Never skip a step because this is "just practice" and these are not "real surgeries" or "real medications." When establishing your work habits, it is important that everything you do be done as realistically as possible.

☐ Respect your instructor's time, but do ask questions as needed. If the instructor is busy observing or assisting other students, write down your questions so you won't forget them.

☐ Understand that there may be more than one correct way to perform a task. Your instructors, as well as future supervisors, may each have different ways of performing a procedure. The important thing is that your technique follows accepted practice and is safe for both you and your patients.

☐ Keep up with your lab assignments. Many health care classes feature "check-off" sheets that the instructor uses to observe student performance of each required procedure. Figure 7-3 shows an example for taking a temperature. Note how each step is listed separately. This is because health care procedures must be done in a certain way (called a *protocol*), with many of the steps essential for the success of the procedure. When the procedure is completed satisfactorily, it is checked off on the sheet. Strive to complete these sheets in a timely way as you progress through each course.

EVALUATION OF COMPETENCY

Procedure 2—1: Measuring Body Temperature—Electronic Thermometer

Name: _____   Date: _____

Evaluated by: _____   Score: _____

Performance Objective

OUTCOME: Measure oral body temperature.
CONDITIONS: Given an electronic thermometer and oral probe.
             Given an oral probe cover.
STANDARDS: Time: 5 minutes
             Accuracy:
             1. The temperature recording must be identical to the reading
                displayed on the digital display screen.
             2. Satisfactory score on the Performance Evaluation Checklist.

Performance Evaluation Checklist

Yes	No	Performance Standards
___	___	Washed hands.
___	___	Assembled equipment.
___	___	Attached oral temperature probe to thermometer unit.
___	___	Inserted probe into the face of thermometer.
___	___	Removed thermometer unit from its rechargeable base.
___	___	Grasped probe by the collar and removed it from the face of thermometer.
___	___	Is able to state what occurs when probe is removed from the face of thermometer.
___	___	Attached disposable probe cover to probe.
___	___	Is able to state the purpose of probe cover.
___	___	Identified patient and explained procedure.
___	___	Correctly inserted the oral probe in patient's mouth.
___	___	Held probe in place until the audible tone was heard.
___	___	Noted patient's temperature reading on the digital display screen.
___	___	Removed probe from patient's mouth.
___	___	Discarded probe cover in an appropriate receptacle.
___	___	Did not allow fingers to come into contact with cover.
___	___	Returned probe to its stored position in the thermometer unit.
___	___	Is able to state what occurs when probe is returned to the face of the thermometer.
___	___	Washed hands.
___	___	Charted the results correctly.
___	___	The temperature recording was identical to the reading on the display screen.
___	___	Stored thermometer unit in its base.
___	___	Is able to state why thermometer unit must be stored in its base.
___	___	Completed the procedure within 5 minutes.

Figure 7-3 Check-off sheets can help you monitor your progress. These are often included in workbooks or may be provided by your instructors. (*Modified from Bonewit-West K: Study guide for clinical procedures for medical assistants ed 7, St. Louis, 2008, Saunders.*)

Lab Follow-Up

It is important to follow up and review what you learned in lab sessions, just as it is for note taking and reading. You can do a number of things to help move what you learn in lab to your long-term memory.

1. Join or organize a study group to practice procedures and quiz one another on the rationale, safety concerns, and supporting theories.
2. Write out the steps of each procedure from memory. Include any safety concerns or rationale.
3. Make flash cards to help you remember important facts—rules and regulations, normal values (blood cell counts, body temperature, purpose of various lab tests, and so on).
4. Make charts, using color and illustrations to highlight important points about each procedure.
5. Recite the steps out loud, or record them and review by listening.
6. Rehearse the steps for each procedure in your mind. Act them out. Develop mental checklists of the steps. Some students find it helpful to use mnemonics (techniques to help the memory). For example, RICE is a popular way to remember the immediate first aid treatment for sprains:
   R = rest
   I = ice
   C = compression
   E = elevation

 Go to page 205 to complete Prescription for Success 7-1

MATH SKILLS

Math is necessary for performing many health care tasks. Examples include measuring a child's height, calculating the correct amount of medication to give a patient, conducting tests, and determining how much to bill an insurance company. It is not necessary to be a math genius, but there are a few basics you must understand to safely carry out the responsibilities of your job.

Many students think math is difficult and dread the idea of having to deal with it in any form. You may be in this category. The truth is, with practice, almost everyone can master the fundamentals. Some common reasons why students have trouble with math are itemized in the following list. Do any of them apply to you?

1. They either didn't learn or forgot how to perform basic operations, especially those involving fractions, decimals, percentages, ratios, proportions, and simple equations.
2. They don't understand the metric system, which is heavily used in health care as well as the sciences. Many Americans don't know what metric measurements refer to—how big, how much, or how long—because they don't typically use them in daily life.
3. They don't know the meaning of the many strange-looking signs and symbols called *notations*.
4. They have trouble visualizing math operations in their minds.
5. They memorize formulas without really understanding them or knowing how to apply them to solve problems.
6. They avoid taking math classes. When this is impossible, they may skip class and/or not do all the homework.

PERSONAL REFLECTION

1. Describe your previous experiences with math classes. Were they positive or negative?

   _____

   _____

   _____

   _____

   _____

2. Think how you use math (or could use it) in your everyday life. For example, do you understand how interest on loans and credit card balances is calculated? Do you balance your checkbook each month? Can you double a recipe or calculate how much paint to buy for a home-improvement project?

   _____

   _____

   _____

   _____

   _____

Some Truths about Math

Knowing the truth about something can be helpful. For example, if you are told that "math is really easy" and you find it difficult, you might worry that you are not smart enough to understand it. It would be better to hear that although it may not always be easy, it can be mastered with persistence and practice. So, let's talk about some truths about math.

The first is that it is not always easy or fun. Learning math is like learning to use a computer. The strange symbols and unfamiliar language make it seem difficult, but once you learn to use it, it helps you perform many tasks quickly and efficiently.

Another truth you can use to your advantage is that math knowledge builds on itself. You must master each principle and skill before moving on to the next. Walter Pauk,[1] a noted expert on study skills, believes that the most common reason students have difficulty with math is that they didn't understand an earlier principle or process. This means that getting behind in class can really trip you up. Failure to understand one concept can lead to failure in the next. The self-fulfilling prophecy can occur: you get behind and don't understand what's going on, so you avoid the subject because you don't understand it. This leads to failure, and you "prove to yourself" that you can't do it.

Finally, math is a subject in which memorization is helpful, but understanding is essential. In order for math to be useful on the job, you must be able to apply it to new situations. You can do this only if you understand how concepts, operations, and formulas work.

Relieving Math Anxiety

Although many students cringe at the thought of having to deal with numbers, some become downright panicky. They may do very well in other academic subjects but feel completely helpless and even stupid when faced with math. These feelings have been labeled **math anxiety**. Stanley Kogelman and Joseph Warren[2] developed a series of workshops to help people of all ages approach math with confidence. They firmly believe that math problems are more emotional than intellectual. The material in this section was adapted from their book *Mind over Math*.

Kogelman and Warren suggest that you start by accepting your feelings of anxiety and realizing that many students experience the same feelings. By being aware of and experiencing your emotional reactions, you are in a better position to handle them. The next step is to develop a positive attitude about learning and using math. Having confidence in yourself is one of the most important factors in developing math ability. As an adult student, for example, you have more life experience than you did in grade school. Research has shown that most adults can learn arithmetic in a relatively short time.

Avoid saying, "I can't do math," because doing so prevents you from even trying. Negative self-talk defeats you before you even start! Get rid of unrealistic expectations that only leave you feeling discouraged. The fact is that almost no one, not even most mathematicians, can work all problems quickly or "in

 with a Health Care Professional
Debbie Sholter

Debbie is a medical assistant in a single-physician office. Debbie describes the use of math in her everyday duties.

Q Can you tell me about how you use math and numbers in your work?

A Sometimes we have to convert kilograms and pounds from one to the other. This happens when we get medical records and the patient's weight has been recorded in kilograms. These are usually out-of-country records. We use the English measurement system—pounds—so I have to change them. I need to make them uniform so we can track things like weight gain and loss. This is important because weight changes can provide clues to a patient's condition. An unexplained weight gain, for example, might mean that a cardiac patient is retaining water.

Q Are there other kinds of conversions you have to make?

A Yes, with medications. Lots of them come in doses for adults, so I have to cut them down for children. You have to calculate by the patient's weight, so you may have to divide or multiply carefully—you can't make any mistakes here! Too much medication can do real harm to the patient.

Another thing with medications is taking health history information. If a patient is taking medications, we have find out what these are and accurately record the dosages. So we have to understand metric measurements and units and know abbreviations mcg, mg, etc. Thyroid, for example, comes in micrograms. It's important to understand how diagnostic test numbers relate to medication doses.

Q How about business uses of math?

A I keep a price sheet and collect money from patients. Everything has to add up correctly. For certain insurance companies, we have to calculate percentages to know what patient should pay—their copay, that is.

Then we have to track payments and make change. Many people use credit cards, but some do use cash. So we have to make change accurately.

Some offices do their own billing. The staff has to prepare statements for insurance, calculate write-offs, add daily intake of money, prepare deposit slips, and take the money to the bank.

Q Do you help with any purchasing?

A Yes, I buy supplies for the office, both front and back. I try to get the best deals by comparing prices. I do this by calculating the price per unit, per test, etc. This also helps the physician determine how much to charge patients. I go through prices at least annually because they change and new suppliers become available. Some employees are paid bonuses, so saving money affects everyone.

their head." And know that there is usually more than one way to think through and solve a math problem. Your way may be just as correct as the next person's.

It is very difficult to concentrate and focus, which are essential to learning math, when you are anxious and nervous. In other words, math anxiety itself, not your lack of ability, can be a major cause of your problems with math. Relax and take your time. Read and work through math books and problems slowly and carefully. Don't worry if you have to go over a concept many times before you get it. That's okay! If you do feel really stuck, take a short break. The unconscious part of your mind will continue to work, and you may find that the "impossible" problem you left is not so difficult after all.

Finally, don't make the situation worse by avoiding math. Attend all classes, do the studying, and complete all assignments. Ask questions in class. Failure to make an effort adds pressure on yourself and will only add to your anxiety and stress. Stay with it. Work all the examples in your book and do lots of practice problems. Explanations often don't make sense until you've actually worked with the problems yourself.

Success Tips for Mastering Math

Choose from among the following study techniques the ones that best fit your preferred learning styles:

- ☐ Make flash cards for learning "math facts," such as the multiplication tables, formulas, and common conversions.
- ☐ Draw pictures of concepts to help you understand them.
- ☐ Use paper plates, clay, blocks, and other materials to make shapes and help you see how parts relate to the whole in fractions and decimals.
- ☐ Look for examples of math applications in everyday life: shopping, bills, bank statements, recipes, weights, measurements, taxes, and interest on loans.
- ☐ Read math explanations aloud. Be sure you understand each word or idea before moving on.
- ☐ Try to translate math concepts into words you are familiar with.
- ☐ Mark your book with questions or your own explanations.
- ☐ If you don't understand the explanations in your own books or materials, look for others in the library or bookstore or ask your instructor for resources. Sometimes a different approach helps.
- ☐ Buy or borrow a book with exercises and answers.
- ☐ Be proactive. Ask questions about anything you don't understand.
- ☐ Write down any calculations the instructor does in class. Be sure to include each step so you can review it later.
- ☐ Join or form a math study group.
- ☐ Learn how to check your work for correctness. For example, use multiplication to check division problems.
- ☐ Try explaining important concepts to someone else. By having to say it, you may clarify and understand it better.
- ☐ Explain concepts and processes in writing. Pretend you are writing a letter to a friend in which you describe what you are learning in class.
- ☐ When studying math, plan to concentrate fully. Remove as many distractions as possible, and try to spend at least 30 minutes of focused time before taking a break.

Math Review

"Most of the fundamental ideas of science are essentially simple, and may be, as a rule, expressed in a language comprehensible to everyone."
—*Albert Einstein*

Math has its own special language. For example, when referring to a fraction, it is awkward to say "the bottom half" or "the number underneath." Its proper name is "denominator," and knowing this makes talking about it easier. Knowing the vocabulary of any subject, including math, can help you better understand your teachers and textbooks. See Table 7-1 for the definitions of common math terms.

Table 7-2 contains more math vocabulary along with a brief review of some of the operations commonly used in health care—and commonly forgotten by students! The purpose of the table is to help you recall math skills you have already learned, not to teach new material. As you are reading the explanations and looking at the examples, keep in mind that there are different "right ways" to work a problem. For example, division problems are not set up the same way in every country—or even in every part of the United States. As you go through the material in Table 7-2, try working the examples. Sometimes explanations don't make much sense until you work with the numbers yourself.

The Multiplication Chart

Knowing the products of all possible combinations of the numbers 1 through 12 is a great time saver. This is not a substitute for learning how to multiply but a way to increase your efficiency. It is also a good study aid for learning the multiplication tables. To use the chart in Box 7-1, find the intersection of the two numbers you wish to multiply, one from the row across the top and the other from the far left

TABLE 7-1	The Language of Math	
Word or Phrase	**What It Means**	**Examples**
Digit	Any of the numerals 0-9.	The number 834 has three digits: 8, 3, and 4.
Whole number	A number that has no fraction or decimal.	5, 67, and 1893 are whole numbers
Mixed number	A number that has two parts: a whole number and a fraction.	$1\frac{1}{3}$, $4\frac{1}{2}$, $17\frac{2}{5}$ are mixed numbers
Factors	The numbers being multiplied in a multiplication problem.	$8 \times 10 = 80$ 8 and 10 are the factors
Product	The answer to a multiplication problem.	$8 \times 10 = 80$ 80 is the product
Dividend	In a division problem, the number to be divided.	$72 \div 8 = 9$ 72 is the dividend
Divisor	The number by which the dividend is divided in a division problem.	$72 \div 8 = 9$ 8 is the divisor
Quotient	The answer to a division problem.	$72 \div 8 = 9$ 9 is the quotient
Cubic measurement	Measure of volume, or the amount of space that something takes up. Medications are sometimes measured in cubic centimeters. (See Table 7-3 for an explanation of the centimeter.)	To calculate the volume of a box, multiply the height times the width times the length. A box that is 3 feet long, 2 feet high, and 5 feet wide = $3 \times 2 \times 5 = 30$ cubic feet.
Place value chart	A chart that shows the unit values of the places that follow the decimal point.	Tenths 0.1 Hundredths 0.01 Thousandths 0.001 Ten thousandths 0.0001 Hundred thousandths 0.00001

Volumes measure space, such as in a box or containers of various shapes.

column. For example, to multiply 3 times 4, find the 3 in the top row and the 4 in the first column. Move down the column from the 3 and across the row from the 4 until the lines meet at 12. This is the answer. Study the chart in Box 7-1, or make flash cards for any combinations you need to memorize. You can also use graph paper to set up blank tables to fill in to review and quiz yourself.

The multiplication table can also be used as a tool to reduce fractions if the numerator and denominator appear in the same column. For example, for $\frac{12}{96}$, follow both 12 and 96 to the far left column: 12 becomes 1 and 96 becomes 8; $\frac{12}{96}$ = $\frac{1}{8}$. The fraction may need to be reduced further. For example, $\frac{24}{48}$ = $\frac{2}{4}$; $\frac{2}{4}$ can be further reduced to $\frac{1}{2}$.

TABLE 7-2	Math Operations

FRACTIONS

The Language of Fractions

Word or Phrase	What it Means	Examples
Fraction	Represents equal parts of a whole. Always written as two numbers, one on top of the other.	½ represents 1 of the 2 equal parts into which a whole of something has been divided. 5/12 represents 5 of the 12 equal parts into which a whole has been divided.
Numerator	The top number in a fraction. It tells you how many pieces of the whole you have.	In the fraction ½, 1 is the numerator. In 5/12, 5 is the numerator.
Denominator	The bottom number in a fraction. It tells you into how many equal pieces a whole has been divided. The larger the number, the smaller the pieces.	In ½, 2 is the denominator. In 5/12, 12 is the denominator.
Proper fraction	A fraction in which the numerator is smaller than the denominator.	¾ 3 is smaller than 4.
Improper fraction	A fraction in which the numerator is larger than the denominator.	4/3 4 is larger than 3. This represents a whole number and a fraction: 1⅓. (There are 3 thirds in a whole, which equals 1. ⅓ represents the additional—or fourth—third.)
Lowest common denominator	The smallest number that can be evenly divided (leaving no remainder) by all the denominators in a series of fractions. It is necessary to find this number when you want to add or subtract fractions.	The lowest common denominator for ⅙, ¾, and ⅝ is 24.
Simplest form	A fraction in which the numerator and denominator cannot be evenly divided by the same number.	½ is the simplest form of the following fractions: 2/4, 3/6, 4/8, 5/10, 25/50.

Working with Fractions

Operation	What to Do
Reduce fractions to their simplest form	**Problem: Reduce 18/30 to its simplest form.** **Step 1.** Find a number that divides evenly into both the numerator and the denominator. Both 18 and 30 can be divided evenly by 2, resulting in 9/15. **Step 2.** Ask yourself if the fraction can be reduced further. Is there another number that divides evenly into both the numerator and denominator? If not, you're finished! If so, identify that number. In our example, both 9 and 15 can be divided evenly by 3, resulting in 3/5. **Answer:** 3/5 is the simplest form of 18/30. **Note:** This could also have been done in one step by dividing 18 and 30 by 6.
Change fractions so they share the lowest common denominator. You need to do this before adding or subtracting fractions that have different denominators.	**Problem: Find the lowest common denominator for ⅙, ¾, and ⅝.** Step 1. Test various numbers to find the smallest number that can be evenly divided by all the denominators in a series of fractions. Hint: Multiply the denominators by one another to find at least one common denominator. This may not be the smallest common denominator, but it gives you a starting point. By trying several possibilities, we find that 24 is the lowest common denominator for ⅙, ¾, and ⅝. **Step 2.** For each fraction, divide the new denominator by the original denominator. For ⅙: 24 ÷ 6 = 4 For ¾: 24 ÷ 4 = 6 For ⅝: 24 ÷ 8 = 3 **Step 3.** Multiply each product from step 2 by the numerator of the corresponding fraction. This number is the new numerator. For ⅙: 4 × 1 = 4 New fraction is 4/24 For ¾: 6 × 3 = 18 New fraction is 18/24 For ⅝: 3 × 5 = 15 **Answer:** 15/24 You can now add and subtract using this fraction.

TABLE 7-2	Math Operations—cont'd
Operation	**What to Do**
Converting improper fractions to mixed numbers. You will sometimes get an improper fraction after performing a calculation, such as adding two fractions. Improper fractions must be changed because it isn't correct usage to record them.	**Problem: Convert ¹⁰⁄₄ to a mixed number.** Step 1. Divide the numerator by the denominator. 10 ÷ 4 = 2 R 2 Step 2. If there is a remainder (R), it becomes the numerator of a fraction. The denominator is the same as in the original improper fraction. 2²⁄₄ Step 3. Reduce the fraction, if necessary. 2²⁄₄ = 2½ **Answer: 2½**
Add fractions	**Problem: ⅙ + ¾ + ⅝ = ?** **Step 1.** If the fractions do not have the same denominator, find the lowest common denominator. 24 is the lowest common denominator. Convert the fraction(s): ⅙ = ⁴⁄₂₄ ¾ = ¹⁸⁄₂₄ ⅝ = ¹⁵⁄₂₄ **Step 2.** Add the numerators. ⁴⁄₂₄ + ¹⁸⁄₂₄ + ¹⁵⁄₂₄ = ³⁷⁄₂₄ **Step 3.** Simplify the result if it is an improper fraction. 37 ÷ 24 = 1 R 13 **Answer: 1¹³⁄₂₄**
Subtract fractions	**Problem: ⅝ − ¼ = ?** **Step 1.** If the fractions do not have the same denominator, find the lowest common denominator. 8 is the lowest common denominator (recall that this is the number into which both denominators can be divided evenly). Convert the fraction(s): ¼ = ²⁄₈ **Step 2.** Perform the calculation by subtracting the second numerator from the first. ⅝ − ²⁄₈ = ⅜ **Answer: ⅜** **Step 3.** Reduce the fractions, if necessary. **Note:** When subtracting mixed numbers, change them to improper fractions before subtracting the numerators. Here's how: Let's start with 1⅝. **Step 1.** Multiply the whole number by the denominator. 8 × 1 = 8 Add the product to the numerator of the fraction, and use the result as the new numerator. 8 + 5 = 13 The denominator is the same as in the original fraction. **Answer: ¹³⁄₈**
Multiply fractions	**Problem: ½ × ¾ = ?** **Step 1.** Multiply the numerators by each other and then the denominators by each other. Numerators: 1 × 3 = 3 Denominators: 2 × 4 = 8 Create a new fraction with the products: ⅜ **Answer: ⅜** **Step 2.** Reduce the fraction, if necessary.
Divide fractions (everyone's big fear!) What you are figuring out: how many fractions will fit into another fraction	**Problem: ¾ ÷ ½ = ?** **Step 1.** Invert (switch) the numerator and the denominator of the divisor. ½ inverted becomes ²⁄₁. Use this fraction in the following steps. **Step 2.** Multiply the numerators by each other and the denominators by each other. (That's right—you don't actually divide as we know it. This is what makes an otherwise simple operation seem confusing and hard to remember!) Numerators: 3 × 2 = 6 Denominators: 4 × 1 = 4 Create a new fraction with the products: ⁶⁄₄ **Answer: ⁶⁄₄** **Step 3.** Simplify and/or reduce the fraction, if necessary. ⁶⁄₄ is an improper fraction. Simplify by dividing 6 by 4. 6 ÷ 4 = 1 R 2 The proper fraction is 1²⁄₄. Reduce the fraction by dividing 2 and 4 by 2. **Answer: 1½**

Continued

TABLE 7-2	Math Operations—cont'd

Examples of Fractions in Health Care

- Fluid intake and output
  1. Janice drinks 1½ cups of juice, ⅓ cup of water, and ⅝ glass of soda. What is her total fluid input?
- Changes in weight and height
  2. Al weighed 175¼ pounds. After following a recommended diet, he weighs 162½ pounds. How much weight did he lose?
  3. During the first month of life an infant grew ½ inch, ⅝ inch during the second, and ¾ the third. How much did the infant grow in 3 months?
- Units of time
  4. Cassie worked in the front office for 2½ hours, in the back for 3¾, and in the lab for 1⅓. How many hours did she work?
  5. If Cassie earns $16.00 an hour, how much did she earn for the work in the previous problem?
- Quantities and lengths
  6. A patient takes ¾ ounce of a liquid antacid twice a day. How long will a 24-ounce bottle last?

DECIMALS

The Language of Decimals

Word or Phrase	What It Means	Examples
Decimal	Like fractions, decimals represent equal parts of a whole. Decimals are written using a point, the same symbol as a period. When decimals are expressed as fractions, they always have denominators written in units of 10 (10, 100, 1000, 10,000, etc.).	0.3 = ³⁄₁₀. Both represent 3 of the 10 equal parts of a whole.

Working with Decimals

Operation	What to Do
Add decimals	**Problem: Add 3.96 + 4.229 + 6.1.** **Step 1.** Line up the numbers so the decimal points are aligned. 3.96 4.229 6.1 **Step 2.** Use zeros to fill in the spaces to the right of the decimal point so that all the numbers have the same number of digits. 3.960 4.229 6.100 **Step 3:** Add as you would whole numbers. 3.960 4.229 6.100 14.289 **Step 4.** Place the decimal point in the answer directly under the points in the numbers you added. 3.960 4.229 6.100 14.289 **Answer:** 14.289
Subtract decimals	**Problem: Subtract 18.453 from 72.5.** **Step 1.** Line up the numbers so the decimal points are aligned. 72.5 18.453 **Step 2.** Use zeros to fill in the spaces to the right of the decimal point so that both numbers have the same number of digits. 72.500 18.453 **Step 3.** Subtract as you would whole numbers. 72.500 −18.453 54047 **Step 4.** Place the decimal point in the answer directly under the points in the numbers you subtracted. 72.500 −18.453 54.047 **Answer:** 54.047

TABLE 7-2	Math Operations—cont'd
Operation	**What to Do**

Multiply decimals	**Problem: 16.953 × 3.52 = ?**
	Step 1. Multiply as you would whole numbers. (Note: You do *not* fill in with zeros as you did in the addition and subtraction problems.)
	    16.953
	× 3.52
	    33906
	    84765
	   50859
	  5967456
	Step 2. Count the number of decimal places in the two factors. To do this, start at the far right of each factor and count left until you reach the decimal point.
	Next, starting at the far right of the answer, count this number of places to the left. This is where you place the decimal point in the answer.
	16.953—3 places
	3.52—2 places
	Count 5 places to the left: 59.67456
	Answer: 59.67456

Divide decimals	**Problem: 9 ÷ 2.5 = ?**
	Step 1. Set up the problem as you would if you were dividing whole numbers.
	2.5⟌9
	Step 2. If the divisor is a decimal, move the decimal point to the right, placing it immediately after the last digit in the number. Then move the decimal point in the dividend to the right the same number of places, adding zeros if necessary.
	2.5⟌9.0
	Step 3. Divide as you would with whole numbers.
	     36
	25⟌90.0
	   75
	  150
	Step 4. Place the decimal point in the answer directly above the decimal point in the dividend.
	    3.6
	25⟌90.0
	   75
	  150
	Answer: 3.6

Working with Decimals and Fractions	
Operation	**What to Do**
Change decimals to fractions	**Problem: 0.25 = ?** **Step 1.** Write the numbers in the decimal as the numerator (drop the decimal point). Numerator is 25 **Step 2.** Write the unit of the decimal as the denominator. (tenths, hundredths, thousandths, etc. See Placement Value Chart). 0.25 has 2 places (digits) to the right of the decimal point. Therefore the denominator is 100. The fraction is 25/100 **Step 3.** Reduce the fraction, if necessary. Both 25 and 100 can be divided evenly by 25: 25÷25 = 1 100÷ 25 = 4 The reduced fraction is ¼. Answer: 0.25 = ¼

Change fractions to decimals	**Problem: 3/4 = ?**
	Step 1. Set up a division problem in which the numerator is divided by the denominator. 4⟌3
	Step 2. If the dividend is smaller than the divisor, write a decimal point and add one or more zeros to the dividend, as needed. If there is already a decimal point, add the necessary zeros. 4⟌3.00
	Step 3. Divide as you would with whole numbers.
	     75
	4⟌3.00
	   28
	   20
	   20
	    0
	Step 4. Place the decimal point in the answer directly above the decimal point in the dividend.
	   .75
	4⟌3.00
	Answer: 3/4 = 0.75

Continued

TABLE 7-2	Math Operations—cont'd

Examples of Decimals in Health Care

- Temperatures
  1. At 8:15 AM a patient's temperature measures 104.5° F. At 2:30 PM it is 101.2° F. What is the decrease in his temperature?
- Quantities
  2. You are to administer 5.25 milligrams of medication to a patient daily. In the morning, he received 2.5 milligrams. What is the remaining dose for today?
  3. If a patient is to take 4.5 milligrams of a drug and it is available in 1.5-milligram tablets, how many tablets must she take?
- Costs and expenses
  4. If a box of 100 disposable gloves costs $6.50 and a case containing 1000 gloves costs $49.46. Which quantity is the better deal for a large clinic that uses at least 1500 gloves per month?
- Statistical data
  5. In 1 year, the following costs were incurred because of injuries: motor-vehicle crashes, $199.6 billion; work injuries, $132.1 billion; home injuries, $118.1 billion; and public injuries, $82.1 billion. What was the total cost incurred for injuries that year?

PERCENTS

The Language of Percents

Word or Phrase	What It Means	Examples
Percents	A fraction with a denominator of 100 that is expressed as a whole number with a percent sign.	37% represents 37 of the 100 parts of a whole. It is the same as $^{37}/_{100}$ and 0.37.

Operation	What to Do
Change percentages to decimals	**Problem: Change 41% to a decimal.** **Step 1.** Start counting from the decimal point and move it 2 places to the left. Fill in with zeros as needed. If the whole number does not have a decimal point written in, it is understood to be located at the far right side of the number. In this problem, the decimal point is understood to be directly to the right of the 1. Now drop the percent sign. **Answer:** 0.41
Calculate amounts represented by percentages; requires first converting the percentages to decimals	**Problem: Find 65% of 730** **Step 1.** Change the percent to a decimal. 65% = 0.65 **Step 2.** Multiply the number for which you want the percent by the decimal. $$\begin{array}{r} 730 \\ \times\, 0.65 \\ \hline 474.50 \end{array}$$ **Answer:** 474.5 **Note:** Extra zeros to the far right of the decimal point can be dropped in the answer.

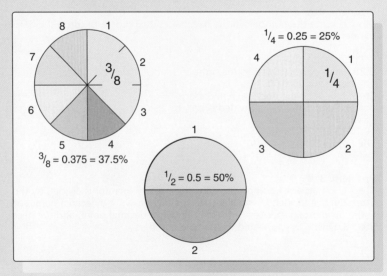

This figure illustrates the relationship between fractions, decimals, and percentages. All three represent parts of whole items or numbers of items

TABLE 7-2	Math Operations—cont'd	

Word or Phrase	What It Means	Examples
	Examples of Percents in Health Care	

- Solution concentrations
  1. If a physician orders a 12% solution of medication to be infused over 1 hour, how many parts of medication should be added to 100 parts of solution?
- Comparisons and changes
  2. In 1 year, General Hospital admitted 5343 patients. Just over 27% were patients with heart attacks. How many patients were admitted because of heart attacks?
  3. The following year the hospital initiated a heart wellness program for the community. That year, 1283 patients were admitted because of heart attacks. What was the percentage decrease in heart attack patients?
  4. Mr. Jaspers lowers his cholesterol number from 243 to 213. By what percent does he lower his cholesterol?
- Purchasing
  5. If a medical office agrees to buy all its computer and printing supplies from the Good Byte Company, it will receive a 20% discount. The office manager just ordered $7314 in goods from Good Byte. How much will the office pay after the discount?

EQUATIONS

The Language of Equations

Word or Phrase	What It Means	Examples
Equation	An equation is a statement that 2 quantities are equal. This equality is represented by an equals sign. Equations help you find values for unknown quantities by using the information you do know. The unknown quantities are commonly represented by letters.	$x \div 12 = 18$ $6x - 4 = 30 + 26$

Working with Equations

Operation	What to Do
Solve simple equations	**Problem: Find the value of x** $5 + x = 12$ Reorganize the equation so that the unknown (x) is by itself on one side of the equals sign. Do this by adding, subtracting, multiplying, or dividing *both* sides of the equation by the same number. Subtract 5 from each side of the equation: $5 + x - 5 = 12 - 5$ Answer: $x = 7$ **Problem: $6x - 3 = 15$** Add 3 to each side of the equation: $6x - 3 + 3 = 15 + 3$ $6x = 18$ Divide each side by 6: $6x \div 6 = 18 \div 6$ Answer: $x = 3$ **Note:** As you see in the second problem, you may have to do more than one calculation to isolate x completely.

PROPORTIONS

The Language of Proportions

Word or Phrase	What It Means	Examples
Ratio	Expresses the relationship between 2 numbers. Ratios can be written several ways.	Most common way to write a ratio: 1:2 Other ways to write ratios: 1 to 2 ½
Proportion	Statement that 2 ratios or fractions are equal (show the same relationship between numbers).	1:2::5:10 ½ = 5/10 "1 is to 2 as 5 is to 10" (Why? Because 1 is half of 2 and 5 is half of 10. The two sets of numbers have the same relationship to each other.)

Continued

TABLE 7-2	Math Operations—cont'd
Working with Proportions	
Operation	**What to Do**
Find an unknown quantity in a proportion.	**Problem: Find the value of X in 1:2::10:X.** **Step 1.** Write each ratio as a fraction. ½ = ¹⁰/ₓ **Step 2.** Multiply the denominators by the opposite numerators. 1 × X = 2 × 10 X = 20 **Step 3.** Solve for X, if necessary. **Step 4.** Write out the completed proportion. Answer: 1:2::10:20 (Say: 1 is to 2 as 10 is to 20) **Problem: Find the value of X in X:12::3:9.** **Step 1.** Write each ratio as a fraction. X/₁₂ = ³/₉ **Step 2.** Multiply the denominators by the opposite numerators. X × 9 = 9X 12 × 3 = 36 Therefore 9X = 36 **Step 3.** Solve for X. 9X ÷ 9 = 36 ÷ 9 X = 4 **Step 4.** Write out the completed proportion. **Answer: 4:12::3:9** (Say: 4 is to 12 as 3 is to 9) **Note:** Another common way to discuss proportions is in terms of the "means" and the "extremes." In the example 1:2 = 10:x, 1 and x are the extremes and 2 and 10 are the means. The product of the means equals the product of the extremes. This is the same operation as cross-multiplying the fractions. Extremes 1:2 = 10:X Means **Problem: Find the value of X in 8:X::14:91.** **Step 1.** Multiply the means. X × 14 = 14X **Step 2.** Multiply the extremes. 8 × 91 = 728 **Step 3.** Set up an equation using the products of the means and the extremes. 14X = 728 **Step 4.** Solve for X. 14X ÷ 14 = 728 ÷ 14 X = 52 **Step 5.** Write out the completed proportion. Answer: 8:52::14:91
Examples of Proportions in Health Care	

- Medications
  1. If 200 milliliters of solution contains 25 grams of pure drug, how many grams are contained in 75 milliliters?
  2. If there are 600 milligrams in one tablet of a drug, how many milligrams are there in five tablets?
- Quantities
  3. If a cup of canned soup contains 650 grams of sodium, how many grams are there in ¾ cup?
- Measurement conversions
  4. If 2.2 kilograms (kg) equals 1 pound and a patient weighs 65 kg, what is his weight in pounds?
  5. A patient is directed to take 2 teaspoons of medication per dose. The bottle of medication is labeled in milliliters. If a teaspoon equals 4.93 milliters, how many milliliters should the patient take per dose?

 Go to page 206 to complete Prescription for Success 7-2

Making Sense of the Metric System

The **metric system** is an obstacle for many students. It is actually a very logical system of measurement based on multiples of 10. Used in most countries other than the United States, it also serves as the measuring system for science and health care. People who come to the United States find it difficult to learn our units of measurement. Our units have names that don't follow any pattern: "inch," "foot," "yard," "pound," "mile," and so on. To make things even more confusing, some of these words—"foot," "yard," and "pound"—have other meanings as well!

Here are some facts to help you better understand the metric system:

1. It works on a base of 10. This means that the units of measurement are created by multiplying to make larger units and dividing to make smaller units by powers of 10 (10, 100, 1,000, 10,000, etc.).

2. Prefixes that designate multiples of 10 are added to the basic units of measurement to make them larger or smaller. The same prefixes are used for all the basic units, so you have to remember only one set. (Examples: *milli*meter, *milli*liter, and *milli*gram are all one thousandth of a unit of measurement.)

micro-	0.00001
milli-	0.001
centi-	0.01
deci-	0.1
deka-	10
hecto-	100
kilo-	1000

3. A knowledge of decimals is important for understanding metric units of measurement. (See Table 7-2 for a review of decimals.)

Americans who don't often use the metric system find it difficult. We know about how far a mile is, but we may be lost if someone asks us if we'd like go on a 5-kilometer walk. The easiest way to begin understanding the metric system is to learn the names of the various weights and measures and then get a feel for what each one represents. Then you can start doing conversions between the two systems, and this requires some math. Figure 7-4 illustrates metric equivalents. Figure 7-5 shows a common application of the metric system found on every grocery store shelf. Table 7-3 contains explanations of common metric units and compares them to the U.S. measuring system.

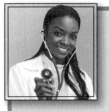

USING MATH ON THE JOB

Reading numbers correctly and performing math calculations accurately are critical to patient safety.

Here are some examples of how health care professionals use math:

- **Calculate the correct amount of medication to administer.** This is one of the most important applications of math in health care occupations. Medications are one of our most effective treatments today. At the same time, medication errors are responsible for thousands of deaths each year. Medications are sometimes ordered by physicians using a different system or dosage (amount) than what is used by the suppliers. It is sometimes necessary to convert from one system to another and then calculate the proper quantity to administer. These calculations require an understanding of the various systems of measurement, as well as how to use proportions and solve equations.

- **Take and record vital signs.** The metric system is sometimes used when patient weight, height, and temperature are recorded. Blood pressure is expressed in millimeters, a metric measurement. Body temperature may be measured using either the Fahrenheit or Celsius system. Figure 7-6 contrasts the readings for normal body temperature.

- **Bill for services.** Patient bills must be calculated accurately and recorded properly to ensure proper payment from insurance companies. Adjustments must be calculated when insurance payments are posted. Some patients pay in cash, so the ability to calculate correct change and track amounts of cash for bank deposits is essential.

| **BOX 7-1** | **Multiplication Chart** |

1	1	2	3	4	5	6	7	8	9	10	11	12
2	2	4	6	8	10	12	14	16	18	20	22	24
3	3	6	9	12	15	18	21	24	27	30	33	36
4	4	8	12	16	20	24	28	32	36	40	44	48
5	5	10	15	20	25	30	35	40	45	50	55	60
6	6	12	18	24	30	36	42	48	54	60	66	72
7	7	14	21	28	35	42	49	56	63	70	77	84
8	8	16	24	32	40	48	56	64	72	80	88	96
9	9	18	27	36	45	54	63	72	81	90	99	108
10	10	20	30	40	50	60	70	80	90	100	110	120
11	11	22	33	44	55	66	77	88	99	110	121	132
12	12	24	36	48	60	72	84	96	108	120	132	144

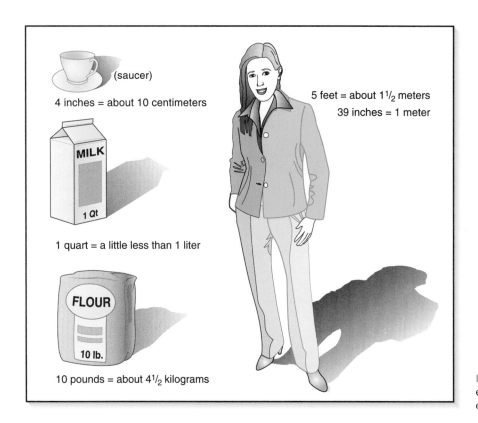

(saucer)

4 inches = about 10 centimeters

5 feet = about $1\frac{1}{2}$ meters
39 inches = 1 meter

MILK
1 Qt

1 quart = a little less than 1 liter

FLOUR
10 lb.

10 pounds = about $4\frac{1}{2}$ kilograms

Figure 7-4 Examples of metric equivalents of common U.S. units of measure.

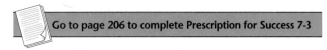

Go to page 206 to complete Prescription for Success 7-3

CLINICAL EXPERIENCE

Your clinical experience, whether it is called an "externship," "internship," "fieldwork experience," "practicum," or some other name, can be one of the most valuable parts of your education. It provides the final link between your education and your future career. Experienced professionals and/or clinical instructors will guide your work in a real occupational setting. This phase of your education provides you with opportunities to do the following:

- Apply the skills learned in class
- Gain confidence in performing these skills
- Learn firsthand about the expectations of employers
- Practice working with patients
- Think and problem solve in real-life situations
- Demonstrate your abilities to a potential employer (students are sometimes hired to work at their clinical site after graduation)

A successful clinical experience requires your full attention and effort. Some students make the mistake of thinking that this part of their education is less important than their academic classes, especially if the clinical experience is graded on a pass-fail basis. But nothing could be further from

the truth! The clinical experience really counts in the sense that you now have an impact on real people and real problems. It is also during the clinical experience that you begin to establish your professional reputation. Your performance at this time can influence your ability to get a job.

Not every clinical experience will be ideal. Things will not always go just as you expected or hoped. At these times it may be necessary for you to adjust your attitude. The truth is, not every work environment will be ideal, either. Act professionally and focus on doing your best to learn and achieve your learning goals. Even difficult situations offer opportunities to practice getting along with others, adapt to a work environment, and solve problems.

Success Tips for Your Clinical Experience

☐ Take advantage of the assistance and advice offered by your school. The staff has experience in setting up clinical experiences so students will have the best chance to succeed.

☐ Strive to have excellent attendance. If you must be absent, call the site before the time you are scheduled to arrive and let them know. Your attendance may have a significant impact on

Nutrition Facts

Serving Size 1 cup (228g)
Servings Per Container 2

Amount Per Serving

Calories 90   Calories from Fat 30

                                    % Daily Value

Total Fat 3g	**5%**
Saturated Fat 3g	**0%**
Cholesterol 0 mg	**0%**
Sodium 300 mg	**13%**
Total Carbohydrate 13 g	**4%**
Dietary Fiber 3g	**12%**
Sugars 3g	

Protein   3 g

Vitamin A 80%	Vitamin C 60%
Calcium 4%	Iron 4%

* Percent Daily Values are based on a 2,000 calorie diet. Your daily values may be higher or lower depending on your calorie needs:

		Calories	2,000	3,000
Total Fat	Less Than		65g	80g
Sat Fat	Less Than		20g	25g
Cholesterol	Less Than		300mg	300mg
Sodium	Less Than		2,400mg	2,400mg
Total Carbohydrate			300g	370g
Dietary Fiber			25g	30g

Calories per gram

Fat 9   •   Carbohydrate 4   •   Protein 4

Figure 7-5   The contents of food are reported in metric units. Understanding what these mean is especially important today, with our increased emphasis on healthy eating. *(Adapted from* Understanding food labels. *Copyright 1997, American Dietetic Association. Used with permission.)*

the site's ability to deliver services. (Most schools require you to notify them, too.)

☐ Be sure you understand what you will be expected and allowed to do. Some facilities have students start with relatively easy tasks before giving them more complex assignments. Others have students jump right in with a full set of duties.

☐ Learn the policies and procedures at the facility. Ask for a copy of any that apply to the work you will be doing. Use your reading skills, discussed in Chapter 5, to read for information and learn all you can.

☐ Ask questions about anything you don't understand or want to learn more about. Try to determine the answers for yourself first, but don't hesitate if you are unsure. This is especially important regarding procedures that have safety consequences for you or the patients.

☐ Ask an appropriate person to check your work if you are unsure about its accuracy.

☐ Follow all rules and dress codes, even if others do not seem to be doing so.

☐ Be courteous to everyone. These are your future professional colleagues, even if your future job is at a different facility.

☐ Learn as much as possible from the staff. Observe them at work and get to know them as people. Do be careful, though, not to get involved in gossip sessions.

☐ Become a contributing member of the health care team. Offer to help without being asked.

☐ Find out how you will be evaluated. Be sure you understand the performance expectations.

☐ Set goals for yourself. Think about why you are there and what you want to learn.

☐ Take advantage of any resources the facility has available. Is there a technical library you can use? Does the facility have reference materials about topics in which you have a special interest? Are there additional opportunities for you to observe and talk with people about their work?

☐ Apply what you learn in Chapter 13, "Success on the Job." The concepts discussed there apply to clinical experiences as well as to paying jobs

PERSONAL REFLECTION

1. Which of your personal characteristics do you believe will most help you have a successful clinical experience?

_____

_____

_____

_____

_____

2. Which personal characteristics do you need to work on to increase the benefits you will receive from your experience (e.g., shyness, impatience, or difficulty being on time)?

_____

_____

_____

_____

_____

TABLE 7-3	How the Metric System Works	
Type of Measurement	**Units of Measurement**	**How it Compares with the U.S. System**
Length or distance	*meter* (m) = basic unit	A little more than 1 yard (1 yard = 36 inches and 1 meter = 39.37 inches)
	millimeter (mm) = 0.001 meter	About the size of the width of a pinhead. There are just over 25 millimeters in 1 inch.
	centimeter (cm) = 0.01 meter	About ⅖ (or 0.4) of an inch, the width of a child's little finger. There are about 2½ centimeters in an inch.
	decimeter (dm) = 0.1 meter	About 4 inches
	dekameter (dam) = 10 meters	A little more than 10 yards
	hectometer (hm) = 100 meters	A little more than 100 yards
	kilometer (km) = 1000 meters	About ⅗ (or 0.62) of a mile
Liquids or volume	liter (L) = basic unit	Approximately 1 quart (2 liters is now a popular size for soft drink bottles; that's about ½ gallon because there are 4 quarts in a gallon)
	*milliliter** (mL) = 0.001 liter	*Very* small drop (commonly used in medicine)
	centiliter (cL) = 0.01 liter	About 2 teaspoons
	deciliter (dL) = 0.1 liter	Between ⅓ and ½ cup
	dekaliter (daL) = 10 liters	About 10 quarts or 2½ gallons
	hectoliter (hL) = 100 liters	About 25 gallons
	kiloliter (kL) = 1000 liters	About 250 gallons
Weight or mass of solids	*gram* (Gm, g) = basic unit	Approximately 1/28 of an ounce. About the weight of a paperclip.
	microgram (mcg) = 0.000001 gram	An incredibly small amount (1 millionth of 1/400 of a pound!!) Don't be fooled, however. This can be a significant amount in health care. The body depends on *very* small quantities of certain substances to function properly. It can also be harmed by *very* small amounts of the wrong substances.
	milligram (mg) = 0.001 gram	Also very small amounts, although they are many times heavier than a microgram.
	centigram (cg) = 0.01 gram	
	decigram (dg) = 0.1 gram	
	dekagram (dag) = 10 grams	5/14 of an ounce
	hectogram (hg) = 100 grams	About 3½ ounces
	kilogram (kg) = 1000 grams	2.2 pounds
Temperature	*Celsius* (commonly called centigrade) 0° C = freezing point of water 100° C = boiling point of water Celsius thermometers are marked in one-tenth intervals.	Fahrenheit is the system commonly used in the United States. In this system, 32° F is freezing and 95° F is a sunny day at the beach. 1° C = 1.8 times 1° F
	Water freezes: 0° C	32° F
	Normal body temperature: 37° C	98.6° F
	Water boils: 100° C	212° F
	Sterilization occurs: 121° C	250° F
	To convert between the 2 systems: Fahrenheit to Celsius: 1. Subtract 32 from the F temperature 2. Multiply by ⅝	98.6° F 98.6 − 32 = 66.6 5/9 × 66.6 = 5/9 × 66.6/1 = 37 Another way to solve for approximate answer: 66.6 ÷ 1.8 = 36.7
	Celsius to Fahrenheit: 1. Multiply the C temperature by 9/5 (or 1.8) 2. Add 32	37 × 9/5 = 37/1 × 9/5 = 333/5 = 66.6 66.6 + 32 = 98.6 Another way to solve: 37 × 1.8 + 32 = 98.6

Note: Units in italics are the most common units of measurement in health care.
*A milliliter is the same amount as a cubic centimeter (cc). This is important to know in health care because these terms are sometimes used interchangeably.

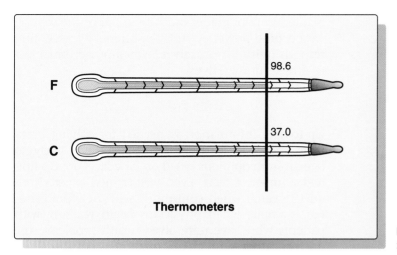

Thermometers

Figure 7-6   You may use both Fahrenheit and Celsius measurement systems when working in health care.

PROBLEM SOLVING AND DECISION MAKING

Every day we are confronted with situations that require us to solve problems and make decisions, both large and small. The quality of your life depends to a great extent on your ability to make good decisions. On the job this ability also affects the lives of your patients and co-workers.

Critical thinking is a term you will hear used a lot in health care. There are many definitions. In this book, it means paying attention to what you are doing; considering whether what you hear or read makes sense; using logic and reasoning to make choices and decisions; and applying what you have learned in class to new situations. An important part of critical thinking is separating facts from opinions. Facts are based on evidence, experience, and observation. Opinions are based on feelings, emotions, and unproven beliefs. Distinguishing between the two requires a foundation of knowledge and the ability to research and find the facts.

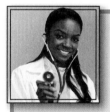

CRITICAL THINKING ON THE JOB

I observed good examples of critical thinking when my husband was in the hospital. The entire hospital had started converting to a new computer system a few hours before he was admitted. All patient information, charting, records of medications—everything—was now being entered on laptop computers the staff wheeled around on small stands.

One problem with the new system was figuring out how to delete information entered by mistake. We observed the physician struggling with medications he wanted to delete from his orders. After he left the room, we commented to the nurse about the increased risk of medication errors for the next few days until everyone learned to use the new system. She responded that the staff would have to pay even more attention than usual to medical orders and double check anything that didn't seem correct. They would have to think critically and apply their knowledge about drugs.

A Six-Step Plan for Problem Solving

Having an organized way to approach problems makes it easier to find effective solutions. Many helpful methods have been developed. Some are specific to certain health care occupations. For example, Box 7-2 contains the steps that make up the **nursing process**. The more general problem-solving method presented in this chapter is organized into the following six steps:
1. Define the problem.
2. Gather information.
3. Develop alternative solutions.
4. Consider possible results and consequences.
5. Choose a solution and act on it.
6. Evaluate the results and revise as needed.

Step One: Define the Problem

"A problem well stated is a problem half solved."
—*Charles F. Kettering*

BOX 7-2   The Nursing Process

1. *Assessment:* Systematically collecting data about the patient.
2. *Nursing Diagnosis:* Describing actual and potential health problems based on the data collected.
3. *Planning:* Setting goals for the patient and establishing a nursing care plan to achieve these goals.
4. *Implementation or Nursing Interaction:* Carrying out actions to assist the patient to promote, maintain, and restore health.
5. *Evaluation:* Measuring the patient's progress toward achieving the goals set in step 2. Determining ways to assist patients who do not reach their goals. Setting new goals for patients who are progressing as planned.

Adapted from O'Toole M, ed: *Miller-Kean encyclopedia and dictionary of medicine, nursing, and allied health,* ed 6, Philadelphia, 1997, Saunders.

You may have what seems to be an obvious problem, but sometimes what we believe to be the problem is only a symptom of a deeper underlying problem. For example, suppose that Kathy, a nursing student, is earning Ds and Fs in her pharmacology class. She may define the problem as "getting low grades in class." Grades, however, are only a symptom of the problem, not the problem itself. Asking questions is one way she can start to identify the real problem.

- Do I understand the textbook? The lectures?
- Do I use good study habits?
- Do I put off studying for this class? If so, why?
- Do I attend all class sessions?
- Am I able to follow the instructor's presentations?
- Does the subject require background knowledge that I don't have?
- Am I having difficulty understanding what is asked for in test questions?
- Do I complete all homework assignments and projects?
- Do I have the math knowledge and skills needed to understand and perform the necessary calculations?

Suppose that Kathy identifies the problem as a weakness in math. She makes lots of mistakes when calculating dosages, converting between systems of measurement, and working with proportions. Her poor grades are a symptom of her problem, which, now identified, she can start to solve.

It isn't always easy—or comfortable—to uncover real problems. Many of us tend to avoid tough issues by ignoring them, or we blame circumstances or other people for our difficulties. But when we fail to recognize our part in causing problems, we also give away our power to find solutions. For example, if we blame our poor grades on the teacher or the school, we become powerless to raise them. By accepting responsibility for ourselves, we empower ourselves to direct our own lives.

Step Two: Gather Information

Up-to-date information is needed for solving problems and making decisions. We are not likely to benefit from opinions based on false facts or on a limited number of facts. Even well-trained experts conduct research when confronted with new problems. For example, when physicians begin working with patients who have unresolved health problems, the doctors gather as much information as possible. They observe the patient, ask questions, and run diagnostic tests. They call on their own knowledge. They may discuss their findings with other physicians and health professionals and consult reference books and recent technical articles. In summary, they gather as much information as possible from a wide variety of sources.

Gathering facts helps prevent emotional and nonproductive reactions to life's problems. If Kathy's response to receiving low grades in pharmacology class is, "I'm just dumb and I'll never get this," she will be discouraged from seeking an effective solution. If she passed the admissions requirements for her school and is receiving passing grades in her other classes, the evidence does not support her statement that she is dumb. Insisting that she is "just dumb" becomes a way to escape being responsible for seeking solutions to the problem. It is an excuse to avoid the work of going through the problem-solving process and making needed changes.

Relying on incorrect opinions and emotional responses can also negatively influence the health care professional's work with patients. For example, if you assume you know what patients are thinking or feeling, believe you know what is best for them, or react emotionally when confronted with difficult patients, you may fail to ask appropriate questions and collect the information necessary to help them resolve their health problems.

There are many sources of information for help in addressing problems:

- Your own knowledge and observations—what you know that relates to the problem.
- The knowledge and opinions of others, such as experts and people with special knowledge.
- Books, journals, and the Internet. There are many reader-friendly books about handling personal and professional problems.
- Classes, workshops, and conferences.

The number of resources you consult depends on the size, complexity, and importance of the problem. Some situations require only your current knowledge and a quick observation. Others require extensive research. (Review the section on research in Chapter 5.)

A good professional practice is to keep up-to-date in your field by reading and pursuing continuing education opportunities. This will give you the background needed for making sound decisions. It will also enable you to more effectively judge the quality of the information you gather. Not all published information or material from the Internet is based on thorough research. It can have errors or be biased by the opinions of the writer. Up-to-date knowledge of the fundamentals of your area will help you distinguish fact from opinion, an important component of critical thinking.

Here are some potential sources of information to help Kathy with her problem:

- Her math or pharmacology instructor
- Math tests that diagnose weak areas of knowledge
- Books, articles, and workshops about math anxiety
- Basic math textbooks
- Math books for health care students
- Measurement and dosage practice problems
- Online math help (the Internet)
- The resource center and library at her school

Step Three: Develop Alternative Solutions

There may be several effective solutions for a given problem. Use a technique called **brainstorming** to think of as many ideas as possible. Write them all down, even silly or impractical ideas. Don't discard anything, because even ideas that seem foolish can lead to ones that work.

Here is Kathy's list:

☐ Drop the class and hope to become smarter over time.
☐ Drop out of school. What's the use?
☐ Stay in the class, keep trying, and repeat the class if I don't pass.
☐ Drop the class and take it later. Use the extra time to work on math skills.
☐ Stay in the class and spend extra time developing math skills.
☐ Work through a basic math textbook.
☐ Use learning software.
☐ Work with a tutor.
☐ Form or join a study group.
☐ Ask the instructor to work with me after class several times a week.
☐ Ask a friend or relative who is good at math to help.
☐ Go to a hypnotist who specializes in helping people overcome anxiety problems.
☐ Use positive self-talk and visualizations.
☐ Borrow my children's math books.
☐ Ask my children for help.

☐ Go to a learning supply store and buy math games and toys.

 Go to page 206 to complete Prescription for Success 7-4

Step Four: Review Possible Results and Consequences

Now is the time to use critical thinking skills to evaluate your ideas. Review each option and ask yourself, "What would happen if I took this action?" You may find that you need to ask more questions and gather more information. Look for ideas that can be combined or that suggest other workable solutions. Let's review a few of Kathy's ideas from step three.

Drop out of school. What's the use?

This is an emotional response that's perfectly natural when a person feels frustrated and discouraged. Possible results and consequences:

☐ Disappointment at not reaching her goal of a career as a nurse.
☐ Missed opportunity to help others.
☐ Feelings of failure and depression.
☐ Student loans to repay and no job to help her financially.
☐ A feeling of relief. This just wasn't for her.

New questions Kathy can ask:

☐ How can I find out if I really am capable of learning the necessary math?
☐ How did I do in past math classes?
☐ Did I learn these skills at one time and just need to review, or did I never learn them at all?
☐ Do I have review materials, tutors, friends, and/or family members available to help me?
☐ What other career possibilities are open to me? Do I really want to change directions now?
☐ How much has my education cost so far? What would my student loan payments be each month if I were to drop out now?
☐ What other jobs am I qualified to start immediately? How much would they pay?

Stay in class and spend extra time developing math skills.

Possible results and consequences:

☐ She masters the math skills and does well in the class.
☐ She understands just enough to get by and passes the class.
☐ She tries but just never gets it and fails the class.
☐ She neglects her other classes when she spends extra time working on math skills.
☐ She passes all her classes, including math.

New questions Kathy can ask:

☐ How much math review do I think I need? Have I mastered at least the most fundamental math skills (e.g., multiplication and division of whole numbers)?

☐ What resources are available to help me learn the necessary math skills?

☐ How much extra time can I devote to learning math? (Consider job, family, etc.)

Go to a hypnotist for a cure for math anxiety.

Possible results and consequences:

☐ It works! She now looks forward to working with numbers.

☐ It doesn't work. She still experiences mental paralysis when faced with a problem that involves numbers.

☐ She still doesn't love math, but she can get through it to accomplish what needs to be done in her classes and on the job.

New questions Kathy can ask:

☐ Do I think that math anxiety is the problem, or have I just forgotten or never learned the necessary skills?

☐ Do I believe in hypnosis?

☐ Would I be comfortable trying hypnosis?

☐ Is there a good, reputable hypnotist in the area?

☐ How much does it cost? Can I afford it?

Although Kathy decides not to see a hypnotist, just considering this idea helps her realize that math anxiety may be a real problem for her. She decides to seek help from her school counselor and read a book about conquering math anxiety.

Step Five: Choose a Solution and Act on It

"It is common sense to take a method and try it. If it fails, admit it frankly and try another. But above all, try something."
—Franklin Roosevelt

After weighing the various alternatives, select the one that best fits your own mission and goals. It's easy to spend a lot of time thinking and then be afraid to take action. Think positively, make a plan, and do your best to implement the solution you have chosen. You may decide to combine several alternatives and attack the problem from different directions to increase your chance of success. Kathy decides to stay in the math class. She finds a math tutor and asks her sister to watch her children two afternoons a week to give her the extra time needed for meeting with the tutor and studying. She also decides to use positive self-talk to work on eliminating her negative feelings about math.

Step Six: Evaluate the Results and Revise Your Plan as Needed

Did you achieve the desired results? Were there unknown facts or circumstances that resulted in unexpected consequences? How can you revise your plan to get the results you want?

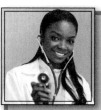

PROBLEM SOLVING ON THE JOB

Examples of common daily problems encountered by health care workers include the following:

• A man calls Dr. Beck's office complaining of chest pain. The medical assistant takes the call and must ask appropriate questions, apply what she knows, and decide whether the man should speak with the doctor, come to the office, or call 911 for emergency assistance.

• Dr. Beck is unhappy with the poor service he is receiving from the office's current supplier of certain medical supplies. The office manager contacts suppliers, compares prices and services, and uses the information collected to choose a new supplier.

• Rhonda is a nursing assistant at an extended-care facility. She has small children at home and must make childcare arrangements at least 1 week in advance. Several times during the past few weeks her supervisor has changed her schedule with only a day's notice. Rhonda wants to keep her job but cannot continually find childcare at the last minute. She must find a way to work out this problem with her supervisor.

• Carla, a medical biller, needs to learn a new billing software system as soon as possible to avoid getting behind in her work.

After working with the tutor for 3 weeks, Kathy realized that this person, though well-meaning, was unable to explain the concepts so she understood them. She decided to work on her own and bought a math software program that her math instructor recommended. She also joined a study group to share ideas and gain support from other students. The results of her revised plan were positive. She learned the skills she needed, gained self-confidence, and passed her pharmacology class.

 Go to page 207 to complete Prescription for Success 7-5

CREATING A PERSONAL REFERENCE GUIDE

After graduation, it's possible that you'll use your textbooks, lecture notes, and completed assignments as resources. Putting together your own reference guide adds even more value to your education by providing storage for useful information that might otherwise be lost. Collecting information, however, is not useful if you can't find it when you need it. It can make life more difficult, rather than help, if it becomes simply another pile of stuff that gets in your way. Design your guide to be an organized, easy-to-access source of information. Select a medium or large three-ring binder and buy a package of index dividers. Start with a few categories and add to them as you proceed through your program. Include a table of contents to help you see what you have at a glance.

You may find it helpful to incorporate building your guide as part of your study sessions. For example, writing new vocabulary lists can be part of your review for a terminology quiz. You can do the same thing when learning abbreviations, the steps in procedures, and other facts. These lists can then be included as part of your references. You will be applying the art of effective time management by accomplishing two things at the same time: creating a useful reference guide at the same time you are studying and reviewing.

The contents of your guide will vary according to your career area and personal preferences. Here are some suggestions. Put a checkmark next to the ones you think would be useful to include.

_____ Names, phone numbers, and addresses of instructors and classmates with whom you want to keep in touch. Include a sentence or two about each one for recall in the future.

_____ Spelling words from Tables 6-8 and 6-9 in Chapter 6 and other words you are learning and want to review periodically.

_____ New vocabulary words and their definitions.

_____ Important health care abbreviations. (When you become employed, your facility will have its own set of abbreviations you can add to your guide.)

_____ Useful Internet addresses.

_____ Names, titles, organizations, phone numbers, and addresses of professional contacts. Make a few notes about each person to refresh your memory later.

_____ Titles of interesting books and journals. Also, titles of reference books that might be useful on the job. There are pocket-sized guides for many occupations that contain frequently used measurements, formulas, summaries of common procedures, and so on.

_____ Inspiring and helpful quotations.

_____ Names and addresses of professional organizations (see Appendix A).

_____ Sources of equipment and supplies that were used in your school. (This list may be useful on the job if you are asked to make recommendations for purchases.)

_____ Summaries of the procedures you have learned. If check-off sheets are used in your classes, consider including them.

_____ Fact sheets that list measurement systems, test values, and so on. Your textbooks may include these within the body of the book or at the end in the form of appendices.

_____ Potential employers you learn about from your instructors, graduates, guest speakers, job fairs, newspaper articles, and so on.

_____ Completed Prescriptions for Success from this book.

_____ The Resume Building Block forms from Chapter 2:
1. Career objective
2. Education
3. Professional skills and knowledge
4. Work experience
5. Licenses and certifications
6. Honors and awards
7. Special skills
8. Community service and volunteer work
9. Memberships in professional and civic organizations
10. Languages spoken
11. References

Continue to add to these building blocks, as suggested in each chapter. When it is time to write your resume (see Chapter 10), you'll have all the information you need in one place.

Finally, think of your reference guide as a "living document." Add to it as you progress through your program and career. Your guide will be useful while you are in school, during the job search, and on the job.

⇨ SUMMARY OF KEY IDEAS

1. Practicing hands-on procedures forms a bridge between school and the world of work.
2. The ability to learn math is based as much on our emotions as on our intelligence.
3. Math anxiety can be overcome if we accept our feelings and are willing to find out what we need to learn.
4. Preparation, not panic, is the key to success in your program.
5. The clinical experience is your opportunity to enter the real world of health care.
6. Learning to think critically and solve problems effectively can improve the quality of your life.
7. Creating a personal reference guide can add to the value of your education.

⌨ Positive Self-Talk for This Chapter

1. I am perfecting my skills by the work I do in lab sessions.
2. I am overcoming math anxiety and learning what I need to know for health care applications.
3. I am presenting myself competently and professionally in my clinical experience.
4. I use problem-solving techniques to make sound decisions.

To Learn More

Benjamin-Chung M: *Math principles and practice: preparing for health career success,* Upper Saddle River, NJ, 1998, Prentice-Hall.

Kennamar M: *Math for health care professionals quick review,* Clifton Park, NY, 2004, Cengage Delmar.

Kogelman S, Warren J: *Mind over math,* New York, 1978, McGraw-Hill.

Although published 30 years ago, this book is still in print. It is a classic on the subject of overcoming fear of math.

MindTools

www.mindtools.com

This website offers help for developing problem solving and practical creativity (using creativity to succeed on the job).

Palau SM, Meltzer M: *Learning strategies for allied health students,* Philadelphia, 1996, Elsevier.

This book includes study techniques for various topics including math concepts used in health care occupations.

Pauk W, Owens RJQ: *How to study in college,* ed 8, New York, 2005, Houghton Mifflin.

This classic on how to study has good suggestions for mastering math in addition to reading and other skills.

Simmers L: *Practical problems in mathematics for health occupations,* Clifton Park, NY, 1996, Cengage Delmar Learning.

In addition to easy-to-understand explanations, this book has many practice problems that apply to a variety of health care occupations.

Study Guides and Strategies.

www.studygs.net

This website includes excellent sections on math, problem solving, and critical thinking.

REFERENCES

1. Pauk W, Owens RJQ: *How to study in college,* ed 8, New York, 2005, Houghton Mifflin.

2. Kogelman S, Warren J: *Mind over math,* New York, 1978, McGraw-Hill.

BUILDING YOUR RESUME

1. Copy (or tear out) the Building Your Resume forms from Chapter 2 and place them in your personal reference guide.
2. Think about any lab classes you have taken or practical exercises you have completed for your classes. Are there examples of skills you can list on Resume Building Block 3: Professional Skills and Knowledge?

INTERNET ACTIVITIES

For active links to the websites needed to complete these activities, visit **http://evolve.elsevier.com/ Haroun/career/**

1. The Centers for Disease Control and Prevention has developed guidelines for health care workers who come into contact with blood and other body fluids. Explore this site for information about diseases transmitted by blood, and write a short report about practices you can apply in school lab sessions.
2. Math.com contains links to explanations of math operations, sample problems, games, and quizzes for a whole range of math topics. Use the information on the website to learn more about a function you find difficult, and report on what you learned.
3. St Louis University maintains a site called Success in Mathematics that contains good information for students. Using the information you find, explain the difference between active and passive learning; explain how studying math is different from studying other subjects; and list two helpful hints you think might help you with math.
4. The Study Guides and Strategies website has published an excellent explanation of problem solving. Write a brief report summarizing what new information you learn about problem solving from this study guide.

Prescription for Success 7-1
Making the Most of Lab Assignments

1. Describe any previous experience you have had with lab courses. How well do you learn from practical sessions?

   _____

   _____

   _____

   _____

   _____

   _____

2. Which study and learning techniques do you think will work best for you in the lab?

   _____

   _____

   _____

   _____

   _____

   _____

3. Describe how you think working on the job will be different from the practice sessions you do in school.

   _____

   _____

   _____

   _____

   _____

   _____

Prescription for Success 7-2
What's Your Math Status?

1. Based on your review of Table 7-2, how would you rate your knowledge of math?

_____ Excellent _____ Very Good _____ Good _____ Fair _____ Poor

2. What math skills are required in your future profession?
3. If you don't know what math skills you will need, where can you find out?
4. If you rated yourself as "fair" or "poor," what plans do you have for improving?

_____ Take classes at school

_____ Use special services at school, such as computer lab or tutoring

_____ Study on my own

_____ Use workbooks with math problems

_____ Use math software

_____ View videos

_____ Other

Prescription for Success 7-3
Learn With Practice

Practice learning the metric system by using it at home. It you don't have a measuring stick or ruler that is marked in centimeters and millimeters, buy an inexpensive one. Measure and make labels for common items. For example, the height of a doorknob is about 1 meter from the floor. As you see them over and over, you will start to incorporate metric equivalents into your thinking.

Prescription for Success 7-4
More Solutions

List at least five more ideas that Kathy might consider.

1. _____

2. _____

3. _____

4. _____

5. _____

Try Something!

Choose a real problem you would like to solve and go through the six-step process.

1. Define the problem.

_____

_____

_____

2. Gather information.
   A. Sources

_____

_____

_____

   B. Facts, ideas, opinions

_____

_____

_____

3. Brainstorm alternative solutions.

_____

_____

_____

4. Consider possible results and consequences.

Results and Consequences   *Additional Questions or Information Needed*

_____   _____

_____   _____

_____   _____

5. Describe the solution you chose and the action you took.

_____

_____

_____

6. Describe and evaluate the results, and describe any needed revisions.

_____

_____

_____

Developing Your People Skills

OBJECTIVES

The information and activities in this chapter can help you:

- Explain the importance of good people skills.
- Describe ways to better understand people whose backgrounds and beliefs are different from yours.
- Explain the meaning of empathy and its importance in health care work.
- Improve your effectiveness when speaking.
- Become an active listener.
- Use various types of questions effectively.
- Become aware of how you and others communicate nonverbally.
- Prepare and present effective oral presentations.
- Practice good teamwork skills.
- Identify the teaching styles of your instructors, and describe what you can learn from each.
- Apply effective strategies when dealing with difficult people.
- Explain the role of criticism in the learning process.

KEY TERMS AND CONCEPTS

Debate: Formal discussion in which two people or teams take sides on an issue, and each tries to persuade the audience to accept its point of view.

Diversity: The differences that characterize people, including native language, religious beliefs, values, and everyday customs.

Empathy: Awareness and understanding of how another person feels and experiences the world.

Feedback: Techniques used in spoken communication to check your understanding of what you hear another person say.

Nonverbal Communication: Facial expressions, gestures, nondeliberate movements, and body position.

Organizational Cultures: The customs and practices of organizations that influence all aspects of how work is accomplished and what is considered appropriate behavior.

Teamwork: Working with other people to accomplish a common goal. Modern patient care depends on teams of professionals working together.

THE IMPORTANCE OF PEOPLE SKILLS

The last few chapters focused on you as an individual and the personal attitudes, habits, and skills that influence your academic and career success. In this chapter, we shift our focus to other people and how you relate to them. You can expect to work closely with many kinds of people in your career, and your ability to create and maintain mutually beneficial relationships will be an important factor in your career success.

The quality and consistency of patient care are affected by how well health care professionals communicate among themselves as well as with patients and their families. Poor communication with patients contributes to the growing number of malpractice lawsuits. When patients feel they are listened to and understood, they are less likely to sue. This is true even if their treatment outcomes are negative.

At the same time, one of the most frequent complaints from employers today is that their employees lack good people skills. They don't know how to work well with others. More people fail on the job because of poor interpersonal skills than because they lack the necessary technical qualifications.

Good interpersonal skills are also important for academic success. Throughout your studies, you will have opportunities to learn from both your instructors and your fellow students. Your ability to communicate effectively will influence how much and how well you learn. Activities such as working on teams, practicing hands-on skills with other students, and joining study groups are ways you can start now to practice working with others. Most of life's activities take place in relation to other people, and improving the quality of these relationships can improve the overall quality of your life.

RESPECTING OTHERS

"Be kind. Remember, everyone you meet is fighting a hard battle."

Plato

By choosing a career in health care, you have accepted the responsibility to serve others. Your duties may range from performing an uncomfortable medical procedure to explaining a complicated bill for a hospital stay. It will be your obligation to serve all patients or clients with an equal level of care and concern, regardless of their appearance, behavior, level of education, and economic status. Not everyone will look, act, behave, or even smell as you would like. They will not all express appreciation for your efforts. People who feel sick may

be irritable and cranky. The satisfaction you obtain from your work must be based on what you can give to others, not on what you receive from them.

Good health care practice is based on the principle that all human beings deserve to be treated with respect and dignity. The need to treat all patients equally and fairly has been recognized and endorsed by professional organizations such as the American Hospital Association (AHA). The AHA formalized this belief in "The Patient Care Partnership" mentioned in Chapter 1. Specifically, it states that patients have the right to "be treated with compassion and respect."

It is also important to demonstrate respect toward your supervisor and co-workers. The quality of work produced in any organization depends on the quality of the relationships among the people who work there, and good relationships are based on mutual respect.

Guidelines for Respectful Behavior

☐ **Be courteous.** Many observers today have noted that as a society we are moving away from the practice of common courtesy. Many people fail to use expressions like "please" and "thank you." These are powerful words that improve the quality of both personal and professional relationships.

☐ **Maintain professionalism.** As a student and on the job, it is important to display maturity and competence. Examples of inappropriate communication behaviors are chewing gum, arguing, swearing, and yelling.

☐ **Acknowledge the other person.** No one likes to be ignored. If you are busy working with someone else or talking on the telephone when a patient arrives, use eye contact and a quick nod to let the person know you are aware of his or her presence.

☐ **Don't interrupt.** Avoid breaking in when another person is speaking. Some people need extra time to compose their thoughts or express themselves. Avoid the habit of finishing sentences for others. This frustrates the speaker, and your assumption about what they planned to say may be incorrect.

☐ **Show interest.** Look at the other person when you are talking and listening. Show you are listening by nodding or using confirming sounds or phrases such as "uh, huh," "I understand," "okay," and so on. Don't turn your body toward the door as if to say, "Hurry up. I need to move on to something else."

☐ **Guard privacy.** This is good practice in your personal life. In health care, patient privacy is protected by law. It is illegal to discuss patient information with anyone who is not working directly with the patient. Make a habit of never sharing anything told to you in confidence by family members, friends, or classmates. (Patients must even give written permission before information can be given to insurance companies, other health providers, and so on. More information about patient confidentiality is given in Chapter 13.)

☐ **Avoid gossip**. Gossip can be a very serious problem in the workplace. It serves no useful purpose and can lead to hurt feelings, broken trust, and strained relationships. If it involves confidential patient matters, it can lead to a lawsuit.

☐ **Remain calm**. It is important to behave and speak calmly when you are dealing with situations such as emergencies and angry patients. A calm demeanor both reassures others and enables you to focus on doing what can best help the situation.

Take a look at the people in Figure 8-1. Do they appear to be showing respect for one another?

 Go to page 231 to complete Prescription for Success 8-1

APPRECIATING DIVERSITY

"Commandment Number One of any truly civilized society is this: Let people be different."
—David Grayson

The population of the United States is made up of people from all over the world, as illustrated in Figure 8-2. Immigration has increased dramatically

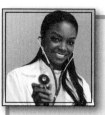

SHOWING RESPECT ON THE JOB

The book *Health Professional and Patient Interaction* includes a conversation from a student who was finishing his clinical experience:

"This might surprise you," John said, "but do you know what I'd say is the most important thing I've learned in the last several weeks of my experiences in the clinics? I'd call it learning that little things mean a lot! Do you think that's ridiculous? For instance, I have learned the importance of pouring a glass of water for a thirsty patient, listening to the ninth inning of a baseball game between parts of a treatment, laughing at something the patient says, wiping a nose. Perhaps these things sound silly to you, but I know that I could not be getting the good results I am seeing if I had not mastered these skills along with my technical ones!" After a pause, he added with a smile, "I guess I have learned to nurture my patients a little!"

It is often the small things that show patients you care about them, and this can have a very positive effect on their health outcomes.

(From: Purtilo R, Haddad A: *Health professional and patient interaction*, ed 7, Philadelphia, 2007, Saunders.)

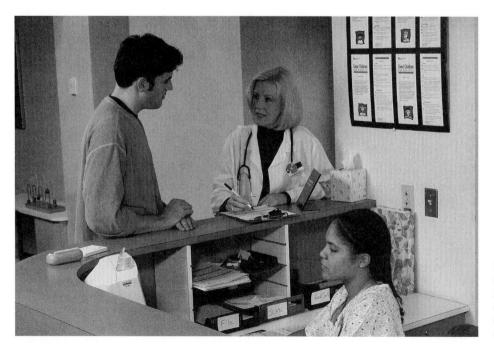

Figure 8-1 Respectful interaction is a critical component of good health care. How are the health care professionals in the photo demonstrating respect as they communicate?

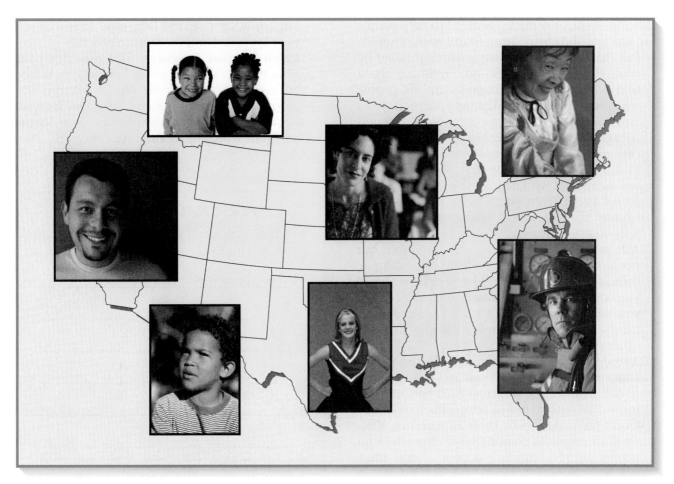

Figure 8-2 It is likely that you will work with people, both patients and co-workers, from a variety of cultural backgrounds. Their differences may include ethnicity, age, and educational levels.

in recent years, and Americans now more than ever represent a wide variety of races, religions, lifestyles, languages, and educational and economic levels. These variations are known as **diversity.**

Diversity also refers to differences not related to cultural background or race. These include age, sexual orientation, disabilities, and appearance. People who are different are sometimes ignored or treated inappropriately, sometimes even cruelly. This may not be done intentionally, so you must think about what you are doing and how it might be interpreted. For example, it is not uncommon for health care professionals to speak to younger relatives who accompany elderly patients as if the patients were not present. Other examples are using "baby talk" with the elderly or shouting at them if they were hard of hearing.

Our society can benefit from the contributions of people with different customs and ideas. By drawing from a variety of viewpoints, we increase our chances of solving the complex problems encountered in modern society. Learning from our differences can be beneficial. Many Americans, for example, find pain relief from the ancient Chinese practice of acupuncture, the insertion of very small needles into specific points on the body. Unfortunately, differences in values and beliefs about life can cause misunderstandings and even lead to violence. Learning to take advantage of the differences and to peacefully work out misunderstandings is one of the major challenges the world faces today.

Work in health care will give you opportunities to interact with people from many different backgrounds. Your personal actions and efforts to understand and serve others can contribute to a more harmonious society. The students in your school probably come from diverse backgrounds. Initiate communication with them. And if your own background is different from that of your classmates, you can serve as a source of information about your culture.

Promoting Understanding

When we learn about others, we also learn about ourselves and what it means to be human. You can enrich your life by accepting diversity and seeking opportunities to learn about different ways to view the world. Here are some suggestions to help people of all backgrounds better understand each other:

☐ **Put fear aside.** Many people are frightened by what they don't understand. Some are afraid that acknowledging differences among people will result in negative changes in society. In fact, the contributions of people from different backgrounds have resulted in the economic success and political stability of the United States.

☐ **Listen to other points of view.** Seek opportunities to interact with people whose backgrounds are different from yours. Encourage them to express their ideas and opinions. Listen carefully to what they say.

☐ **Ask questions.** Use questions to learn more, but not to challenge the other person. For example, instead of asking, "Why do you believe that?" you could say, "That sounds interesting. Could you tell me more about that?" Your goal is to learn and understand, not to imply that the other person is wrong.

☐ **Avoid stereotypes.** Don't make assumptions about people because of their age, race, gender, or other categories. Consider each person as an individual with a unique set of characteristics.

☐ **Don't judge people by their appearance.** Outward appearances do not always represent who people are. To truly know people, you must talk with them and observe their actions. If you immediately dismiss them based on how they look, you may lose the opportunity to form a friendship or a beneficial working relationship. Assuming that patients "are what they look like" may detract from the care you give them.

☐ **Explore different cultures.** Many schools and communities sponsor activities that highlight the cultures represented in the local population. Check your local library and the Internet for other sources of information about the backgrounds of your classmates and future patients.

☐ **Learn about other value systems.** People are defined by their values and beliefs about how they should live. Culture is much more than typical foods and daily customs. Develop a deeper level of knowledge and understanding through conversation and by learning about the religions and important beliefs of the people in your area. See Table 8-1 for examples of cultural and personal beliefs.

☐ **Look for commonalities.** As human beings, we share many of the same needs, concerns, and goals for our lives. Explore what you have in common with people who seem different.

☐ **Offer to help others.** Expand your attitude of caring by looking for ways to help others. For example, offer to help a classmate who has trouble speaking or writing English. Or if English is your second language, offer to teach your language and customs to others.

☐ **Learn another language.** You may not have time now to study another language formally, but you can learn a few key phrases of any major cultural groups in your area. This can increase your effectiveness as a health care professional and your worth to an employer.

PERSONAL REFLECTION

1. Which cultural groups are represented where you live?

_____

_____

_____

_____

_____

_____

2. How much do you know about their customs and beliefs?

_____

_____

_____

_____

_____

3. How can you learn more?

_____

_____

_____

_____

_____

_____

TABLE 8-1	Examples of Cultural and Personal Beliefs
Time	It is important to always be on time for meetings and appointments. Appointment times are just estimations of when they might take place. Time is valuable and should not be wasted. Time is not a resource over which we have control. It just is. Planning and using time productively are important. If something is important, it will eventually get done; there is no reason to rush. The present is more important than the future. The present should be used for planning and preparing for the future.
Personal Space	The distance comfortably maintained when people are talking ranges from a few inches (when you can feel the breath of the other person on your face) to over a foot away.
Age	Youth is valued. People should try to maintain a young appearance and lifestyle as long as possible (exercise, wrinkle creams, and hair dyes). Older people are valued for their wisdom and are shown great respect. When elderly people are no longer able to care for themselves, it is appropriate to place them in nursing or retirement homes. Older people should live with and be cared for by family members until they die.
Touching	Shaking hands is okay for everyone. Only members of the same sex can shake hands with one another. Hugging is okay for everyone, even members of the same sex. Kissing is okay between women. When meeting a new person, only a slight bow is permitted, not touching.
Gender	A woman cannot be treated by a male physician. Women and men are equal. Men are dominant. Women act as the head of most families. Women have no economic or political power.
Eye Contact	Direct eye contact is a sign of sincerity, honesty, and interest in the other person. It is a sign of disrespect. Sustained eye contact communicates hostility and aggression or sexual interest.
Personal Control	Each person is in control of his or her own life. Luck, fate, or the will of God determines how things turn out.
Spiritual Practices	There is one God. God helps those who help themselves. God punishes those who sin. God answers all prayers. There is uncertainty about the existence of God. There is no God. Witchcraft and magic can both help and hurt us.
Definition of Success	Personal and professional achievement. Acquiring material possessions. Living a spiritual life. Achieving inner peace. Raising many children. Being a kind person and helping others.
Health Care Beliefs	Disease is caused by germs, environmental conditions, and personal habits such as smoking. Good health is a gift or reward from God. Illness is a punishment sent by God. Illness happens when the body's energy or humors get out of balance. Science has the best answers for preventing and curing disease. The body can heal itself naturally. Herbs are the best remedies. Only God can heal. Good health is a balance among the mind, body, and spirit. Individuals are responsible for their own health and healing.
Beliefs About Death and Dying	Death is a natural part of the life cycle. Death should be avoided at all costs. Dying is up to God. Death means the health care system has failed. Autopsies destroy the soul. Cremation frees the soul. Everything possible should be done to save life. People who are terminally ill or suffering should be assisted to die if this is their wish. Families should take care of the dying. Hospitals or other health care facilities should take care of the dying.

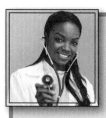

DIVERSITY ON THE JOB

Everything we do is influenced by our cultural background. Being aware that differences exist can help you to better understand the people you will encounter on the job. Beliefs that many of us take for granted, such as, "It is important to always be on time," are not important to everyone. Making assumptions can result in misunderstandings. Let's look at an example. A patient has to wait 15 minutes before you can perform his lab test. In an effort to respect his time and not add to the delay, you keep conversation to a minimum and complete the procedure as quickly as possible. You believe you have been considerate. The patient, from a culture that does not consider time in the same way, is insulted. His interpretation of your behavior is that you obviously have more important things to do than work with him, so you are rushing along. The "right thing" in your eyes was the "wrong thing" in his. Of course, it is impossible to know and accommodate every cultural difference that you encounter. You can, however, be aware of what types of differences exist and strive to be sensitive to them. Ask questions if you are unsure about a person's feelings or understanding of a situation. Table 8-1 lists common areas of differences among cultures.

Go to page 232 to complete Prescription for Success 8-2

Go to page 232 to complete Prescription for Success 8-3

EXPERIENCING EMPATHY

"Don't judge a man until you've walked a mile in his shoes."

Empathy means attempting to see the world through the eyes of other people in order to understand their feelings and experiences. Prescription for Success 1-7 in Chapter 1 asked you to imagine yourself as a patient with a broken arm. Putting yourself in the place of someone else is an important part of experiencing empathy. This is not always easy to do because we are all influenced by our own beliefs, values, and previous experiences. Being empathetic requires listening carefully to others without judging what you hear. You then think about what you hear and, if

necessary, ask for clarification or more information. What is the person trying to communicate or trying to hide? What clues are you getting from the person's body language? What is important to this person?

Health care professionals must have empathy with patients to understand their needs and learn how best to help them. Being empathetic sends the message, "You are important and worth my time and respect. I will make every effort to know who you are and what you need."

A key part of empathy is letting the other person know that you are trying to understand his or her experience. It is best, however, not to say that you know exactly how he or she feels. This sounds insincere because, in fact, it is impossible to know precisely how another person feels. In trying to be helpful, we may be tempted to share and compare our own stories—for example, saying, "Oh, I know just what you mean. The same thing happened to me…" and then launching into a detailed explanation about what happened to us. This shifts the focus to us and away from the person who needs the attention.

Learning to experience empathy improves all interpersonal relationships, including those with friends, family members, classmates, instructors, co-workers, and supervisors. Your relationships can be more harmonious when you make an effort to see the views of others. Here are some ways to increase your practice of empathy at home and in school:

- When you talk with your classmates, listen carefully. How are their views different from yours? What experiences have they had that explain these differences?

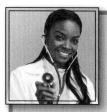

EMPATHY ON THE JOB

A medical office manager shared the following story: The receptionist, Grace, was a very efficient woman who treated all patients courteously. One of the patients, William, was a gay man with AIDS. Grace was courteous but stiffened visibly whenever he came for appointments. She had trouble accepting his lifestyle. One day William learned that Grace's son had been a missionary in Africa. On his next visit, William brought in a scrapbook that showed his experience working with missionaries in Africa. After that, Grace was warm and friendly to William. When asked why seeing the scrapbook had changed her behavior, she said that now she was able to see William as a person and not simply as a gay man with AIDS.

TABLE 8–2	Examples of Spoken Messages		
Purpose	**School**	**Job Search**	**Career**
Provide information	Help a classmate who missed an important lecture	Describe your training to a potential employer	Give instructions to a co-worker
Demonstrate knowledge	Give a presentation in class	Describe your qualifications, using examples, to a potential employer	Report to your supervisor about a workshop you attended
Persuade	Convince a friend not to cheat on a test	Present yourself successfully at a job interview	Inspire a patient to follow her exercise program
Gather information	Ask questions in class	Ask a professional contact for career information	Conduct a patient interview
Acknowledge others	Greet classmates and instructors	Thank interviewers for their time	Express interest in your patients

- Are there students who exhibit poor behavior? Why do you think they behave in this way? What are some clues that might explain their actions?
- Why do family members sometimes "act out"?
- What kinds of experiences have shaped the opinions of your friends?

 Go to page 233 to complete Prescription for Success 8-4

ORAL COMMUNICATION: CREATING THE PEOPLE CONNECTION

Many people believe they are good communicators because they are friendly and like to talk. But the ability to speak is only one part of effective communication. There are four other essential parts of effective communication: listening, thinking, requesting feedback, and using and interpreting **nonverbal communication** (body language, expressions, and gestures). Successful oral communication takes place when the receiver (listener) receives and understands the intended message of the speaker. We all know this is not always the case! Let's look at how you can increase the effectiveness of your communication.

Speaking

Speaking consists of creating and sending messages. The first step in creating a clear message is to determine your purpose. In Chapter 6, we discussed the importance of determining your purpose when writing. It is the same with speaking: you need to know your communication goal. Table 8-2 contains examples of reasons for sending a message.

Effective messages match the purpose of the speaker with the needs of the receiver. These needs are determined, in part, by the characteristics of the receiver. Figure 8-3 contains examples of characteristics you should consider in order to create appropriate messages.

Success Tips for Sending Effective Messages

☐ Speak from a base of sincerity, caring, and respect for others.

☐ Choose a level of language that is appropriate for the receiver. If a person is heavily medicated, for example, use simple words and short sentences.

☐ Choose appropriate vocabulary. Using medical terminology is an effective way to be precise when speaking with co-workers, but it can be confusing for patients. They may hesitate to tell you they don't understand because they don't want to seem dumb. However, ensuring that patients understand your questions and explanations is critical for their health outcomes. The inability to understand health care providers is a major patient complaint.

☐ Avoid slang and nonstandard speech. These are often characteristic of certain age and social groups and can cause misunderstandings with people outside those groups. Speech that is appropriate among friends and at social gatherings may not be correct for school and work. For example, the current use of the word "goes" to mean "says" is understood by many young people but may be confusing to others.

☐ Speak clearly and at a moderate speed—not so quickly that you are difficult to understand or so slowly that the receiver's mind wanders. (We hear and comprehend many times faster than we speak.)

☐ Avoid speaking in a monotone. Speak naturally, but with expression in your voice. Make sure it is appropriate for your message. For example, speak with respect when asking questions in class,

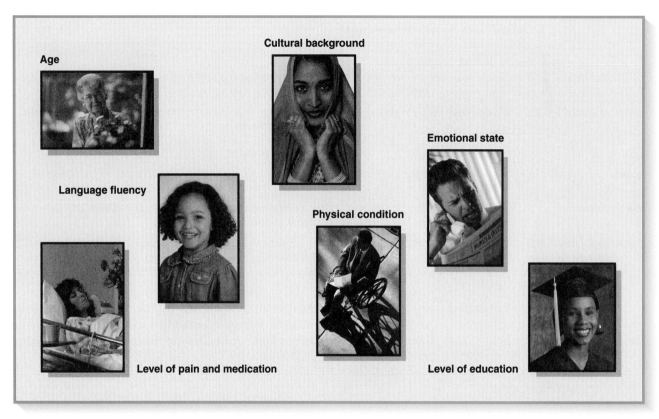

Figure 8-3   Consider who your listener is when creating your spoken message. What do they already know about the topic? Why might they be interested in knowing about what you are saying?

friendliness when greeting a new student, reassurance when calming fears, and firmness when giving instructions that affect patient safety.

ACTIVE LISTENING

"To listen well is as powerful a means of communication as to talk well."
—*U.S. Supreme Court Chief Justice*
John Marshall

Active listening, as was discussed in Chapter 5, should not be confused with hearing. Listening requires effort, whereas hearing is more passive. To listen well, you must pay attention, focus on the speaker's words, and reflect on what you hear. Active listening demonstrates respect for the speaker. It is an essential skill for the health care professional because all patients want to work with someone who listens to them and makes every effort to understand their needs. In fact, patient satisfaction surveys show that patients highly value providers who are excellent listeners and take what they say seriously.[1] The health care professional in Figure 8-4 is demonstrating active listening skills.

Think for a moment about your own listening skills. Do you sometimes catch your mind wandering and thinking about other things? Do you think about what you are going to say next? Do you argue mentally when you disagree? These habits can interfere with your attention and prevent you from hearing the speaker's message. Look over the following checklist of techniques designed to improve listening skills. Are there any you'd like to try?

☐ Prepare yourself mentally to listen by clearing your mind of other thoughts.

☐ Control the noise level of your environment as much as possible. Turn off the radio or television, look for a quiet place to talk, or move out of the busiest part of the office.

☐ Focus on the other person and concentrate on following what he or she is saying. Sometimes when we think we are listening, looking at the speaker, and perhaps even nodding in agreement, we are actually thinking about something else. Practice being aware of where your attention is directed.

☐ If you disagree with what you are hearing, try not to engage in mental arguments. Internal self-talk interferes with your ability to listen. It is usually easy to understand people we agree with. It takes more effort to hear people we disagree with, but only by listening carefully can we begin to understand another's point of view.

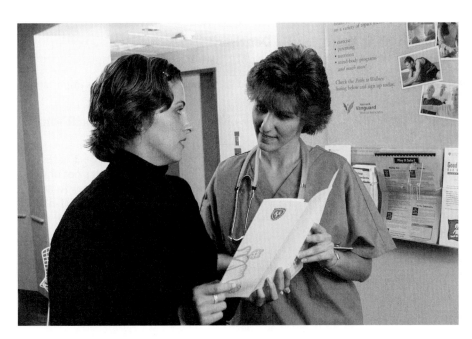

Figure 8-4   Listening well is as important as speaking well. In what ways does this health care worker's body language demonstrate active listening skills?

☐ Practice making quick mental notes about points you need to clarify Work on being able to do this without losing track of what the person is saying.

☐ Focus on what is being said rather than how it is said. Move beyond the speaker's appearance, manners, language level, or even odor. Try not to let unpleasant factors about the person interfere with your ability to concentrate on what he or she has to say.

☐ Acknowledge the person even if you are taking notes or performing a test or procedure while he or she is talking. Look at the person from time to time and make eye contact.

Listening effectively is one of the most valuable skills you can develop for both personal and professional success. It can increase your learning, your effectiveness in helping others, and even your popularity. At the same time, it is a skill many people neglect because they assume they know how to listen. Working to improve your listening skills is one of the most important actions you can take to work well with others.

FEEDBACK

Feedback is a communication technique used to check your understanding of what a speaker says. Even when you listen carefully, there may be times when what you hear is not what the speaker intended. We have all experienced the misunderstandings that occur when we assume we understand the speaker's message—and then learn that the intended message was quite different!

There are several methods for giving and requesting feedback. Here are three of the most common kinds of feedback:

1. **Paraphrasing**. This means saying what you heard in your own words so that the speaker can confirm or correct your statement.

2. **Reflecting**. This is similar to paraphrasing, but you repeat what the other person says using words as close as possible to his or her own words. This gives the person the opportunity to confirm or add additional information.

3. **Clarifying**. This means asking the speaker to explain what he or she means.

See Table 8-3 for examples of each kind of feedback.

ASKING QUESTIONS

"No man really becomes a fool until he stops asking questions."
—*Charles P. Steinmetz*

Scientific discoveries and technologic advances are the result of people asking questions. What causes…? What would happen if…? How can we…? Asking questions is a powerful tool for learning. You can increase your knowledge and understanding in school by asking questions. Yet many students sit through hours of classes and never ask a single question. Take advantage of your opportunities to learn and get ready to ask good questions in class. Here are some tips to get started:

• **Prepare ahead for class.** If you haven't read the assignment or completed the other homework,

with Health Care Professionals Staff at Bend Family Dentistry

The staff at Bend Family Dentistry discusses the importance of communication in the workplace.

Q What can you tell me about communication in this office?

A Simply put, communication is everything. It's even more important than what we actually *do*.

Q Can you explain what you mean by that?

A We've found that the most common reason patients transfer here from other dentists is miscommunication. It wasn't the quality of the dental work. They just didn't understand what was going on or didn't feel that the staff really cared about them. We know we need to explain things to patients—what we're doing and why. Why they need seven fillings. Why a crown costs $1200. And we have to do this in a nice way. We can't tell them it's their fault that they don't brush well and never floss. We can't lecture them. But we can treat them kindly and explain what we've found and what we believe needs to be done.

Q What part does inter-staff communication play?

A A big one. Patients pick up on poor inter-staff communication, and it makes them uncomfortable. You never want them to feel there is any friction or that their information didn't get passed along to the person who needed it.

You should speak to your co-workers as you would like to be spoken to. You really have to value them and consider their input and their feelings. And remember that there is always more than one way to do something, so be accepting of differences among staff. When you're talking with the dentist, you have to think about what you're saying. Identify the important points, summarize, and communicate clearly. Share any information about patients you think will help the next person who is going to work with them.

Q Besides good communication, what else is important?

A Doing your share of the work—and maybe a little extra. Know your job and what your responsibilities are.

Help others, clean up, answer the phone if necessary. Look for things to do—sometimes it's not obvious, but learn to observe and see what needs to be done. Think to yourself, "What could I do to fill in and help the situation?"

Dr. Hester always says that he wants the work environment here to be "like a waltz where everything is smooth, cool, and okay." This means that our goal is to make everyone's job easier. We want the dentists to be able to focus on clinical work and the patients. The dental assistants learn to know what the dentists want and need.

Q People don't usually enjoy going to the dentist. How do you handle this as dental professionals?

A We start with ourselves. One of our sayings here is "leave your stress at the door." We can't expect patients to feel okay about being here if we aren't. So we try to be calm and reassuring. We listen to patients. They may be nervous and talkative—they may express views we don't agree with. When this happens, we are respectful and keep our personal views to a minimum. Patients who are really afraid may be angry, arrogant, or just grumpy. Again, we listen and try to be attuned to their needs. Maybe they need more explanations. They may need to know exactly what's going to happen and what they will feel. If they have had trouble in the past, we ask them went wrong, how they felt, and what we can do to help the situation. Our goal is to establish confidence and trust so they can be more comfortable.

you won't have the background information on which to base a question.

- **Write questions down.** Suppose you did the reading and remember that there were several points you didn't understand, but you didn't write them down, and now you can't remember what they were! Don't let this happen to you. During lectures, write down questions as you think of them so you can ask them at the appropriate time.

- **Don't be embarrassed.** No one wants to ask what they think is a dumb question. But if you already knew everything, you wouldn't be in school, right? Instructors welcome questions in class and are usually pleased when students take an interest in the subject. (Exception: You

don't pay attention in class and/or don't read the assigned material and then ask lots of questions that force the instructor to repeat what he or she just finished saying.)

- **Ask the questions later.** If all the class time is taken up with the lecture or the instructor never gets around to your lab group, arrange a time to ask your questions later. Be willing to make the extra effort to get the information you need.

- **Be brave.** Have you ever found yourself so confused in class you can't even phrase a question? This is exactly when you should ask a question. Try something like, "I'm lost here. Could we go back to...?" Avoid waiting until you're so far behind that you don't have a chance of catching up.

TABLE 8-3	Examples of Feedback	
	What the Speaker Says	**Feedback**
PARAPHRASING		
School	This week's assignment is on page 83 of your workbook. Complete exercises 3 through 8.	Let me make sure that I have it right. We're to do exercises 3 through 8 on page 83 in the workbook and turn them in on Friday.
Job search	We really need employees we can rely on to be here on time every day. It's also essential they can get along with their co-workers.	It sounds like two of the most important characteristics you are looking for are punctuality and the ability to work well with others.
Career	It really hurts most when I get up in the mornings. I feel a little better as the day goes by.	It sounds like the pain is much worse when you first wake up in the morning but decreases during the day.
REFLECTING		
School	Well, I don't have any time for a study group because of my work schedule.	You said that you don't have time to join our study group because of your work schedule? (You suspect there may be another reason, and if it is known, arrangements could be made for the person to join the group.)
Job search	Here is a copy of the job description. It has most of the duties required for this position, although there are some others.	The job description has most of the duties required, but there are a few others? (The interviewer has given the impression that more may be expected than just what is listed on the job description.)
Career	I haven't lost any weight because the diet the doctor gave me isn't working.	You haven't lost any weight because the diet isn't working? (There may be other reasons, such as not following the diet exactly, lack of exercise, and so on.)
CLARIFYING		
School	The tests in this class are really tough. You'll see!	You said the tests in medical terminology are really hard. Can you give me an example of a question?
Job search	It's easy to find. We're really close to the Cross Town Shopping Center.	You said you are close to the Cross Town Shopping Center. Can you tell me about how many blocks that is?
Career	I give him the medication on schedule, but ever since he's been taking it his behavior has been kind of strange.	Can you explain what you mean when you say your son has been acting "strangely" since he started taking the medication?

Types of Questions

There are four basic types of questions, as follows:

1. **Closed-ended**. Can be answered with a "yes" or "no" or in one or two words. They are used for getting specific facts.
2. **Open-ended**. Require a longer answer and request explanations, descriptions, examples, and other details.
3. **Probing**. Based on what the other person has already told you. The purpose is to acquire additional information.
4. **Leading**. Question is worded to provide a possible answer. These questions should be used with great care because they may encourage the other person to simply agree because he or she doesn't really understand the question or thinks you have provided the correct answer. Leading questions can be helpful with people who find it difficult to communicate because of injury, language barriers, shyness, or other problems that make communicating difficult.

See Table 8-4 for examples of each kind of question.

 Go to page 235 to complete Prescription for Success 8-5

Success Tips for Asking Effective Questions

☐ **Choose the right place**. Some important questions are personal, embarrassing, or potentially difficult to answer. A question for the instructor about a low grade you believe to be unfair is best asked in private, not during class. An interview with a patient with acquired immunodeficiency syndrome (AIDS) must be conducted out of the hearing of others.

TABLE 8-4	Examples of Questions
Type of Question	**Examples**
Closed-ended	What is the date of the math test? Can we use our calculators? Have you ever had surgery?
Open-ended	How would you recommend that we study for the math test? What was your understanding of why you needed surgery?
Probing	Could you give us an example of the kind of question that will be on the test? Can you describe how you found it easier to walk after you had the surgery?
Leading	Did you decide not to do the exercises at home because you didn't understand the instructions?

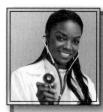

ASKING QUESTIONS ON THE JOB

On the job it will be important to know how and when to ask questions. For example, never proceed with a task if you are unsure about any part of it. It is smarter to ask than to take safety risks, waste supplies, or make it necessary for someone else to redo your work. Questions are also a good way to show interest in your job and gain a better understanding of your duties.

Gathering information from patients is an important part of most health care occupations. In order for physicians and others to make diagnoses, they need information about family history, symptoms, lifestyle habits, and anything else that affects health.

□ **Choose the right time**. Asking your supervisor a question about your performance when he or she is ready to leave the office isn't fair to either of you.

□ **Avoid challenging or judgmental questions**. Your choice of words and tone of voice can communicate the negative message, "You are wrong, and I demand an explanation." For example, questions like, "Why did you do that?" or "What were you thinking?" may draw a defensive reaction or no response at all. A major goal of communication should be to encourage discussion so that issues can be resolved.

□ **Know what not to ask**. There is a difference between showing interest in others and asking questions that are too personal and may offend. To show concern without prying, you can say something like, "You seem really upset. Is there some way I can help?" This allows the person to reveal as much information as is comfortable. If you must ask potentially embarrassing questions, explain why you are asking them and how the information will be used. Assure patients that anything they say will remain confidential, as required by law.

□ **Know what's legal**. Some questions, especially when asked in hiring situations, are illegal. These include asking about age, marital status, number of children, and other matters that are not related to job performance. (See Chapter 11 for more information.)

□ **Allow silence**. Some people need more time than others to think and prepare a response. Unless it is obvious they don't understand the question, don't feel that you must speak to fill the silence.

NONVERBAL COMMUNICATION

More than half of the content and meaning of our messages is communicated nonverbally through our movements, posture, gestures, and facial expressions. In fact, nonverbal communication is often more revealing than verbal communication because we are usually not aware we are doing it—it is not completely under our control. For example, telling a friend that you are "fine" when you have a worried expression on your face sends a mixed message. The friend is more likely to believe your face than your words. Nonverbal communication can either emphasize or distort the content of verbal messages. See Figure 8-5 for an example of common nonverbal language.

Use the following questions as a starting point for becoming more aware of your own nonverbal language.

1. Do you have nervous habits, such as jiggling your leg or playing with your hair, that distract from or distort your messages? These habits can give the impression that you would rather be somewhere else.

2. Is your general posture upright or slouching? Do you face the person you're talking with or partially turn away, as if looking for escape? Leaning slightly toward the other person communicates interest.

3. Do you assume an accepting body position? Crossing the arms, for example, can be a sign of being closed to what the other person is saying.

4. Do you use gestures to emphasize or add meaning to your words? Or are they routine habits

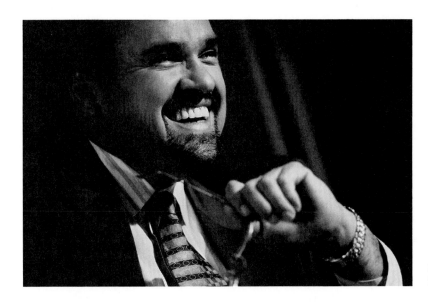

Figure 8-5   What messages are being expressed by this man's nonverbal communication?

that add nothing to your message? Gestures are especially helpful when used for demonstrations and to communicate with people who have limited ability to understand spoken language. Examples include very young children, non-English speakers, and the hearing impaired.

5. Does your face express interest or boredom? In class, do you usually face the instructor or look out the window? When an activity is announced, do you roll your eyes and exchange pained looks with other students? Poor attitudes are easy to read and can negatively affect the quality of the class by annoying the instructor or putting him or her on the defensive. Learning to control facial expressions is important because as a health care professional you will need to maintain expressions that convey caring and reassurance even in difficult situations.

6. Do you smile when it is appropriate? Does your face send the message "I'm glad to be here talking with you"?

7. Do you maintain appropriate eye contact? Failing to look at the other person while you are speaking tends to communicate a lack of sincerity, interest, or respect. (Exceptions to this include cultures that interpret eye contact in different ways.)

In addition to monitoring your own nonverbal communication, practice observing it in others. This will be important when working with patients who may be unable or unwilling to fully communicate with you verbally. Learn to "listen between the lines." Do the speaker's words and actions match? Are there nonverbal signs of confusion, fear, or anger that you should take into account? Does

your instructor give any of the nonverbal messages, discussed in Chapter 5, that communicate what is most important for you to learn?

Ask for clarification if verbal and nonverbal messages seem to conflict. Use the feedback and question techniques discussed previously. Be willing to take the time and make the effort to get the true message. You can improve the interpersonal relationships in all areas of your life by combining an understanding of nonverbal communication with active listening and feedback.

 Go to page 235 to complete Prescription for Success 8-6

 Go to page 236 to complete Prescription for Success 8-7

GIVING PRESENTATIONS WITH CONFIDENCE

Many students find speaking in front of a group to be a frightening experience. This is a fear worth conquering, because the ability to speak with confidence can increase your opportunities to grow professionally and advance in your career. Proper preparation and a lot of practice can take the terror out of public speaking. See Figure 8-6 for examples of self-talk that affect confidence.

Preparing an oral presentation requires some of the same skills you use when writing, such as conducting research and organizing your material. It is said that an excellent way to learn something is to explain it to someone else. Try making oral presentations positive experiences by focusing on how you can learn from them.

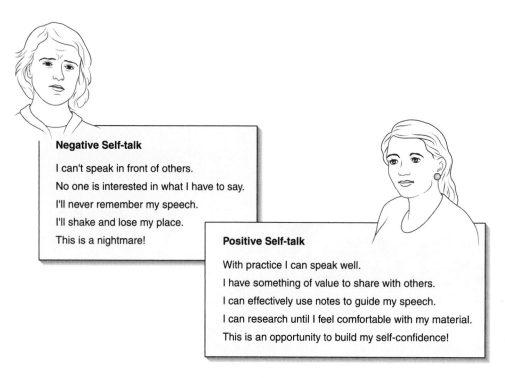

Negative Self-talk

I can't speak in front of others.

No one is interested in what I have to say.

I'll never remember my speech.

I'll shake and lose my place.

This is a nightmare!

Positive Self-talk

With practice I can speak well.

I have something of value to share with others.

I can effectively use notes to guide my speech.

I can research until I feel comfortable with my material.

This is an opportunity to build my self-confidence!

Figure 8-6 You can use positive thinking to turn public speaking monsters into friends. Preparation and practice can give you the confidence you need to make successful presentations.

Preparation

The six steps for preparing a presentation listed here are similar to the suggestions given in Chapter 6 for writing a paper.

Step One: Choose your topic early. It should be something you want to know more about or something you have strong feelings about. (Note: If you must speak on a topic with which you disagree, as sometimes happens in a **debate** on a controversial subject, this is a chance to practice seeing other points of view and experiencing empathy.)

Step Two: Be clear about your purpose: inform, persuade, demonstrate, encourage people to take action, entertain.

Step Three: Find out about your audience. What is their background? How much do they know about the topic? What are their beliefs? What is their interest level?

Step Four: Identify what you need to find out, and then do your research. Make sure you have accurate, up-to-date facts. Health care is constantly advancing and changing. Start now to develop the habit of verifying all information you use or distribute to others. In this sense, preparing for a presentation is like preparing for a test: master your material so you'll "know that you know."

Step Five: Organize your information using one of the techniques suggested in Chapter 6 for use when writing. These include idea sheets, note cards, the brain dump, questions, and mind maps.

Step Six: Divide your presentation into the following three parts:

1. **Part One: Introduction:** "Tell the audience what you're going to tell them."
   - Engage your listeners with an interesting story or fact. Give them a reason to pay attention. Why is this topic important to them? What should they know about it? How does it relate to their lives? Approach your audience with the attitude that you have something to offer them. This helps put both you and them at ease.

2. **Part Two: Body:** "Tell them."
   - This part takes up the most time. In it you explain and develop your ideas; give supporting facts, details, and examples; narrate events; and tell stories. This is the "meat" of your presentation.
   - Put the body of your speech together so it flows smoothly. For example, you might number your major points. Tell your audience how many points there will be and then announce each one as you come to it, for example:
   - "The kidneys have five important functions. The first is the regulation of fluid and electrolytes." (You then explain how they do this.)
   - "The second function is regulation of blood pressure." (More explanation.)
   - "The third is…" (etc.)

3. **Part Three: Conclusion:** "Tell them what you've told them."
   - Briefly review your major points, show how they tie together, and summarize why they are important. Tell the audience what action you want them to take or how they can use what you have told them.

It is especially important that oral presentations be put together in a logical, organized way. With written material, readers can take their time and go back if they miss a point or don't understand something. Listeners don't have this advantage. You continue talking whether they are following what you're saying or not. You can lose them entirely if you jump from topic to topic, fail to support your ideas, or don't provide clear and complete explanations of the material.

Memory Joggers

It is usually a bad idea to read directly from your paper when giving an oral presentation. You may be tempted to look only at your paper instead of at the audience. Presentations that are read lack the warmth of human interaction and are less interesting for the audience. It is better to become familiar with your material and then use one of the following prompts to help you remember what you plan to say:

1. *Note cards* with key points.
   A. **Advantages:** Small and easy to handle. Prevent you from reading directly from your paper. Encourage you to practice beforehand and become familiar with the material.
   B. **Watch out for:** Having too many cards and getting them confused. Failing to number the cards and getting them out of order. Fiddling with them, which can distract the audience. Not including enough information on them and forgetting what you meant to say about each point.
2. *Outline* on full sheets of paper.
   A. **Advantages:** Includes more information than note cards and may increase your confidence in remembering what you plan to say.
   B. **Watch out for:** Rattling the paper while you speak. Looking at the paper instead of the audience. Holding the paper with both hands and failing to use natural gestures while you speak.
3. *Mind map* with major topics and supporting points in graphic form.
   A. **Advantages:** Easy to see major points at a glance. Especially helpful if you are a visual or global learner and don't need a lot of notes to remember what you plan to say.
   B. **Watch out for:** May be less room on the page to include detail, so be sure you know your material. Sometimes mind maps have words written at angles and are difficult to read quickly. Make sure you set it up in an easy-to-read format so that you don't get lost. Nonvisual learners are not likely to find mind maps helpful as memory prompts.
4. *Key points* written on PowerPoint slides, overhead transparencies, or charts or listed on the board. Figure 8-7 contains examples. These can serve both as visual aids for the audience and as a guide for you.
   A. **Advantages:** You and the audience are working together and sharing the experience of looking at the same materials. Listeners may become more involved if they are both listening and seeing. This technique also helps visual learners (the majority) follow your presentation. Take care, however, to explain each point, rather than simply reading the list. The audience can do this for themselves!
   B. **Watch out for:** Poorly prepared visual aids that have too much information or lettering that is difficult for the audience to see. Equipment failures such as a balky computer, burned-out light bulbs, or no extension cord (or discovering at the last minute that the equipment you need is being used by another class!). Prior planning and consulting with the instructor are critical to prevent being tripped up during your presentation.

Practice

"The audience is not the enemy. Lack of preparation and practice is."

Give yourself the best chance possible to make a smooth presentation by practicing it a few times in advance. Run through your presentation in front of a mirror, and then try it on friends and family members. Use the materials that will serve as your prompts to make sure they are clear and easy to follow. Time yourself to find out if you need to lengthen or shorten your presentation. Rehearsing will give you the reassurance that comes from being familiar with your materials and knowing you have anticipated potential problems before you stand in front of an audience.

Should you memorize what you plan to say? Unless you are entering a formal speech contest or it is part of the assignment, this is usually not necessary or even a good idea. First, it is time consuming. Second, it can make you sound stiff and unnatural. Finally, and perhaps most important, if you forget

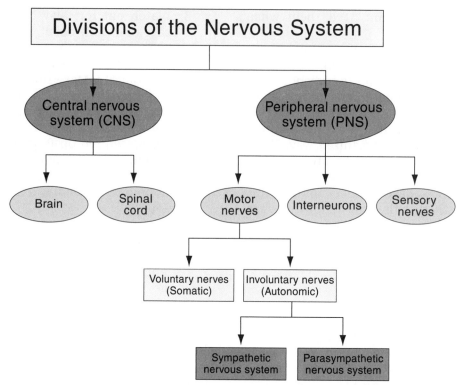

Figure 8-7 Examples of effective visuals for presentations. Keep them clear and simple to highlight and illustrate major points. *(From Gerdin J:* Health careers today, *ed 4, St Louis, 2007, Mosby.)*

a line or lose your place, it can be hard to get back on track. Rather than continuing to talk as you would with natural speech, you are in the uncomfortable position of trying to remember exactly where you are. The resulting long pause is very uncomfortable for both you and your audience.

Whenever possible, check the room where you'll be giving your presentation for details like the following:

- ☐ Is there a place to set down your cards or outline, or will you have to hold them as you speak? If you are short (like me), can you see over the podium?
- ☐ Do you know how to operate the computer or overhead projector? In which direction should the transparencies be placed? How do you adjust the image? Is the machine in working order? Are there extra bulbs available? Can the people in the back row read the material?
- ☐ Is there chalk or a pen available for the blackboard or white board? Will you have time to write out what you need? Is there an eraser?
- ☐ Is there a place to hang your charts, graphs, and other illustrations? Will you need tape, tacks, and so on?
- ☐ If you have models, samples, or other objects to show, is there a place to set them? Will the audience be able to see them? Will you pass them around?

Success Tips for Making an Oral Presentation

- ☐ Before you start to speak, take a breath, smile, and look at your audience. Even if you don't feel glad to be there, act as if you are. Try putting yourself and everyone else at ease.
- ☐ Look at the audience while you are speaking. Make eye contact with them. Look around the audience, not just in one direction. Catch the eyes of people who appear to be listening attentively and are "with you" to increase your feelings of support.
- ☐ Pause briefly if necessary. Some speakers even use pauses for dramatic effect. If you need a moment to gather your thoughts, stay calm. It is better to pause than to nervously ramble on or repeat filler words ("uh") that, if overused, are distracting. Pauses also give the audience time to reflect on what you have said.
- ☐ If you do lose your place or blank out a whole portion of your talk, stop and take a breath. Try not to panic. Acknowledge the audience with a smile or a nod (they may be as nervous as you are), and then concentrate on getting reorganized.
- ☐ Shift your focus from yourself to the audience. Remember that you have prepared well and have something of value to share. The audience needs this information, and you are being of service by sharing it with them.

☐ An old trick used by speakers is to imagine the audience in a funny situation: dressed in silly costumes, wearing big fake noses, standing on their heads—anything to change your perception of them as a threat.

☐ Consider organizing a buddy system. If you are already in a study group with classmates, that might do the trick. Practice your speeches with each other and offer constructive suggestions. Ask them to "cheer you on" by making eye contact when you are speaking, signaling when your time is almost up, and letting you know if you need to speak louder. Ask them to help you with handouts or visual aids. You will feel less alone.

DEVELOPING YOUR TEAMWORK SKILLS

If you are in a study group like the one suggested for giving speeches, you are already working on a team. Modern health care delivery relies on specialized professionals who work together. Look through the help wanted ads for health care jobs and you will see "team player" and "teamwork" mentioned in many of them. **Teamwork** refers to the efforts of individuals to coordinate their work to achieve common goals. High-quality patient care depends on how well people communicate and function as team members.

People do not always work together easily and naturally. Competition, rather than cooperation, is built into many aspects of our educational system. As a student, for example, you may be competing for grades, especially on tests that are scored on a curve. On the job, there can be competition for pay raises, bonuses, and recognition by the supervisor. But competition can get in the way of providing good care. The focus in the workplace must be on serving patients, not on competing with co-workers. Teamwork is so important in health care that National Healthcare Foundation Standards 8 is devoted entirely to teamwork criteria.[2]

President John F. Kennedy's famous statement is often quoted: "Ask not what your country can do for you, but what you can do for your country." Kennedy encouraged Americans to work together to reach goals that ranged from establishing the Peace Corps to putting a man on the moon. Americans achieved both, proving that when people work together, they can accomplish amazing things.

You can begin practicing teamwork in school. Group activities assigned by instructors and lab sessions provide excellent opportunities to prepare for real work situations. You can practice cooperating in study groups. Many students report disliking group activities, saying they much prefer being responsible for their own work. If you feel this way, be aware that learning to work together and knowing how to encourage group members who fail to do their part are essential job skills. Welcoming opportunities to work with others while you are still in school is a good strategy for future career success.

Differences among Team Members

When team members support one another, work becomes a pleasant experience. On the other hand, teams in which members don't get along can slow down the work process and make life difficult for everyone. People have differences that can interfere with communication, cause hurt feelings, and disrupt the workflow. Understanding and taking advantage of these differences can help teams flourish rather than fight.

Just as we all have different learning styles, we also have different work styles. Identifying and taking advantage of the styles of each team member can help prevent misunderstandings and allow each one to make useful contributions. There are no right or wrong work styles. Ignoring styles, however, can decrease the effectiveness of the team and reduce the satisfaction of the people on it.

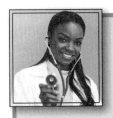

GIVING PRESENTATIONS ON THE JOB

Health care professionals who belong to professional organizations may be asked—or may volunteer—to give presentations at meetings and conferences. They may share information about innovative practices at the organization where they work, new products their employer is exploring, or something they have learned in a workshop or by conducting their own research.

Providing patient education is becoming more important, and sometimes this takes place in groups. Shorter stays in hospitals and larger numbers of outpatient surgeries mean more patients need to learn self-care techniques they will use at home. Some facilities offer group classes presented by nurses and other professionals. For example, all prospective knee-replacement candidates may be required to attend a class about the surgery, what to expect, how to prepare, and postoperative recovery.

Here are some common work preferences. As you read the list, check the ones that apply to you.

☐ Work methodically and complete one task or part of a task before moving on to the next.

☐ Work on several projects at the same time.

☐ Work alone and are responsible for your own work.

☐ Work with others in situations in which cooperation determines the success of the project.

☐ Work with details. Enjoy striving for accuracy and neatness.

☐ Think of ideas, but prefer to let someone else carry them out.

☐ Receive assignments with clear deadlines.

☐ Know exactly what is expected.

☐ Receive general instructions and a final due date. Figure out yourself how to get it done.

☐ Generate new ideas, products, and ways to work. Like to be creative.

☐ Receive a lot of guidance. Have someone check and approve your work as it progresses.

☐ Work with little supervision. Ask questions when you need help.

☐ Prefer quiet and order.

☐ Find noise and activity stimulating.

After reading this list, you can see how work styles are not only different, but even contradictory! It is not surprising that people sometimes find it difficult to work together. Attempting to understand the views and needs of your co-workers and supervisors is part of empathy, discussed earlier in this chapter. Applied in the workplace, empathy contributes to establishing good relations among staff members and creating a positive work environment.

Success Tips for Being an Effective Team Member

☐ **Understand the ground rules and agreements.** These may not be formally stated or written down, but they are important for keeping communication open and preventing misunderstandings.

☐ **Be clear about the purpose and goals of the group.** Everyone should know what is to be accomplished. Have you been assigned a specific project? Or is the goal an ongoing effort related to your role as a student or an employee?

☐ **Do your part—and then some.** Follow through and complete any work you have been assigned or have volunteered to do. Let the group know if you run into problems. Ask for help. Someone may be willing to pick up the slack. Letting things go can result in serious consequences, such as affecting the group's grade, endangering patient safety, or costing the facility money.

☐ **Listen to what others have to say.** What can you learn from them? What are their ideas about how to accomplish the work? What are their needs? What can they contribute?

☐ **Speak up.** Share your ideas and opinions.

☐ **Take advantage of differences.** Maximize group efficiency by assigning tasks that are appropriate for each member.

 Go to page 237 to complete Prescription for Success 8-8

UNDERSTANDING ORGANIZATIONS

Organizations, such as schools and dental offices, have their own personalities, just as individual people do. These personalities are known as **organizational cultures,** and they include the goals, rules, expectations, and customs of the organization as a whole. Schools have cultures, too. For example, some are very formal and emphasize respect for authority. Students are required to address their instructors by title and last name. Uniforms must be worn, and rules are strictly enforced. At other schools, the atmosphere is more casual, with students and instructors on a first-name basis. At some health care facilities, people eat lunch together, celebrate birthdays and holidays, and meet after work. At others, there is a clear distinction between work and social life. Some organizations stress orderliness, engage in detailed planning, and have clear work assignments. Others move at a fast pace, with informal job descriptions and planning done "on the run."

It is important to be aware of the culture you are in—or plan to enter—to see if it matches your preferences or if you can at least adapt to it. Sometimes we can learn from a culture that has values we would like to develop in ourselves. For example, if you have poor study habits and find yourself in a strict school, this can be a great opportunity to get the encouragement you need to develop new habits.

UNDERSTANDING YOUR INSTRUCTORS

We have discussed how people have different learning and working styles. Another factor that can influence your academic success is teaching and classroom management styles. Instructors are individuals who have their own ideas about education, teaching methods, and the proper roles of teachers and students. Understanding what is important to your instructors will help you benefit fully from your classes. You will use these same skills to identify the characteristics of your future supervisors so you can work with them more effectively.

Following are some common characteristics of instructors, along with suggestions for what you can learn from each:

1. **Strict**. Rules are emphasized. They are clearly explained, and there are consequences if they are broken.

   You learn: Good habits for health care work situations in which rules must be followed to ensure patient and worker safety.

2. **Value appearance**. Students must be neat, with clean, pressed uniforms and polished shoes. Points may be deducted from grades for infractions. Students who arrive out of uniform are sent home to change. (In a work environment, improperly dressed employees may also be asked to leave.)

   You learn: To practice the habits of excellent hygiene and correct professional appearance that are critical in health care work. (Remember: Your professional career began when you started school.)

3. **Believe students should be responsible for their own learning.** Instructors with this philosophy may allow you to go all term without ever mentioning that you haven't handed in all your homework assignments. You interpret this as meaning that it's not important and are shocked to receive a final grade of D or F. Never assume that no nagging means "not important." The same can happen at work. An employee may not be told about unsatisfactory work performance until the day of a formal evaluation or the initiation of a disciplinary process.

   You learn: To take responsibility for yourself and what you must do. On the job, supervisors won't have time to remind you constantly about your tasks. It will be up to you to get them done.

4. **Believe they must monitor students closely.** Some instructors believe it is their responsibility to prompt students to complete their work. They give constant reminders, check their progress frequently, call students who are absent, and generally provide "super-support." They are like those supervisors who are very organized and nurturing and are willing to tell employees what's to be done. They provide a lot of feedback.

   You learn: To work with frequent deadlines and a hands-on manager and how to meet deadlines and avoid falling behind in your work. Be careful, however, that you don't become dependent on continual help, because you can't always count on it being there for you.

5. **Value order.** The classroom is neat and tidy, lectures follow a clear pattern, and class activities are well planned.

   You learn: To practice orderly habits when necessary. Although your home may be comfortably chaotic, order is necessary in the health care environment. Forms must be filled out in a very specific way, tests performed in a prescribed order of steps, and disinfecting procedures carried out precisely. Tidying up the classroom or lab before you leave is a good habit to develop, and your instructor will certainly notice and appreciate your efforts.

6. **Value creativity over order.** Classes may seem disorganized. Lectures are mixed with interesting stories and don't follow an orderly plan. Group activities and creativity are emphasized over doing things the instructor's way.

   You learn: To be creative and think for yourself, to work with classmates, and to practice the teamwork skills discussed in this chapter.

The teaching styles chosen by instructors are often reflections of their own learning styles or the way they remember being taught themselves. Instructors may rely on lectures to teach because they are auditory learners or because they believe that their role is to tell students what they know. You can take advantage of different teaching styles to help you improve your weak areas. For example, if an instructor uses a lot of group activities and you prefer to work alone, you now have an opportunity to increase your ability to work with others, something you might not choose to do if it weren't required.

If you have difficulty with an instructor, the first step in resolving the problem should be to speak privately with him or her. If you go straight to a school administrator, neither you nor the instructor has a chance to explore the problem and try to work out a solution. Furthermore, the administrator doesn't have personal knowledge of the situation. The problem has been moved away from its source. If speaking with the instructor fails to resolve the situation, inquire about the proper procedure to follow at your school. If you have problems with your supervisor at work, it is expected that you speak with that person first. How to properly handle interpersonal difficulties with a supervisor is discussed in Chapter 13.

When meeting with an instructor or supervisor to discuss a problem, it works best if you are prepared in advance. Think about what you want to discuss. It might be a good idea to prepare some notes in advance of the major points you want address. At the meeting, let the other person know that your goal is not to complain, but to resolve the issue. Find out their views and listen carefully and nondefensively. Express your own view of the situation, and then discuss the problem in terms of possible solutions.

Most instructors decide to teach because they want to share what they have learned about their profession. They are motivated by concern for their students. This does not necessarily mean they strive to be liked by their students, because this is not the purpose of teaching. Their job is to train students to be excellent health care professionals. You may not like all your instructors, but given a chance, they all have something of value to share with you. And although you may not like all your supervisors, you can still find satisfaction in your work.

PERSONAL REFLECTION

1. How would you describe each of your instructors?

_____

_____

_____

_____

_____

2. What can you learn from each of them?

_____

_____

_____

_____

_____

DEALING WITH DIFFICULT PEOPLE

"One of the best ways to persuade others is with your ears—by listening to them."

—*Dean Rusk*

People problems cannot be avoided entirely. There will be classmates who annoy you, who don't do their share of the work on a group project, or who take up a lot of class time with questions because they never read the assignments. Family members may criticize you because they are upset about the amount of time you spend studying. Friends may be jealous of your future career possibilities. Some of your future patients, clients, co-workers, and supervisors will be challenging, too. Learning to get along with difficult people helps make life more pleasant and productive.

In difficult situations, do your best to separate your health care role from you as a person. It is often your position with which the other person has a problem. For example, your family may be annoyed with your role as a student because of the time it takes away from them. Or a patient may take his anger out on you as a representative of the clinic with which he has a problem.

Empathy, which we discussed earlier in this chapter, can help. Listen carefully to the other person. Try to see the world from his or her point of view. What might explain the behavior? Might there be personal problems you don't know about? Is there a chance you have unintentionally done something to hurt his or her feelings? It can be helpful to acknowledge the other person's feelings without agreeing to feel the same way. For example, you might begin your discussion like this: "I can see why you feel that way, but…" and then state your view. Recognizing the validity of the other person's feelings often decreases the negativity. Remain calm and courteous. Reacting negatively only makes the situation worse. (This does not mean you have to take verbal or physical abuse. If this occurs, seek the assistance of your instructor, other school personnel, or your supervisor.)

Seek solutions to interpersonal problems by being honest and "up front." Tell the other person what you see as the problem and explain how it affects you. For example, with a lab partner who is never prepared to practice the assigned procedures, you might say, "I feel really frustrated when you continually come unprepared. I'm worried that I'm losing the chance to learn, and I can't afford to do that." Simply venting or arguing won't solve the problem; it might even make it worse. Work for a mutually acceptable agreement. Using the lab partner example, you could ask, "Can you agree to come to class prepared?" When there are serious consequences at stake, such as your grades or work performance, let the other person know what you plan to do if the situation is not resolved. Tell your lab partner, "If I can't depend on you to come prepared to work with me, I'll have to ask the instructor to let me change lab partners." As you attempt to find a solution, try to keep a positive attitude. Recall from our discussion about attitude in Chapter 3 that it doesn't make sense to give an unpleasant person the right to ruin your day. Do what you can to seek a positive solution and then move on.

We learn and develop professionally when we engage in all types of relationships, both positive and negative. Expressing kindness toward a troublesome classmate or giving an instructor the benefit of the doubt are signs of maturity. It's easy to be professional when things are going well. True professionals can also deal effectively with challenging situations.

Dealing with Criticism

Criticism and constructive suggestions about your work present you with opportunities to learn. In school, you are paying for instruction that includes correction of your work. Your teachers would not be acting responsibly if they awarded inflated grades or withheld criticism to avoid hurting students' feelings. It would be unfair to allow students to perform work incorrectly, because this would only set them up for failure on the job, where the consequences are more serious.

You may receive criticism for behaviors or work results when you are on the job. This might come from your supervisor, a co-worker, or even a patient. No one likes to be criticized, and it is natural to react strongly. Dismissing the criticism as unfounded, becoming angry, or taking the criticism to heart and feeling worthless are common reactions. These feelings are natural but not very helpful. A more constructive response is to pay attention to the message, examine the criticism, and consider it carefully. Then decide if any or all of it actually applies to you. If it does, you can choose to benefit from it and engage in self-improvement. If it does not, consider talking over your feelings with the person who gave the criticism to see where the misunderstanding lies.

If you receive criticism that seems harsh, try to focus on the content and not on the way it is delivered. Not all instructors and supervisors are skilled at giving suggestions. If you don't understand what you did incorrectly, ask for clarification. It is your responsibility to learn as much as possible. Feelings must be put aside, if necessary, to ensure that you attain the skills necessary to be a competent health care professional.

Giving Constructive Criticism

The purpose of constructive criticism is to provide the person receiving the criticism with the means for improvement. It is based on the assumption that behavior can be changed for the better. It is important, when giving constructive criticism, to focus on the problem behavior rather than on the person. Suppose you have a co-worker who frequently fails to return equipment to its designated storage space, causing you to waste time looking for needed items to do your work. State the problem behavior clearly: equipment is not being returned and this is affecting your efficiency. Avoid negative statements about the other person such as that she is inconsiderate, a poor co-worker, disorganized, and so on. Judgmental statements about personal characteristics tend to put people on the defensive and make them less willing to examine their behavior and make positive changes.

Here are a few more suggestions for giving criticism that helps rather than hurts:

☐ Choose a private location to talk, and allow enough time for the other person to respond and ask questions.

☐ Use empathy and show respect for the other person's feelings.

☐ Include positive statements along with the criticism.

☐ Be clear when explaining the problem. Give specific examples that illustrate the problem.

Neither giving nor receiving criticism is easy, but done well and taken in the spirit in which it is intended, it contributes to our learning and growth.

⇨ SUMMARY OF KEY IDEAS

1. The ability to get along with others is essential for career success.
2. All human beings deserve to be treated with respect.
3. We are all people, in spite of our differences.
4. Empathy is essential for the caring health care professional.
5. The ability to listen well is as important as the ability to speak well.
6. The keys to effective oral presentations are preparation and practice.
7. Understanding the work, learning, and teaching styles of others will increase your ability to work with them effectively.
8. You can learn from difficult situations.

Positive Self-Talk for This Chapter

1. I respect other people and try to learn something from everyone I meet.
2. I value differences and strive to promote understanding among people.
3. I practice empathy with others.
4. I have good communication skills.

5. I prepare well and speak confidently in front of groups.
6. I work well with others and make valuable contributions to teams.

To Learn More

Hildebrand V, Phenice LA, Gray MM, Hines RP: *Knowing and serving diverse families,* ed 2, Upper Saddle River, NJ, 2000, Merrill, Prentice-Hall.

This book offers a good introduction to diversity, then covers a different ethnic group in each chapter. In addition, a variety of family structures are discussed, including single teenage parent and step families. Recommendations are given for serving each group.

Luckmann J: *Transcultural communication in health care,* Clifton Park, NY, 2000, Thomson Delmar Learning.

From this book you can learn about the cultural values and beliefs of a wide variety of people, including Latinos, Muslims, Native Americans, and Hasidic Jews. The author's purpose is to help students increase their self-awareness and become more sensitive to cultural differences.

Mears P: *Healthcare teams: building continuous quality improvement,* Boca Raton, 1994, St Lucie Press.

Although written for group facilitators, this book can help you understand the importance of teamwork in health care settings.

Milliken ME: *Understanding human behavior: a guide for health care providers,* ed 6, Clifton Park, NY, 2004, Delmar Cengage.

This reader-friendly book gives practical information to assist health professionals understand and effectively work with their patients.

Purtilo R, Haddad A: *Health professional and patient interaction,* 7th ed., Philadelphia, 2007, Saunders.

Good discussions and examples of how to empathize and communicate with patients.

Tamparo CD, Lindh WQ: *Therapeutic communications for health care,* ed 3, Clifton Park, NY, 2008, Delmar Cengage.

Easy to read and full of specifics and examples.

REFERENCES

1. Anderson R, Barbara A, Feldman S: What patients want: a content analysis of key qualities that influence patient satisfaction. www.drscore.com/press/papers/whatpatientswant.pdf (Accessed 2/9/09)
2. National Consortium on Health Science and Technology Education: National Healthcare Foundation Standards and Accountability Criteria. www.nchste.org/cms/wp-content/uploads/2008/03/foundation_standards_ac_rev_01_08. (Accessed 2/13/09)

BUILDING YOUR RESUME

1. Think about how you will use your communication skills to ask questions about jobs of interest, to listen actively to learn about jobs and the needs of employers, and to orally explain your education, work history, and other qualifications.
2. Using Resume Building Block #4: Work History, in Chapter 2, to list any transferable skills related to communication, interpersonal, and teamwork skills you acquired during previous employment. These are skills all employers look for in future hires. Are there specific examples you can use during interviews to support your qualifications in these areas?

INTERNET ACTIVITIES

For active links to the websites needed to complete these activities, visit **http://evolve.elsevier.com/Haroun/career/.**

1. The University of Washington Medical Center has developed a cultural diversity training course. Although some information applies to this medical center, most of the material addresses cultural diversity in general. Read the online presentation, and write a summary of what you learn about diversity in health care.
2. The purpose of the Southern Poverty Law Center is to fight hate and promote tolerance (the acceptance of differences among people). Review the sections entitled "10 Ways to Fight Hate" and "101 Tools for Tolerance." Choose five suggestions from the lists and describe how they could be applied to work in health care.
3. *Listen Up! Enrich Your Relationships through Active Listening.* Read the article about the important but often neglected skill of listening. Write a short report explaining why listening can be difficult for many people. List techniques for improving one's listening skills.
4. The *Physician's News Digest* contains an excellent article on communication in health care. The author suggests that communicating effectively with patients can be broken down into a process that includes the following communication tasks: engagement, empathy, education, and enlistment. Read the article, and write a summary of each of these communication tasks.
5. Rice University's Online Writing Lab includes information on designing effective oral presentations. Read through the material and then choose a section to summarize in the form of advice for someone preparing an oral presentation.

Prescription for Success 8-1
Showing Respect

1. List three ways, in addition to those listed in the text, you can show respect to others.

_____

_____

_____

_____

_____

2. Describe a situation in which someone made you feel that you were respected. How was respect communicated to you?

_____

_____

_____

_____

_____

3. Explain why showing respect to patients is an important part of providing good health care.

_____

_____

_____

_____

_____

Prescription for Success 8-2
Getting to Know Yourself

The first step toward understanding others is knowing ourselves. Fill in the chart below with your own beliefs about each concept. You may use any of those listed in Table 8-1 or you can write your own.

Concept   *My Beliefs*

Time   _____

Personal space   _____

Age   _____

Touching   _____

Gender   _____

Eye contact   _____

Personal control   _____

Spiritual practices   _____

Definition of success   _____

Health care beliefs   _____

Prescription for Success 8-3
Your Health Care Beliefs

1. What is your personal definition of "health"?

_____

_____

_____

2. How much responsibility do you believe people should have for their own health?

_____

_____

_____

Prescription for Success 8-3 (Continued)

3. What do you believe are the main causes of health problems?

_____

_____

_____

4. What are the best ways to take care of health problems?

_____

_____

_____

5. How do you think your own beliefs about health may influence your future work?

_____

_____

_____

Prescription for Success 8-4
What Would It Be Like to Be . . . ?

Answer the questions that follow for patients in the following conditions:

- Paralyzed

- In pain

- Unable to work

- Blind

- Mentally ill

- Poor and without health insurance

- Elderly and living alone

- Unable to speak English

- Having a terminal illness

Continued

Prescription for Success 8–4 (Continued)

1. What emotions might they be experiencing?

   _____

   _____

   _____

   _____

2. What might be their concerns and fears?

   _____

   _____

   _____

   _____

3. What are their major needs likely to be, both physical and emotional?

   _____

   _____

   _____

   _____

4. How are their conditions likely to affect their quality of life?

   _____

   _____

   _____

   _____

5. How could you learn more about each person?

   _____

   _____

   _____

   _____

Prescription for Success 8-5
And the Question Is . . . ?

Write two examples of each of the four types of questions.

   1. Closed-ended

_____

_____

   2. Open-ended

_____

_____

   3. Probing

_____

_____

   4. Leading

_____

_____

Prescription for Success 8-6
What Does It Mean?

Choose a time and place to observe people (politely!) as they are communicating. The exercise works best if you cannot hear what they are saying.

   1. Give at least three examples of nonverbal behaviors you observed.

_____

_____

_____

   2. What do you think they mean?

_____

_____

_____

Continued

Prescription for Success 8–6 (Continued)

3. How can you become more aware of your own nonverbal communication?

_____

_____

_____

4. Are there gestures you often use when speaking? If so, describe what they are and what they mean.

_____

_____

_____

Prescription for Success 8-7
Rate Your Communication Skills

1. Do any areas need improvement?

   a. _____ Sending clear messages

   b. _____ Listening actively

   c. _____ Requesting feedback

   d. _____ Asking good questions

   e. _____ Understanding nonverbal communication

   f. _____ Demonstrating appropriate nonverbal communication

2. If so, what can you do to improve them?

_____

_____

_____

3. What resources, including people, can help you improve your communication skills?

_____

_____

_____

Prescription for Success 8-8
Go, Team!

1. Describe at least three teams to which you belong or have belonged at work, school, church, etc.

_____

_____

_____

_____

2. Describe your role on each team.

_____

_____

_____

_____

3. How is or was the work assigned?

_____

_____

_____

_____

4. How are or were group decisions made?

_____

_____

_____

_____

5. How could each team be or have been more effective?

_____

_____

_____

_____

CHAPTER 9

Beginning the Job Search

OBJECTIVES

The information and activities in this chapter can help you:

- Understand how a positive attitude contributes to a successful job search.
- Know what skills you have to offer an employer.
- Identify your employment goals and income needs.
- Use a variety of organizational techniques to conduct an effective job search.
- Use a variety of resources effectively to locate health care job leads.

KEY TERMS AND CONCEPTS

Cover Letter: Letter of introduction sent along with your resume to a potential employer.

Fax Machine: Device that allows you to send documents over telephone lines.

Job Lead Log: An organized list of the information you gather about various job leads.

Job Lines: Recorded lists of available jobs you can access by telephone.

Mailing Lists: Subscription services that send messages on specific topics via e-mail. (Also called *Listservs*.)

Newsgroups: Online discussion groups in which participants post information about topics of interest.

Reference Sheet: A written list of your references that includes their titles and contact information.

Web Forums: Discussion groups accessed via the World Wide Web in which interested individuals can take part. Also called *online communities* and *message boards*.

THE SEARCH IS ON

"Employment is nature's physician, and is essential to human happiness."

—*Galen*

Congratulations! All the studying, assignments, labs, and clinical experience are about to pay off. You are now ready to focus on the job search and reaching your goal of working in the health care field. Completing your education and graduating represent important personal achievements. Your attitude played a large part in your success. In the same way, attitude will play an important role in helping you get the right job.

The Big A: Attitude

"Remember that your own resolution to succeed is more important than any one thing."

—*Abraham Lincoln*

Attitude is the single most important factor in determining whether a student finds a job. In Chapter 3, we discussed how we have control over our attitudes and noted that any situation can be approached either positively or negatively. For example, some people are nervous and fearful about looking for a job. They worry about lacking the qualifications needed by employers and see each interview as a chance to be rejected. A more positive approach is to look at the process from the employers' point of view. Think about it: health care facilities cannot function without good employees. Employers must fill positions with well-trained individuals who can help them serve their patients. *You* are a recently trained person ready to fill one of these positions.

In Chapter 2, we compared starting a new career with marketing a new product. You are now ready to begin marketing yourself to prospective employers. Knowing what skills and competencies you have is the first step in presenting yourself successfully as the person who fits an employer's needs. Students sometimes don't realize just how much they have learned. They tend to underestimate their abilities and the amount of practice they have had in applying their skills. Being aware of your accomplishments will build your self-confidence and help you present yourself positively at interviews. Take some time now to review what you have learned, your self-ratings in Prescription for Success 1-4, and to give yourself credit for what you have to offer.

 Go to page 255 to complete Prescription for Success 9-1

Focus Your Search

"To find out what one is fitted to do, and to secure an opportunity to do it, is the key to happiness."

—*John Dewey*

Knowing where to market yourself is the next step in carrying out a successful job search. This means identifying the type of job and facility in which you would prefer to work. In Prescription for Success 1-4 you began to identify your job preferences. As you worked through your educational program, you may have changed your work preferences.

 Go to page 256 to complete Prescription for Success 9-2

As we discussed in Chapter 1, it is sometimes necessary to set short-term goals to achieve long-term career success. When seeking an entry-level position, you'll do better if you are open to a variety of possibilities. School career services personnel report seeing students lose good opportunities by setting limits that are too restrictive. For example, some students don't want to have long commutes. But passing up a good position at an excellent facility by refusing to consider jobs just outside your immediate area may not be a good career move. Driving an extra 10 minutes may, in the long run, be worth the inconvenience.

MAKING A COMMITMENT TO THE JOB SEARCH

"You can't try to do things; you simply must do them."

—*Ray Bradbury*

Obtaining a job has been compared to actually working at a job. It can take a lot of time and effort. You'll be most successful if you dedicate a portion of each day to your search and be on call to follow up quickly on leads. Employment professionals recommend that job seekers spend between 20 and 40 hours per week on job-search efforts. In this and the following chapters, you will learn about the many activities necessary to conduct a successful search, such as the following:

- Preparing skill inventories and examples
- Networking
- Finding leads
- Conducting searches on the Internet
- Writing and revising your resume
- Assembling your portfolio
- Writing letters
- Contacting references
- Creating a **reference sheet**
- Preparing for and attending interviews
- Writing thank-you notes

Failure to spend adequate time on these activities is one of the major reasons why people fail to get hired. You can apply many of the time-management tools and techniques suggested in Chapter 3 to your job search (Figure 9-1).

PERSONAL REFLECTION

How strong is my commitment to finding a job?

_____

_____

_____

How much effort am I willing to put forth?

_____

_____

_____

Time Management Tips for Your Job Search

☐ **Prioritize.** The job search should be your main focus, apart from your family. Dedicate sufficient time and attention to achieving this goal. Looking for a job *is* your job. Determine which search activities are most productive, and spend the majority of your time on them.

☐ **Keep a calendar.** Missing—or even being late for—an interview is a sure way to lose a job even before you are hired. Take care to note all appointments and follow-up activities accurately, and check your calendar daily. If you haven't developed a calendar system yet, now is the time to start.

☐ **Plan a weekly schedule.** Decide what needs to be done each week, and create a to-do list to serve as a guide to keep you on track. It's easy to reach the end of the week and discover you've accomplished only half of what needed to be done.

☐ **Plan ahead.** This is very important. Suppose that one morning you are notified that a hospital where you want to work is scheduling interviews for later the same day. You don't want to miss out because you haven't completed your resume or don't have a clean shirt to wear. Being prepared leads to being hired. Make sure your car is in good running order or that you have other reliable transportation.

☐ **Plan for the unplanned.** The unexpected tends to strike at the worst possible moment. Keep an extra printer cartridge on hand. Have extra copies of your resume printed. Leave early for interviews in case you get lost. (Better yet, take a dry run a day or two in advance to learn the route. Check out alternate routes in case of traffic.)

SETTING UP JOB SEARCH CENTRAL

Create a personalized employment headquarters by designating a space for job-search activities. Save time and prevent the loss of important information by gathering your resources and supplies in one location. Check the list in Box 9-1 to see if you have what you need.

Your Job-Search Records

Each person's job search is unique. Creating personalized job-search records will help you focus your efforts and keep track of phone numbers, website

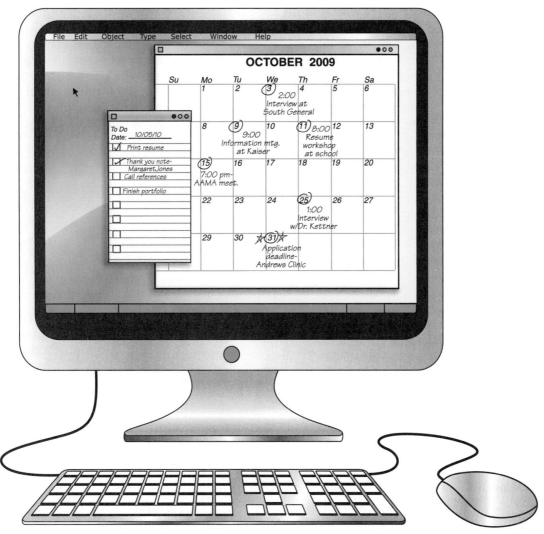

Figure 9-1 Apply your time management skills to conduct a successful job search.

| BOX 9-1 | Job Central Checklist |

- Telephone
- Telephone directories, including Yellow Pages
- Computer, printer, and supplies
- Dictionary
- Good-quality paper for resume and **cover letters**
- Matching envelopes
- Extra copies of resume
- Note paper or thank-you cards
- Calendar, planner, or electronic planner
- Job-search notebook

addresses, and the name of the office manager at the clinic where you last interviewed. A three-ring binder gives you the flexibility to add pages and keep everything organized. If you prefer, create computerized folders and files. Choose content that

will best support your efforts. The purpose of this resource is to save you time and effort. Here are suggestions for information you might find useful to include:

☐ List of professional contacts (from your Personal Reference Guide, discussed in Chapter 7)

☐ List of professional organizations (also from your Personal Reference Guide; see Appendix A for a list of health care organizations)

☐ Copies of Prescription for Success 9-1 and 9-2

☐ Resume Building Block forms from Chapter 2

Job Lead Log

A **job lead log** consists of pages, either paper or computerized, on which you record all job leads and contacts. An example of a job lead log is on the following page. Copy the log on page 242 or create your own.

If you have more than one version of your resume (for example, different objectives to match specific jobs), indicate on your lead log which version you sent, place a copy of the resume on the next page in your binder, or refer to the computer file name. This way you'll know how to respond if you get a call for an interview. It will also ensure that you take the correct resume to the interview. (Chapter 11 contains more information about interviews and what to take with you.)

Students who prefer to use a computer for tracking can set up an Excel spreadsheet or other form, such as a table in Word, to record their job-search activities. Regardless of the method you choose, design something that is easy for you to use and be sure to keep it up-to-date.

JOB LEAD LOG

Source of Lead

☐ Personal contact   ☐ Printed ad   ☐ Referral from school   ☐ Internet

☐ Other

Facility Name: _____

Contact Person: _____

Address: _____

Telephone Number: _____

Fax Number: _____

Website Address: _____

Contacts and Follow-up Action

Date	Action (Called, sent resume, sent thank-you note, etc.)
_____	_____
_____	_____
_____	_____
_____	_____
_____	_____
_____	_____
_____	_____
_____	_____
_____	_____
_____	_____
_____	_____

Dialing for Jobs

The telephone provides a vital link with potential employers and job lead sources. The telephone can be one of the job seeker's best friends. It can also be a barrier if not used properly. Employers form an impression of you based on your telephone manners, so be sure they hear you at your best. The following suggestions for making calls will apply to your telephone habits on the job as well as during the search to get a job:

1. Be prepared with pen and paper for taking notes.
2. Prepare what you plan to say ahead of time, and be as brief as possible without rushing and speaking too quickly.
3. Be courteous, never pushy. If the receptionist cannot connect you to the person you wish to speak with, leave a clear message and ask for a good time to call back.
4. Speak clearly and distinctly. Don't mumble or use slang or nonstandard speech that the listener may not understand.
5. When making appointments or gathering important information, listen carefully and repeat (use feedback) to make sure that you have the correct date and time, address, suite or office number, and so on.
6. Always thank the other party and end the call graciously.

It is *critical* that your school, potential employers, and other contacts be able to reach you in a timely way. Be sure the telephone number you distribute is accurate and includes your area code. If you have an answering machine, call your number to make sure it is working properly. The outgoing message should be simple and professional. Avoid the use of music, jokes, and clever remarks, such as "You know what this is and you know what to do." (This also applies to your e-mail address. If it's too cute or strange, it may send the wrong message to any potential employer who sees it.) Instruct everyone who might answer the telephone about proper telephone manners and how to write down a message. Every contact represents you, and employers don't have time to deal with rude adults or untrained children. If you are away from the telephone during office hours and don't have a cell phone or an answering machine, give out an alternate number where someone reliable can take messages for you. You might consider getting an inexpensive cell phone with prepaid minutes. Don't lose out on jobs because you can't be contacted.

Communicating by Fax

Some employers want you to fax your resume. If you don't own a **fax machine** or a computer that has fax capability, find a print, postal, or business supply store that provides this service. Some schools will fax student resumes to potential employers. When sending documents by fax, the print on the original should be clear and dark for maximum-quality transmission. Be sure there is at least a 1-inch margin on all sides so nothing gets cut off.

When faxed resumes are requested, it is best to follow the employer's instructions. Mailed resumes may arrive too late to be considered. Demonstrate that you are resourceful and can follow instructions. If you don't hear from the employer in a couple of days, call to make sure your resume was received.

SETTING UP A SUPPORT SYSTEM

Your job search will be easier and more pleasant if you have people available who care about your success and are willing to help you. They can provide technical support or offer friendly encouragement. Could you use some help with any of the following tasks?

☐ Proofreading your resume and other written materials (more than one person should proofread).
☐ Role-playing with you to practice interviewing.
☐ Discussing postinterview evaluations. (Postinterview evaluations are covered in Chapter 12.)
☐ Acting as a cheerleader.
☐ Helping you to keep things in perspective and not get discouraged.

You may want to work with just one other person who is qualified to help you in many areas. Or you might enlist the help of several "specialists." Be sure the people you choose are qualified to spot spelling and grammatical errors and are comfortable giving you constructive feedback. They should know when you need a push and when you need a hug. Consider drawing from friends, family members, classmates, school personnel, and health care professionals. If you have a mentor, this person might be an excellent choice.

Most people will be happy to support your efforts to secure employment. Take care to keep your support system intact. Be considerate of everyone's time, be prepared when you have meetings with them, and show appreciation for their help.

The career services department at your school provides specific help and support to students as they conduct their job search. Find out what services are provided. In addition, some schools and communities have job clubs or support groups for people seeking employment. Consider using these resources to supplement your support system. They can offer additional viewpoints, encouragement, and helpful suggestions.

Go to page 257 to complete Prescription for Success 9-3

UNDERSTANDING THE JOB MARKET

Employment conditions vary from one geographic location to the next. And economic conditions change over time. Think about the following factors when planning your job-search strategies:
- Local employment customs
- Current economic conditions
- Current employment rate
- Trends in health care delivery
- Medical advances
- Changing government regulations

Local customs vary regarding what is considered acceptable dress for the workplace. In some parts of the country, health care providers dress casually, with men sporting long hair and even wearing an earring. In other areas, anyone who showed up for work looking like this would be sent home to change—or worse, sent home for good!

Local and national economic conditions affect the job seeker. When the economy is strong and unemployment is low, job seekers have the advantage. When the economy slows down, competition heats up and it becomes more difficult to find a position. At the same time, some health care occupations are experiencing of shortages of applicants, and this will make finding a job easier for qualified candidates.

Health care occupations are also affected by state and federal laws. The demand for certain occupations is influenced by the reimbursement (payment for services) policies of both government and private insurance carriers. Knowing what's happening in your local area as well as being aware of national trends is important when planning both your initial job search and your long-term career strategy. Your local newspaper is a good source of information. Look in the business section for articles about the economy and local employment trends. Health care trends and major facilities are often featured. For example, a state law that increased the required nurse-to-patient ratios in California hospitals was reported in the newspaper. The predicted result was (and will be for the next few years, at least) a shortage of registered nurses to meet employer needs. This information is valuable for the recent nurse graduate or a student who is considering nursing as a career. Articles about major health care employers can give you an edge when choosing where you want to work. Knowing about the facility to which you are applying enables you to present yourself at interviews as a candidate who has taken the time to learn about the employer.

Many newspapers publish a special weekly or monthly section dedicated to employment. These are good sources of information. They contain articles about resume writing, lists of local agencies that assist job seekers, and announcements of job fairs. News magazines such as *Newsweek, Time, U.S. News and World Report,* and *Business Week* contain many articles about health care topics. The Internet provides access to a wide variety of topics from literally millions of sources. For example, the Bureau of Labor Statistics maintains a website with reports on employment trends and the national labor market. Apply the research techniques discussed in Chapter 5 in conducting your job search.

Go to page 257 to complete Prescription for Success 9-4

LOCATING JOB LEADS

There are many ways to find job leads, ranging from talking with people you know to searching the Internet. You can increase your chances of finding the job you really want by using a variety of lead sources. Don't limit yourself to the one or two methods you find easiest or most comfortable to use. People who work in sales know that it usually takes many calls to make a sale. In the same way, the more sources you use in your job search, the greater your chances of finding the right job for you. Employment experts recommend that no more than 25% of your time be spent on any one job-search method. See Figure 9-2 for a look at the wide variety of sources available.

When the economy is slow and there are few job openings, networking and developing personal contacts can be the most effective methods for finding a job. It's possible you won't find the "perfect job" under these economic conditions. Looking for an opportunity to gain experience may be the best strategy. When the economy is booming or there is a shortage of qualified workers in your field, you are likely to have a larger selection of opportunities. Under these conditions, you may find that responding to job postings and directly contacting potential employers are very effective methods. It is a sure thing that you will experience all types of job markets during your career. The economy and employment levels run in cycles, and you must be prepared to deal with changing conditions.

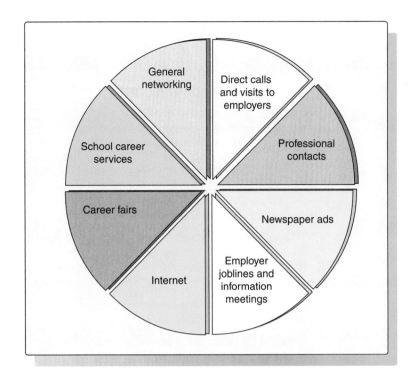

Figure 9-2 Use a variety of job lead sources to increase your chances of finding the right job for you.

Career Services at Your School

The staff at your school wants you to succeed. The goal of health care educators is to train future workers, and a sign of *their* professional success is when a graduate becomes satisfactorily employed. Schools have special personnel who are trained to help students find jobs. These people work to develop relationships with local employers. Your school may be contacted about job openings before they are even advertised. It is time-consuming for employers to review resumes, set up appointments, and interview large numbers of applicants. The success of a health care facility depends on the quality of its employees, so it is important that they find and hire the right people. Considerable time, expense, and doubt can be avoided if employers know they can count on local schools to provide qualified candidates. So how can you be among those who are recommended by your school?

☐ Get to know the career services staff. Introduce yourself early in your program. Don't wait until you are beginning the job search. Seek their advice about how you can best prepare ahead for successful employment.

☐ Treat school staff with the same courtesy and respect you would an employer. They cannot risk the school's reputation with employers by recommending students who are rude or uncooperative.

☐ Maintain an excellent attendance record. Schools report that this is the question asked by nearly every employer about students. It ranks far above inquiries about grades. (Even great skills are no help to anyone if you aren't there to use them!)

☐ Participate fully in any career development classes or workshops that are offered. Attend every session and complete all assignments. Conduct yourself in practice interviews as if they were the real thing.

☐ Follow up on any leads you are given, even if you don't think the job is for you. Attend all interviews scheduled for you. Failure to show up embarrasses the school and may result in the employer refusing to consider candidates from your school in the future. Take advantage of all opportunities to meet potential employers. You will get valuable confidence-building interview practice. Even if the job isn't the one for you, the employer may know about one that is.

☐ Keep the school informed about how to contact you. If you move and career services can't find you, they can't help you.

☐ Let the school know when you are hired. Many agencies that regulate and accredit schools require annual reports to monitor graduation and job placement rates. These act as school report cards and are important for schools to stay in good standing. If the staff has taken the time to help you, return the favor by giving them the information they need to complete their reports.

with a Career Services Professional
Melva Duran

Melva is the Director of Career Services at Kaplan College in San Diego, California.

Q With so many job seekers out there, how can graduates increase their chances of being noticed by employers?

A I think many graduates make the mistake of simply submitting a resume or application. When using the Internet, they may believe that once they've pushed the send button, it is up to the employer. But I have found that this just isn't enough. Graduates need to follow up. Unless requested otherwise in the job posting, this might be a phone call. It can be brief—something like, "I noticed your job posting on the Internet and I've sent an application online. I wanted to let you know I'm very interested in the job and am wondering when you'll be making a hiring decision."

I even had a major health care employer tell me that after he receives resumes, he waits a day or two to see if he receives any follow-up. Then he only reviews the resumes of applicants who have followed up!

Q You mention the Internet. Are you finding that many graduates are getting jobs by posting their resumes?

A Actually, the large job sites often attract too many resumes—there is just so much competition. So I recommend to students that they browse the job postings to identify where the jobs are and find potential employers. Then they should go in person with their resumes.

Q So you believe applicants should go personally to places of employment?

A Oh, yes, I think that's even better than a phone call—and certainly better than simply sending a resume electronically. They should do both—send a resume and then follow up. If they notice a large, local employer that seems to have jobs available, they should go to the facility. When talking to a contact person, they should state their interest in employment, ask about current hiring and other jobs that might be available, and if there is anything else they should do to apply for jobs.

Q How about cold calling—do you recommend it?

A Absolutely! In fact, I've had good success with this method when graduates have trouble getting hired. I advise them to dress professionally and go to buildings that have potential employers. This is a better and faster approach than calling on the phone. Employers may be looking to hire, and this saves them time and money spent on posting the job. Even if they don't have an opening, they often take the resume and call later.

This should be a soft sell—that is, don't be pushy and don't ask for an interview on the spot. On the other hand, do be prepared for an interview because that can happen!

Q Are you suggesting that job seekers should not make telephone calls to seek openings?

A No, not at all. With the telephone, you can obviously contact more potential employers.

Q What is the best way to conduct a phone search?

A It's critical when calling to conduct yourself professionally. Second, it's important to speak with someone who has hiring authority. In a physician's office, this is not likely to be the receptionist, so you need to ask for the office manager.

Q Many of us are nervous when making these calls. What is the best way to go about it—what should graduates say?

A First state your name and say that you are a graduate of the _____ program at _____ school. Then say something like, "I would like to get my resume to you for any jobs you might have now or in the future."

If they are willing to receive your resume, it is best if you drop it off in person. This gives you a chance to see the facility, even if briefly and only the front office, and it gives someone there the chance to see you. (Be sure to dress professionally!) So before hanging up, ask for the address and any special directions.

Government-Sponsored Resource Centers

The government has established a program of "one-stop" resources for job seekers. These may be called One-Stop Resource Centers, County Career Centers, or possibly another name in your area. The U.S. Department of Labor sponsors them, and their purpose is to provide a wide variety of information and services for the public. Staff members are well informed about employment conditions, as well as specific employers, in their local areas. Ask your school about these resources or go to www.careeronestop.org for the location of your nearest center.

Direct Employer Contacts

Calling or visiting employers to inquire about job openings can be a successful strategy. These actions demonstrate motivation and self-confidence, the very qualities that can help win you a job. They are also a way to discover the estimated four fifths of jobs that are never advertised—the "hidden job market." There are two ways to make contact: in writing and by telephone. If you are sending a cover letter and resume, it is necessary to find the name of the person who makes the hiring decisions for his or her department. If you are calling a small medical office, this may simply mean getting the name—with correct spelling!—of the physician. In the case of a large facility, you may have to do more inquiring by phone to find the right person. When calling, use your best telephone manners.

Craft a letter that explains why you would be a good employee for this particular employer. The letter should demonstrate enthusiasm, interest, and a desire to help the employer. Of course, this means that you know something about the employer: specialty or services offered, typical patients, etc. Include your resume with the letter, which is directed to a specific person. Follow up in a few days with a phone call.

Calling employers by phone to inquire about job openings can be helpful if you are relocating. Phone calls provide an efficient way to contact a large number of employers. Explain that you will be moving and are unfamiliar with the area. If the facility contacted has no openings, ask whether they can refer you to anyone else in the area.

Dropping in on employers gets the word out that you are looking for a job. Visiting all the offices in a large medical facility can be a productive way to spend a day. It gives you a chance to introduce yourself to at least one staff member and personally distribute your resume. If the person who greets you has time, ask for information about the facility. If this is not possible, ask who does the hiring, leave your resume, and express your appreciation. Although you should be dressed as if you were attending an interview, *do not ask* for one at this time if you don't have an appointment.

Large medical facilities, such as hospitals, often coordinate hiring through their human resources office. All resumes and applications must be submitted to this office. It can be worthwhile to also contact or visit the department where you wish to work. Ask for the supervisor and, if he or she is available, let him or her know that you have applied for work through human resources and are very interested in working in that department. Explain why you want to work there and ask that your application be given consideration. If the supervisor is not available, ask to make an appointment. Don't be discouraged, however, if you are unable to make direct contact. Health care professionals today are extremely busy and simply may not have the time. If they don't, send a letter or e-mail that expresses your interest.

Networking

Many people learn about job openings and become employed through personal contacts. In Chapter 2, it was recommended that you start early to meet people in the health care field. Professional organizations were suggested as an excellent source of contacts. In addition to providing you with useful information about your occupational area, they can be a source of job leads and referrals. If you have already met people through professional networking, let them know that you are launching your job search. Don't be shy about asking for their advice about where you might apply, as well as about the job search in general. People who are successful in their careers are generally happy to help newcomers. Do show consideration for their time, and send a thank-you note when they put forth effort on your behalf. It is critical that you follow up on any leads given to you by professional contacts. Failure to do so is not only rude, it may result in the withdrawal of their support.

In addition to professional contacts, general networking can be an effective way to get the word out about your search efforts. I once learned about a job opening for a school director—a position I got and enjoyed for a number of years—from a friend who had seen the ad in the newspaper. Let the people in your life know you are seeking employment. By telling 10 people who each know 10 other people, you create a network of 110 people who know you are looking for a job. Of these 110, it is likely that a few work in health care. And most people use health care services. There is a chance that someone will know someone or something that can help you. Keep in touch with your classmates. Once they have jobs, they may be willing to pass on your name to their employers (Figure 9-3). When speaking with others about your career goals, present yourself positively and express enthusiasm about your field. People want to feel confident about passing your name along.

PERSONAL REFLECTION

Do I conduct myself professionally at all times, including in the classroom? _____

Based on my daily behavior, will people who know me feel confident recommending me for jobs? _____

Are there habits or behaviors I need to improve so people will recommend me?

_____

_____

_____

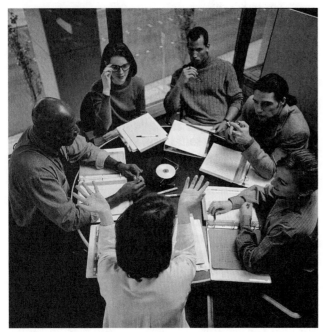

Figure 9-3   Contribute to your career success and that of others by staying in touch with friends from school.

Your Clinical Site

Students who perform well during their clinical experience are sometimes offered jobs at the site. Some employers even create new positions for graduates who impress them with their attitude and skills. Although it is *not* appropriate to ask your clinical site for employment before completing your training there, you should work as if this were your goal. Even if the site is unable to offer you a position, your clinical supervisor can serve as a valuable reference and may recommend you to another employer.

Career and Job Fairs

Some schools, community agencies, and large health care facilities organize activities to connect job recruiters and job seekers. In a single day, you can meet dozens of potential employers. You can gather information, ask questions, and submit your resume. Check your local newspaper for events in your area. Inquire if large health care organizations in your area have career fairs or open houses. You can also find upcoming career fairs across the nation on websites such as nationalcareerfair.com.

Here are some suggestions for taking full advantage of job fairs:

☐ Dress as you would for an interview. If the event takes place at school and you will go directly from class in uniform, be sure it is clean and pressed.

☐ Prepare a list of questions in advance. It's easier to think of them beforehand than to remember them all in a noisy room. Good questions to ask include the following:
  1. What types of jobs does your facility offer?
  2. How can I get more information?
  3. What are the most important qualifications you look for when hiring employees?
  4. Can you give me a written job description?
  5. What is the application procedure?
  6. Who do I contact to set up an interview?
☐ Take copies of your resume. Carry them in a large envelope or folder to keep them clean and neat.
☐ Smile, make eye contact, and introduce yourself to recruiters. Your goal is to get information about the types of jobs they have and what they are looking for in applicants. Thank them for any information they give you. Leave graciously by telling them it was nice meeting them, you appreciate their help, and you look forward to speaking with them again.
☐ Take something in which you can collect brochures, job announcements, and business cards. A small notebook is helpful for taking notes.
☐ As soon as possible after the fair, organize what you collected and use your job lead log pages to record information about the people you met and what you learned. Prepare a list of follow-up activities, such as people to call and resumes to send.

Employer Meetings, Websites, and Telephone Job Lines

Some large facilities that do a lot of hiring have public meetings at which they explain their employment needs and application process. Contact personnel departments, watch the local newspaper, and visit employer Internet sites to find announcements. You may not have a chance to meet personally with the hiring staff, but it is still important that you make a professional impression by dressing and acting appropriately. Be prepared to take notes and ask questions.

Many employers, especially large organizations, have jobs listed on their websites. They also accept applications electronically. Read more about this in Chapter 10.

Some employers are still using **job lines**, taped announcements of current openings. These are accessed by telephone and provide information about how to apply for the jobs described. Some help wanted ads and job postings include telephone numbers. Try calling the personnel department at the facility in which you are interested to inquire whether they have this service.

EMPLOYMENT ADs

The help wanted section of the newspaper is one of the oldest and most traditional methods of locating openings. Although the Internet has become popular as a source of job leads, some newspapers still include employment ads that can be a good source of job leads. Writing a cover letter and mailing or faxing a resume is worth the time and expense it takes. Every action you take increases your chance of finding the right job.

In addition to the newspaper, many professional journals contain employment ads. These can be especially useful if you are willing to move to another area.

USING THE INTERNET

The Internet is the newest job-search tool. It greatly expands your job-search possibilities by being available 24 hours a day. It offers a wide range of how-to information, facts about specific occupations and employers, and job postings. So much information is available, in fact, that it's easy to get lost in cyberspace. You may suddenly realize that you've spent 3 hours moving from one interesting site to another without actually adding much to your job-search efforts!

Getting Started

An excellent place to start learning about using the Internet for the job search is the *Riley Guide* (www.rileyguide.com). Developed by a librarian and available both in print and online, it has provided free, updated career and employment information since 1994. The website serves as a gateway to hundreds of other websites on all phases of the job search. Other good sources that have been in business for some time are Quintessential Careers (www.quintcareers.com) and CareerBuilder (www. careerbuilder.com).

General Research

Studies have shown that only a small percentage of applicants are actually hired as the result of posting a resume on one of the large employment websites; there is simply too much competition. There are literally millions of resumes online at any one time. However, the Internet is a valuable job-search tool. It provides a vast and easily accessed source of information. You can read about health care trends, the general economy, and advances in medicine. You can scan job postings to see what characteristics employers mention most, get information about major facilities, and see samples of good resumes. To access general information, use the search engines discussed in Chapter 5 with key phrases such as "health care trends," "future of health care," "health care providers," and "health care employment." Government agencies such as the Department of Labor (www.dol.gov) and the Bureau of Labor Statistics (www.bls.gov) have information about the national job market, laws that affect employees, and resources for job seekers.

Other effective ways to take advantage of "the net" are discussed in the following sections.

Health Care Facility Websites

Many large health care facilities have websites that include photos, maps, information about the services they offer patients, and statements of their goals and overall mission. If you don't know the address, use a search engine such as Google (www.google.com) and enter the name of the company or facility. Many organizations now list their current job openings along with online applications. In fact, some facilities accept *only* electronic applications. (Chapter 10 contains information about submitting electronic resumes and completing online applications.)

Job-Posting Websites

Job openings are listed on hundreds, perhaps thousands, of websites. Although some websites are easier to use than others, most organize jobs by occupational fields, such as health care, and geographic location. Following are six general employment websites that have been operating for several years and are rated well by users:

1. www.indeed.com
2. www.careerbuilder.com
3. www.hotjobs.yahoo.com
4. www.jobbankinfo.org
5. www.jobcentral.com
6. www.monster.com

You can view the job listings on these sites without registering. If you wish to post your resume, however, you must register by supplying information such as your name, address, and telephone number. You then select a username and password to access your account each time you visit the website. A feature available to those who register on these sites is the assistance of a "search scout," an automated search that matches jobs to your resume and e-mails the results to you.

The general websites listed previously include health care categories and job postings. At the same time, there are employment websites specific to health care, such as the following:

1. www.healthjobsusa.com
2. www.healthcaresource.com
3. www.medzilla.com

In addition to these general health care sites, there are dozens of specialty websites that feature jobs in one career area, such as dental assisting. Links are available at www.quintcareers.com/healthcare_jobs.html.

Most professional organizations maintain websites, and some offer placement assistance for members. For example, the American Health Information Management Association (AHIMA) maintains job postings online for members. See Appendix A for a list of professional organizations and their contact information.

Keep in mind that new websites are continually being developed and old ones are merging, being deleted, or being moved to a different "address." Some of the addresses given in this book and in others may have changed by the time you try them. And it is certain that new websites will have been created.

Networking

The Internet provides opportunities for sharing information and ideas with others through mailing lists and newsgroups. **Mailing lists** (also known as *Listservs* and *e-mail discussion groups*) operate through e-mail. Each list is devoted to a specific topic: occupations, hobbies, health conditions, and so on. Once you have subscribed, you receive e-mail messages to which you can respond. Your e-mail is then sent to all other subscribers. Mailing lists offer a way to learn what other job seekers are doing and what's happening in your field around the country. Comprehensive directories of the thousands of mailing lists are available from CataList (www.lsoft.com/lists/listref.html) and Topica, Inc. (http://lists.topica.com). Another source of mailing list groups is available from Yahoo! at http://groups.yahoo.com

Newsgroups offer another way to network online. A newsgroup is basically an online discussion group for a specific topic. Anyone can join and participate by reading and posting messages. Messages that address the same topic are called a "thread," and each time a different topic is introduced, a new thread is started. Most Web browsers have a search capacity called a "newsreader" that organizes the many newsgroups and enables you to post a message.

If you decide to use either mailing lists or newsgroups, it is important to learn the proper "netiquette" for participating. Experts suggest that you read a group's messages for at least 2 weeks before submitting anything. That way, you'll know the type and quality of material that is expected. It is also recommended that you check the "Frequently Asked Questions" (FAQ) section, if available, to avoid asking something that has already been covered. This is because all subscribers, not just you, receive the answer to your question and may find it annoying to receive information they already know and that is available elsewhere. When you do send messages, keep them short and to the point.

Web forums are another form of online discussion group offered through a variety of websites. You only need an e-mail address and Web browser to participate. You can ask questions, such as "How's the job climate in San Antonio?" and someone from that area is likely to answer. Lists of discussion groups are available on the Internet. Using a browser, enter the keyword "forum" and a topic of interest to get a list of ongoing forums.

One important rule is to never send advertising or use these groups to ask for a job. You may, however, find someone in the group whom you can contact personally via e-mail for possible assistance, just as you would other professional contacts. Good people to write to are those who have posted messages demonstrating that they have knowledge of or work in the occupational area you wish to enter. In your e-mail to that person, identify yourself and the interests you have that seem related to what this person has said in his or her electronic messages to the group. Do *not* ask the person for a job. The purpose of this contact is to ask for—or better yet, share—information about something you have in common. Once a relationship is developed online, and this person seems to have useful knowledge and is willing to share it, it is appropriate to ask for information and career advice.

Success Tips for Using the Internet

☐ **Learn more.** If you are not already proficient at using the Internet, take a class, find online help (see To Learn More at the end of this chapter), or get a copy of one of the many books on how to use it. If your school does not offer instruction, look for adult education classes in your community. Many are offered free of charge.

☐ **Be patient.** The Internet is a developing technology and still has a few bugs. You may get bumped offline just as you find what you are looking for.

A promising-sounding website may have disappeared. But the wealth of information available is worth the time it takes to search.

☐ **Monitor where you are.** It's easy to get lost in a maze of links that takes you far from the original site. When you access a major site, write down its name and address so you can find it again.

☐ **Mark favorite sites.** Most Internet-access software allows you to create personalized lists of useful sites so you can find them later. Also, for any online groups you join, save information in your job-search notebook about how to unsubscribe and the name and e-mail address of the person who manages the list.

☐ **Watch the time.** Using the Internet can be addictive. You can wander for hours linking and looking and actually accomplishing very little. If you find sites that look interesting but are unrelated to the task at hand, write down or mark their addresses and return to them later.

☐ **Beware of scams.** Take care when posting your resume or sending private information. If a website makes claims about jobs that seem too good to be true, it may simply be a means of getting personal information about you. Stick with major employment websites and the websites of employers whose existence you can verify in other ways.

☐ **Don't exceed 25%.** Remember, the Internet is only one tool for your job search. Use it wisely as a supplement to other methods. Some experts even recommend spending no more than 10% of your job-search time using the Internet.

☐ **Be careful what you post.** If you have pages on websites such as MySpace and Facebook, be *very* careful about what you post. Photos of yourself that may be amusing but that don't show you at your best may damage your chances for employment. Many employers reportedly search potential employees on the Internet, and some admit not hiring based on what they find.[1] You might consider using the Internet to your advantage. For example, if you have volunteered for a community fundraiser or serve meals at a community center, include photos of yourself participating in these activities.

Internet Tracking Form

If you use the Internet to find information, post your resume, and/or participate in groups, take a little time to record your activities. Use the Internet tracking form that follows to track the job opportunities you find online. Make copies of the form, or set up one of your own to keep in your job-search notebook or on your computer.

RESPONDING TO JOB POSTINGS AND ADS

Regardless of the source—Internet, professional journal, or newspaper—look under every category that might contain jobs for which you are prepared. For example, while "nursing assistants" are likely to appear under "nursing," they may also be listed under "medical" or "health care." If your training has prepared you for a variety of positions, be sure to check all possible job titles. For example, graduates of health information programs may be qualified for the following positions: coding specialist, health information technician, medical records coordinator or supervisor, and patient records technician. New job titles are constantly being created to describe the many activities performed in the modern health care facility. Use the skill inventories you created for yourself to help you identify all the jobs for which you might apply. Don't be discouraged if you find only a few postings or ads—or none—for your occupation. This may actually mean that there is such a shortage of applicants that employers have given up placing expensive ads.

When you respond in writing to a job opening, point out how you meet the employer's needs. You can do this in the cover letter, which will be discussed more fully in Chapter 10. For now, let's look at a couple of sample ads and see how to encourage the employer to read your resume and call you for an interview. Even very short ads contain information you can use. The ad for a medical assistant in Figure 9-4 lists three requirements and shows how they can be addressed in a cover letter sent with a resume. The response to the ad in Figure 9-5 is written in a different format but still addresses the employer's needs. (The same advice applies to electronically posted openings.)

There is not one best way to write an effective response to an employer. Highlight your qualifications with a format that best suits the stated requirements. It isn't necessary—or even desirable—to repeat what's in your resume. A few quick highlights about how you meet the specific requirements are sufficient, along with a fuller description of why you, in particular, can help this employer.

 Go to page 258 to complete Prescription for Success 9-5

INTERNET TRACKING FORM

Name of website: _____

Website address: _____

Purpose of website:

- Job lists
- Resume posting
- Search scout
- Information, articles
- Newsgroup
- Mailing list
- Company website

My username: _____

My password: _____

Date resume posted: _____

Responses: _____

Employers identified: _____

_____

_____

Notes (information you provided the employer, version of resume submitted, etc.)

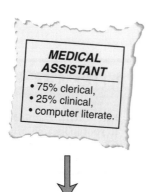

MEDICAL ASSISTANT
• 75% clerical,
• 25% clinical,
• computer literate.

Your Requirements

How I Meet Them

75% clerical

I enjoy and am proficient in front office duties. I received top grades in my administrative classes. I understand the importance of efficiency, accuracy, and confidentiality when performing clerical functions in the medical office. My written and oral communication skills are excellent.

25% clinical

I have up-to-date skills in all medical assisting clinical procedures.

Computer literate

I have basic computer literacy skills, can work in a Windows environment, and am proficient in Medical Manager, Word, and Excel.

Figure 9-4 Example of a direct, point-by-point response to a job posting.

DENTAL ASSISTANT—RDA

We are looking for the best! If you understand quality, modern dentistry, appreciate excellent patient care and are dedicated to true teamwork, please fax your resume to...

Your response:

I am a registered dental assistant who recently completed a program of study at Dental Technical College in Health Town. My training program was patient-focused. In all courses, we learned the importance of considering the needs of each patient and delivering the best care possible. I also understand the importance of teamwork, having worked closely with other students throughout both the theory and lab portions of the program. During my clinical experience with Dr. Frank Samuels, I enjoyed sharing responsibilities with his five-member office staff.

Figure 9-5 Example of a paragraph that addresses the employer's stated needs.

➡ SUMMARY OF KEY IDEAS

1. Know yourself: what you want and need and what you have to offer an employer.
2. Get to know the employment climate.
3. Increase your chance of finding the right job by using a variety of lead sources.

◩ Positive Self-Talk for This Chapter

1. I am confident and competent.
2. I have valuable skills to offer an employer.
3. I am organized and have a good job-search plan.
4. I will find the job that's right for me.

To Learn More

Bolles RN: *What color is your parachute? A practical manual for job-hunters and job-changers,* Berkeley, 2009, Ten Speed Press.

www.thejobhuntersbible.com

Bolles's book has become a classic job-search manual. The ideas are original, well researched, and reportedly very effective. The companion website is also packed with useful ideas, including hints on effectively using the Internet in the job search.

Career Builder

www.careerbuilder.com

Website includes job-search tools, career advice, list of career fairs around the country, and a salary calculator.

Dickel MR, Roehm, F: Guide to Internet job searching 2008-2009, Columbus, Ohio, 2008, McGraw-Hill.

Nemko M, Edwards P, Edwards S: *Cool careers for dummies,* ed 2, Indianapolis, 2001, Wiley Publishing.

This book provides reader-friendly and effective information—even for "smarties."

Riley Guide

http://rileyguide.com

Margaret Dickel is a librarian who has been tracking the Internet as a job-search resource for many years. Her book is excellent, or you can access lots of information from her website.

Quintessential Careers

General job-search and career information: www.quintcareers.com

Health care jobs: www.quintcareers.com/healthcare_jobs.html

This website contains information on every phase of the job search and career development in the form of articles, resources, and tutorials.

U.S. Department of Labor, Bureau of Labor Statistics

www.bls.gov

The BLS website contains information about economic conditions, wages, and unemployment rates. By clicking on "jobseekers," you will find a list of links to other government websites covering industries, including health care, and specific occupations.

REFERENCES

1. Kate Lorenz, Warning: social networking can be hazardous to your job search. www.careerbuilder.com/Article/CB-533-Job-Search-Warning-Social-Networking-Can-Be-Hazardous-to-Your-Job-Search/?ArticleID=533&cbRecursionCnt=1&cbsid=920e95b94af84818bfb7a8e12af99ffd-288916701-R3-4 (Accessed 2/25/09.)

BUILDING YOUR RESUME

Review and fill in the forms for Resume Building Blocks #6, #7, #8, and #9 in Chapter 2, which list activities and skills that support your job search.

INTERNET ACTIVITIES

For active links to the websites needed to complete these activities, visit **http://evolve.elsevier.com/haroun/career/**.

1. Locate an article about using networking to learn about job openings, and write a summary of what you learn.
2. Using websites that list job openings, find and list 10 jobs for which you might be qualified.
3. Read the article "How to Use the Internet in Your Job Search" (http://rileyguide.com/jobsrch.html), and create a list of the suggestions.
4. Explore the website of a professional organization related to your occupation. What kind of information does it contain? Job postings? Opportunities to network? Conference dates? Anything else?

Prescription for Success 9-1
Inventory of Technical Skills

1. Refer back to the Building Block #3: Professional Skills and Knowledge form in Chapter 2, in which you began to list the skills you were learning in school. If necessary, gather additional sources of information to help you complete your inventory: lab checklists, course objectives, clinical performance evaluations, textbooks, and class handouts.

2. Create categories, such as the following, that are appropriate for your occupational area. List your specific skills under each heading:

Equipment I Can Use

Lab Procedures I Can Perform

Tests I Can Perform

Patient Procedures I Can Perform

Administrative Procedures

Computer Skills and Applications

Medical Records

Documentation and Charting

Medical Insurance

Billing

Communication Skills

    Oral

    Written

3. Think of examples that demonstrate your mastery of each skill, such as your performance in the laboratory or classroom, completion of special projects, or work you did during your clinical experience. Are there areas in which you demonstrated particular expertise? You can use these examples to better present your qualifications to potential employers on both your resume and at job interviews.

Prescription for Success 9-2
What Do I Want? An Update

Review Prescription for Success 1-9, and record any changes you have made.

1. **Type of facility:** large, small, urban, suburban, rural, inpatient, outpatient

   _____

2. **Type of population served:** economic status, age range, gender, ethnic groups

   _____

3. **Work schedule:** steady employment, per diem, flexible hours, fixed hours, overtime, days only, evenings and weekends

   _____

4. *Specialty area*

   _____

5. *Type of supervision*

   _____

6. **Work pace:** fast, moderate

   _____

7. *Amount of interaction with others* (All health care professionals are part of a team, although some work more independently than others.)

   _____

8. **Range of duties:** wide variety, concentrate on a few

   _____

Prescription for Success 9-3
My Support System

Think about the people in your life who are qualified to help your job-search efforts. Who can you ask to help you with each of the following?

1. Proofreading your resume and other written materials

   _____

   _____

2. Interview practice

   _____

   _____

3. Postinterview evaluations

   _____

   _____

4. Encouragement

   _____

   _____

Prescription for Success 9-4
What's Going On?

Use your research skills to find answers to the following questions:

1. What is the unemployment rate in your area? _____

2. Who are the major health care employers?

   _____

   _____

   _____

   _____

Continued

Prescription for Success 9–4 (Continued)

3. What are the current hiring trends in health care?

_____

_____

_____

_____

4. How might these conditions affect your occupation?

_____

_____

_____

_____

5. How might they influence your job-search strategies?

_____

_____

_____

_____

Prescription for Success 9-5
Create a Targeted Response

Find an employment ad, either printed or on the Internet. Identify the employer's requirements and write a response that demonstrates how you meet these requirements. (Attach copy of ad or computer printout.)

Your Response

_____

_____

_____

_____

_____

Finalizing Your Employment Presentation Materials

OBJECTIVES

The information and activities in this chapter can help you:

- Write an effective resume.
- Write appropriate cover letters.
- Fill out employment applications correctly and accurately.
- Secure good references who will support your job-search efforts.
- Prepare a reference sheet.
- Create a professional portfolio that supports your qualifications.

KEY TERMS AND CONCEPTS

Applications: Forms containing questions and spaces for information that employers need to make a decision regarding an applicant's qualifications for a job.

Liability: Responsibility, often financial, for damages and losses.

Objective: Your job or career goal.

Portfolios: Collections of items that provide evidence of job-related skills and capabilities.

Resumes: Written documents that summarize professional skills and capabilities.

Targeted Objective: An objective that matches the requirements of a specific employer.

PRESENTATION: PUTTING YOUR BEST PEN FORWARD

"The door of opportunity won't open unless you do some pushing."

Preparing high-quality written materials is an essential part of a successful job search. Some documents are designed to outline your qualifications and let potential employers know what you can do for them. These include **resumes**, cover letters, and **applications**. Other materials serve to support your claims and include reference sheets and **portfolios.**

Anything you submit in your bid for employment is a form of personal advertising. Written materials reflect who you are and what you can do, so apply your best organizing, writing, and spelling skills to their creation. Keep in mind that written materials are, in a sense, permanent. What's on paper stays there. You can't change, correct, or explain, "What I really meant to say was…." Once in the hands of prospective employers, a resume and cover letter are all they have to go by. So prepare all written materials thoughtfully and carefully so they represent you in the best way possible.

 Go to page 283 to complete Prescription for Success 10-1

YOUR RESUME: A PRODUCT BROCHURE

"The resume gets you the interview. The interview gets you the job."

Selling yourself as a qualified job candidate begins with a well-prepared resume. The purpose of a resume is to convince prospective employers to interview you. To accomplish this, you must show them you have the qualifications they need. Health care employers are looking for employees who will contribute to their success in caring for their customers. (Yes, many employers think of their patients as customers.) Your well-constructed resume is one way to show them that you are the kind of person they are looking for.

COMPLETING THE BUILDING BLOCKS OF YOUR RESUME

In the following sections, you will use the information you have been writing on the Resume Building Block forms provided in Chapter 2 to complete the various components of your resume. Then you will go through the steps to pull them all together into a completed resume you can be proud to have represent you.

PERSONAL REFLECTION

Why do you think a resume is referred to as a "product brochure"?

_____

_____

_____

Does thinking about your resume in this way influence how you will write it? If so, how?

_____

_____

_____

Many employers are using the Internet extensively in the hiring process. Some have started scanning all resumes they receive and entering them into a computerized database. Each resume is then reviewed electronically, and key words are identified. When there is a job opening, the computer searches for resumes that contain key words that match those in the job description. Other employers are accepting only electronically sent resumes.

These new practices require thinking a little differently as you write your resume. Because of the key-word element, these are an important consideration as you write the various sections. Start by preparing a list of key words that relate to your job target. Twenty to 60 words are recommended. Consider which key words most nearly describe the jobs for which you want to be considered, as well as the types of skills and qualities employers are seeking. If possible, secure job descriptions from potential employers. Read ads or job announcements, and visit facility websites. The *Occupational Outlook Handbook,* a government publication that contains descriptions of thousands of jobs, is a good source. Good key words are nouns that name specific skills, such as insurance billing, laboratory tests, and patient care.

Building Block #1: Career Objective

The objective you write for your resume may be quite general—"Seeking a position as a licensed practical nurse"—or more specific—"Seeking a position as an administrative or front-office medical assistant in an urgent care facility." The more restrictive the objective, the fewer the positions that are likely to be available. Here are some questions to ask yourself when determining your career objective:

- Am I willing to accept only those jobs that meet my specific requirements?
- Am I more interested in a specific facility or a specific type of work?
- What are the current economic conditions? (If the competition for jobs is great, being willing to consider a variety of positions will increase your chances of being hired.)
- What are the current job conditions for my occupational and geographic area? Are there many applicants? Is there a shortage of applicants?
- What are my skill base and amount of experience? What advantages do I have over other applicants?
- Am I responding to an advertised position? Does my objective match the requirements of the position?

Consider writing a **targeted objective** when applying for a specific job. This type of objective mirrors the employer's language and draws attention to how you fit that particular job. **The following example shows how to write a targeted objective:**

Ad: "X-ray tech with strong patient-relations skills for orthopedic practice. Great opportunity to join an established team environment."

Key words in the ad: "x-ray tech," "patient relations skills," "orthopedic," "team."

Targeted objective: Position as an x-ray tech in an orthopedic office where I can apply my excellent human-relations skills working with patients and fellow professionals.

If you create and print your own resume on a computer, you can change your objective slightly for each job you apply for.

Go to page 284 to complete Prescription for Success 10-2

Go to page 284 to complete Prescription for Success 10-3

Building Block #2: Education

Up-to-date training is likely to be one of the strongest employment qualifications of recent graduates who don't have previous work history in health care. The Education section can contain more information than simply a list of the schools you have attended. The following items are examples of what you can include:

☐ Name of the health care program you completed

☐ Degree, diploma, or certificate earned

☐ Grade point average, if at least 3.0 (on a 4.0 scale)

☐ Licenses, special certifications, and other documentation of preparation

☐ Additional courses, workshops, seminars, and special training you have completed

☐ Special projects that demonstrate your qualifications

Some program titles do not clearly communicate the types of skills acquired by students. For example, the program entitled "Patient Care Assistant" varies in content from school to school throughout the country. In cases like this, it is a good idea to list the courses you have completed. This gives the employer a better idea of your skills. (If this takes too much space on the resume, consider including a list of courses or a copy of the curriculum in your portfolio.)

Following is an example of an education section:

Mental Health Technician Certificate, 2008
Wellness College, Salem, OR
- Graduated with Top Honors
- Grade point average 3.7 on a 4.0 scale
- Received Perfect Attendance Award

Nursing Assistant Certificate, 2009
GetWell Health College, Portland, OR
- Grade point average 3.8 on a 4.0 scale
- Maintained perfect attendance
- Completed CPR training
- Organized musical program presented by students at Christmas to local extended-care residents

Workshops completed 2005-2006
Sunnyville Psychiatric Institute, Salem, OR
- Review of Research on Depression (25 hours)
- Suicide Prevention Measures (20 hours)
- Managing Assaultive Patients (25 hours)

Go to page 284 to complete Prescription for Success 10-4

Building Block #3: Professional Skills and Knowledge

Occupational skills acquired through both training and work history are listed in the Professional Skills and Knowledge section. Recall from Chapter 2 that these may be listed individually or in clusters of related skills. Take a look at the following examples:

Example 1: Creating skill clusters
Medical assistant skills
- Administrative skills
  Schedule appointments, handle telephone calls, greet patients, maintain medical records, code and fill out insurance forms, perform billing and bookkeeping functions

- Clinical skills

Assist physician, prepare and administer medications, perform venipuncture and ECG, take vital signs, practice aseptic technique

- Laboratory skills

Perform urinalyses, hematological tests, various specialty tests

- Computer skills

Medical Manager, Microsoft Word, Excel, PowerPoint

Example 2: Listing individual skills

Medical insurance technician skills

- Abstract medical information from patient records
- Code diagnoses and procedures accurately
- Complete insurance forms correctly
- Submit and monitor insurance claims
- Process payments

If you plan to list your skills and classes in the Education section, you may omit this section from your resume.

 Go to page 284 to complete Prescription for Success 10-5

Building Block #4: Work History

A record of your previous employment, the Work History section can be more than a simple listing of jobs and the duties you performed. As discussed in Chapter 2, your Work History section can be strengthened by including your accomplishments and emphasizing transferable skills that relate to the health care job you want now.

Use action verbs when describing job duties and achievements. For example, saying "taught students of all ages to swim" is a stronger and more effective statement than "Responsible for teaching swimming." Even better is "Successfully taught students of all ages to swim so that 97% passed the Red Cross swim test for their level." See Box 10-1 for a list of suggested action verbs.

Military service and your clinical experience can also be included in this section. Just be sure to make it clear that the clinical experience was an unpaid position and that you were a student. It is not necessary to include very short-term or part-time jobs unless they are directly related to your job target. Do not include your reasons for leaving each job. You may find this question on employment applications, but it should not be part of your resume.

Here is an example of a Work History entry:

Cashier, Petamerica Bigdog, GA

- Assisted customers and informed them about products
- Performed cashier duties
- Closed out registers at end of day
- Named "Most Helpful Employee" for 2007
- Maintained perfect attendance for 2 years
- Promoted to head cashier after 1 year
- Selected to train newly hired cashiers

 Go to page 284 to complete Prescription for Success 10-6

BOX 10-1   Action Verbs for Use on Resumes

Achieved	Educated	Launched	Recorded
Administered	Encouraged	Led	Regulated
Assisted	Established	Maintained	Repaired
Billed	Expanded	Managed	Reported
Budgeted	Generated	Monitored	Represented
Calculated	Greeted	Motivated	Revised
Cared for	Handled	Negotiated	Scheduled
Coded	Helped	Obtained	Secured
Communicated	Hired	Operated	Set up
Composed	Implemented	Ordered	Showed
Constructed	Improved	Organized	Sold
Controlled	Increased	Participated	Supervised
Coordinated	Influenced	Performed	Taught
Created	Informed	Planned	Tested
Demonstrated	Initiated	Prepared	Trained
Designed	Inspired	Presented	Verified
Developed	Instructed	Produced	Word processed
Directed	Introduced	Provided	Wrote
Documented	Justified	Purchased	

Building Block #5: Licenses and Certifications

Include a Licenses and Certifications section on your resume only if this information is not listed in the Education or any other section. Wherever you put it, be sure the dates and numbers are accurate.

Examples of ways to present certifications include the following:

- Certified Occupational Therapist Assistant, 2009 American Occupational Therapy Association
- Registered Nurse California State Nursing License, #123456
- Certified Medical Assistant, 2005 American Association of Medical Assistants

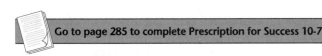

Go to page 285 to complete Prescription for Success 10-7

Building Block #6: Honors and Awards

Honors and awards can be from organizations other than your school. When listing these items, include information about why you received them if this is not clear from their names. (These could be listed under Education or Professional and Community Organizations. Choose where they fit best; just make sure to list them only once.)

Example:

Parent Volunteer of 2010 for James Madison Middle School

Recognition for organizing activities that raised over $150,000 to purchase instructional equipment, such as computers and library books

Perfect Attendance Award, Wellness College, 2009

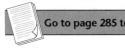

Go to page 285 to complete Prescription for Success 10-8

Building Block #7: Special Skills

Do you have skills that don't fit in any other section but that add to your value as a health care employee? This section gives you the opportunity to include and even highlight them.

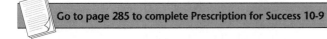

Go to page 285 to complete Prescription for Success 10-9

Building Block #8: Community Service and Volunteer Work

Service and volunteer work do not have to be directly related to health care. For example, work in which you demonstrated responsibility, the willingness to contribute to society and help others, and/or your teamwork skills is appropriate to include. You may have done this at school, through a religious organization, or with any group devoted to promoting the good of the community. Write brief phrases to describe what you did, if necessary. Use action verbs as in the Work History section. Do not list activities you already included in the Education section or elsewhere.

Following are some examples:

March of Dimes, 1999-present
Participated in annual fund drives
Boy Scout Troop Leader, 1997-2003

Go to page 285 to complete Prescription for Success 10-10

Building Block #9: Professional and Civic Organizations

In the Professional and Civic Organizations section, list organizations to which you belong. Briefly describe any organizations that might not be familiar to prospective employers. If you take or have taken an active part, such as serving on a committee or as an officer, state what you are doing or did. On your resume, this heading can also be called "Memberships" or "Affiliations."

Examples include the following:

Florida Association of Medical Assistants, Tampa Chapter

Chair of membership drive, 2002

Member of continuing education planning committee, 2001-present

(**Note:** It is best not to include organizations that are highly political or are generally considered to hold radical views. If you are in doubt about what to include on your resume, check with your instructor or your school's career services' office.)

Go to page 285 to complete Prescription for Success 10-11

Building Block #10: Languages Spoken

If you are able to communicate in a language other than English and have not included it in any other section, it can go in a special Languages section. Include a little information about your skills and level of ability, as in the **following examples:**

Spanish: Speaking and reading, good; writing, fair.

Vietnamese: Very basic conversational ability. Some knowledge of health care terms for conducting patient interviews.

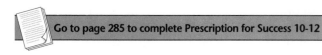

Go to page 285 to complete Prescription for Success 10-12

PULLING IT ALL TOGETHER

You are now ready to gather the information in your Resume Building Blocks to construct a finished product. Just like actual blocks, the content from your Prescriptions for Success 10-3 through 10-11 can be put together in a variety of ways. The steps described in this section will help you create a document that best highlights your qualifications.

You will see as you progress through this chapter that there is no one best way to write a resume. Everyone has different talents and experiences. Even students who complete the same program at the same time come from a variety of backgrounds that can be presented in different ways. For example, a young person who graduated from high school shortly before beginning a dental assisting program will most likely benefit from emphasizing different areas than a classmate who worked in sales for 20 years before entering the same program.

There are also local customs and employer preferences regarding resumes. Seek the advice of your instructors, school career service personnel, and professional contacts. They keep in touch with employers and can offer sound advice.

At this busy time in the job-search process, you may be tempted to use a standard resume format. Filling in the blanks on a "one-type-fits-all" resume may seem to be a fast and easy way to complete this task. However, the time spent customizing your resume can pay off in several ways. For example, you will do the following:

1. Better recognize and review your own qualifications
2. Respond to employers' specific needs
3. Be prepared to support your claims with examples
4. Demonstrate your organizational skills
5. Show your initiative and creativity

Note: Your school may require or recommend that you use a format it has developed. In this case, it is probably best to use what is provided.

An effective way to increase your efficiency when putting together your resume is to use word-processing software. This gives you several advantages because you can:

- Try different layouts and formats
- Change and reorganize content quickly and easily
- Check for (most) spelling errors
- Change your objective or skill clusters to address specific employer needs

- Use special features such as bolding and changing the size and style of the letters
- Send your resume as part of an e-mail and/or post it on the Internet (this will be discussed later in this chapter)

If you don't know how to use a word-process program, now is a good time to learn if you have a little time. Today's software is quite easy to learn and even nontypists can produce great-looking documents by learning a few basic commands. Spacing, bolding, underlining, moving text, and printing can be accomplished with the click or two of a button. If you can spend a few hours to learn the basics of a word-processing program now, it will be a good investment of your time. Not only will this skill support your job-search effort, it will provide you with a valuable workplace skill. Even health care professionals who dedicate most of their time to hands-on patient activities can benefit from knowing how to word process. Today, computer skills are considered essential for most health care jobs.

10 STEPS FOR ASSEMBLING YOUR RESUME

Whether you create your resume on a computer or not, following a step-by-step process can help you assemble a resume to fit your needs. Box 10-2 summarizes the steps that are explained in the following sections.

Step One: Prepare the Heading

It is not necessary to write the word "Resume." Instead, clearly label the top of the page with your name, address, and telephone number. Centering

---

BOX 10-2   A 10-Step Checklist for Assembling Your Resume

1. Prepare the heading.
2. Add the objective.
3. Select the best type of resume for you.
4. Decide if you want to include a Summary of Qualifications section.
5. Choose which Resume Building Blocks to include.
6. Plan the order of your Building Blocks.
7. Decide whether you want to add a personal statement.
8. But…leave out personal information.
9. Plan the layout.
10. Create an attractive and professional-looking document.

your name is good for both appearance and practicality. Placing it on the far left side makes it more difficult for the employer to find if it is placed in a stack of other resumes or in a file. (You might even put your heading justified right.) Capitalizing your name and/or using a slightly larger font (letter) size than the rest of the document helps it to stand out.

JAIME RAMIREZ
3650 Loma Alta Lane
San Diego, CA 92137
(619) 123-4567
jrnurse@aol.com

Capitalize and boldface your name and consider using a larger size font. Include your ZIP code and area code. Be sure all numbers are correct. Include your e-mail address if you have one.

The following format is an option if your resume is long and you are trying to conserve space:

JAIME RAMIREZ
3650 Loma Alta Lane, San Diego, CA 92137
(619) 123-4567 jrnurse@aol.com

Step Two: Add the Objective

The objective, from Resume Building Block #1, should be near the beginning of the resume so prospective employers can quickly see whether there is a potential match between your goals and their needs. This part of the resume may change slightly, as discussed before, if you are trying to match your objective with the stated needs of each employer. Your objective will not change if you have specific requirements you are not willing to change, if you have written a very general objective that meets a number of job targets, or if your objective simply states a job title such as "surgical technologist."

Step Three: Select the Best Type of Resume for You

The three basic types of resumes are chronological, functional, and combination. They provide different ways to present your work history and professional qualifications. Your particular background determines which type you should choose.

Chronological Resume

The chronological resume emphasizes work history. It shows the progression of jobs you have held to show how you have gained increasing knowledge, experience, and/or responsibility relevant to the job you want now. This type of resume is recommended if you have:

☐ Held previous jobs in health care
☐ Had jobs in other areas in which you had increases in responsibility or a strong record of achievements
☐ Acquired many skills that apply to health care (transferable skills)

In the chronological resume, each job you've had in the past is listed, followed by the duties performed and your achievements. The Work section is well developed and likely to be longer than most other parts of your resume. See Figure 10-1 for an example of the Work History section for a nurse's chronological resume.

Functional Resume

The functional resume emphasizes skills and traits that relate to the targeted job but that weren't necessarily acquired through health-care employment. They can be pulled from both work and personal experiences. For example, if you cared for a sick relative for an extended period of time, this is an experience you might decide to include. Review Prescription for Success 1-4 and the transferable skills on Resume Building Block #4 for ideas. Once you have identified and listed qualifications that fit your target jobs, organize them into three or four clusters with descriptive headings. Figure 10-2 shows three clusters developed by a graduate who wants to find a job in health information technology. She has drawn from her experiences as a parent, active member of her community, and bookkeeper.

Functional resumes are advantageous in the following situations:
☐ If you are entering the job market for the first time
☐ If you have held jobs unrelated to health care
☐ If you have personal experiences you can apply to health care work

The Work History section of a functional resume consists of a simple list of job titles with each employer's name, city and state, and your dates of employment. See Figure 10-2 for examples. A functional resume may take more time to develop than a chronological one, but the extra effort can really pay off because it allows you to highlight the qualifications that are your strongest bid for employment.

Combination Resume

The combination resume, as its name implies, uses features of both the chronological and functional types. The details of the job(s) held in or closely related to health care are listed, along with clusters

WORK HISTORY

Registered Nurse III, Surgical Unit
Gladstone Hospital, Happy Valley, OR   2006-Present

- Serve as charge nurse, providing high quality nursing care
  without supervision

- Develop and implement patient care plans based on individual needs

- Evaluate and revise plans as needed

- Conduct patient care conferences with care team members

- Serve as a patient advocate to ensure provision of appropriate
  and high quality care

- Teach and counsel patients and their families to perform
  home care procedures and maximize wellness

- Serve as preceptor for ADN and LPN nursing students

Registered Nurse II, Surgical Unit   2003-2006
Gladstone Hospital, Happy Valley, OR

- Identify patient care problems

- Implement nursing interventions and evaluate the results

- Administer medications without error

- Teach patients preoperation and postoperation procedures

- Carry out procedures as ordered by physician

- Communicate clearly to patients, their families, co-workers,
  and physicians

- Orient new employees

Staff Nurse   1999-2003
Sunnyville Community Hospital, Sunnyville, OR

- Provide direct patient care

- Carry out nursing care plans

- Complete prescribed treatments

- Give medications

- Document all care given on patient charts

- Call physicians as needed in response to patient's conditions

Figure 10-1   Work History section of chronological resume for an experienced applicant seeking a nursing position. The most recent job is listed first. As you read from the bottom up, note the increasing complexity of tasks and levels of responsibility. For example, in his first job he carried out nursing plans; in his most recent job, he developed the plans.

of qualifications or a list of supporting skills. This resume is appropriate in the following situations:

☐ If you have held jobs in health care *and*

☐ If you have related qualifications you gained through other, non–health care jobs and experiences *or*

☐ If you have held a number of jobs in health care for which you performed the same or very similar duties

Let's look at how a recent occupational therapy assistant graduate who worked for 2 years as a nursing assistant and for 3 years as a preschool aide creates a combination resume. She decides to do the following:

☐ Include a list of the duties she performed in the nursing assistant job

☐ Create clusters to highlight her teaching and interpersonal skills, both important in occupational therapy

COMPUTER SKILLS

- Created electronic spreadsheet to track fund-raising for Lewison Elementary School PTA

- Taught self to effectively use leading brand software programs in the following areas: word processing, database, spreadsheets, and accounting

- Set up and managed electronic accounting system for family construction business

- Teach computer classes at Girl Scout summer day camp

ORGANIZATIONAL SKILLS

- Created system to monitor all church collections and fund-raising projects

- Initiated and developed computer career awareness program for Girl Scouts

- Secretary for college HIT student organization

- Completed HIT associate degree program with record of perfect attendance while working part-time and managing family life

CLERICAL/ADMINISTRATIVE SKILLS

- 7 years bookkeeping experience

- Keyboarding speed of 78 wpm

- Excellent written communication

WORK HISTORY

Bookkeeper   2008-Present
Buildwell Construction Company, Yuma, AZ

Bookkeeper   2003-2008
Perfect-Fit Cabinetry, Yuma, AZ

Secretary   1999-2003
Caldwell Insurance Company, Yuma, AZ

Figure 10-2 Work History section of a functional resume for a recent graduate seeking a health information technology (HIT) position. The graduate does not have experience in this field, so she has clustered other skills that support work in HIT, such as bookkeeping and tracking details.

☐ List skills from her teaching and other experiences under each cluster heading

Figure 10-3 illustrates how she organized her material to best show her qualifications.

Choosing the Best Resume for You

Review your skills and experiences and use the guidelines in this section to choose the best type of resume for you. If you decide to use a chronological presentation, copy what you prepared for your Work History in Building Block #3.

If a functional resume would serve you better, use the following guidelines to create the clusters:

1. Consider the current needs of employers. Check your local help-wanted ads and job announcements, the National Healthcare Foundation Standards, and the SCANS competencies for ideas.
2. Think about the skills and traits that will contribute to success in your occupation.
3. Look over your work history, clinical experience, personal experiences, volunteer activities, and participation in professional organizations.
4. Refer to your completed Prescriptions for Success 1-4 and 9-1 for skills and characteristics you can use in clusters.

NURSING ASSISTANT   2005-2010
GoodCare Nursing Home, Denver, CO

- Encourage patients to achieve their maximum level of wellness, activity and independence

- Demonstrate interest in the lives and well-being of patients

- Assist patients with prescribed exercises

- Organize and participate in activities with patients

- Help patients carry out basic hygiene and dressing

TEACHING SKILLS

- Teach swim classes to all ages at YMCA

- Conduct CPR instruction for the American Heart Association

- Organize holiday programs and outings for nursing home residents (volunteer)

- Planned and supervised craft and play activities for preschool children

- Tutored ESL students at Salud College while in OTA program

INTERPERSONAL SKILLS

- Provided daily care for parent with Alzheimer's disease for 18 months

- Answered telephone, directed calls, and took messages for busy sporting goods manufacturer

- Received Connor Memorial Award for graduating class for making positive contributions and assisting classmates at Salud College

WORK HISTORY   **Preschool Aide** 2002-2005
Bright Light Preschool, Denver, CO

Swim Instructor 2002-Present
YMCA, Denver, CO

Receptionist 1999-2002
Sportrite Manufacturing Co., Denver, CO

Figure 10-3   Work History section of a combination resume for a recent graduate seeking an occupational therapy assistant position. She details the one health care–related job she has held while organizing other skills that support the new career into clusters.

5. Create three or four headings for clusters that support your job target and give you an opportunity to list your most significant qualifications. The following list contains examples of appropriate clusters for health care occupations:
   - Communication Skills
   - Organizational Skills
   - Teamwork Skills
   - Interpersonal Relations
   - Computer Skills
   - Clerical Skills

6. List appropriate specific skills under each heading.

Step Four: Summary of Qualifications

Decide whether to include a Summary of Qualifications Section. This is an optional section. Its purpose is to list skills that support you as a product but that don't fit well in other sections. It can also serve to highlight how you will benefit the employer and encourage the reader to look over the rest of your resume. In other words, it can serve as an appealing introduction to you and your resume.

You may have decided to use a chronological resume but have additional experiences that don't belong in the Work History section. Or maybe you have designed a functional resume but have single experiences worth mentioning that don't fit any of the headings, as in the following examples:

- Excellent time-management skills
- Work calmly under pressure
- Proven problem-solving ability
- Cost conscious
- Enthusiastic team player
- Work well without supervision
- Enjoy learning new skills

A Qualifications section can also serve as a summary of highlights to draw attention to your most significant features. Such a summary might look like this:

- ☐ Eight years' experience working in health care
- ☐ Up-to-date administrative and clinical medical assisting skills
- ☐ Current CPR certification
- ☐ Fluent in spoken Spanish
- ☐ Excellent communication skills

Review the same information sources recommended in Step Four for preparing functional clusters. The difference in preparing the Qualifications section is you can combine different kinds of characteristics. They don't have to fall into neat categories but only have to demonstrate capabilities, traits, and special skills that relate to the job you want.

Note: If you have created clusters and are using them in a functional or combination resume, you may not need a Qualifications section. The important thing is not to repeat information in your resume. Step Five talks more about deciding what to include.

Step Five: Choose Which Resume Building Blocks to Use

You want your resume to be comprehensive, but at the same time you don't want to repeat information. For example, if you are using a functional format and have listed a special skill in one of your clusters, don't repeat it under another heading. Group as much as fits well into each Resume Building Block instead of having many headings with just one item listed. Think about which items fit together. The following are the most appropriate to combine:

1. Licenses and certifications can be placed in their own section, can be listed in the Education section, or can be listed as a Professional Qualification.

2. Honors and awards earned in school can be listed under Education. If you have a variety of awards, it might be better to highlight them by listing them in their own section.

3. Memberships can go under Education if they are related to school groups or your health care professional organization. If you have been active in the organizations and want to state what you've done or are involved in several organizations, they might better go in their own section.

4. Clinical experience can be listed under either Education or Work History. Wherever you place it, include some information about the duties you performed. For career changers and recent graduates, this may be a significant part of work history. Be sure to indicate clearly, however, that the work was unpaid and part of an educational program.

5. Languages you speak other than English can be listed under Qualifications, Special Skills, or Languages Spoken.

Deciding which headings to use and where to place content depends on the amount of content, how directly it relates to the kind of job you want, and your own organizational preferences. Suppose you speak two languages other than English. If they are spoken by many people in your geographic area, they are likely to be valuable job qualifications and might be listed in a Summary of Qualifications. If they are not commonly spoken in your area, they might best be listed under Languages—skills you want to show but that may not be directly related to the job. Think about the relative importance of your content as you decide how best to organize and label it.

Step Six: Plan the Order of Your Building Blocks

Place the sections that contain your strongest qualifications first. For example, if you are changing careers and recent education is your primary qualification, list that section before Work History.

Step Seven: Decide If You Want to Add a Personal Statement

In their book *Career Planning*, Dave Ellis and coauthors suggest adding a positive personal statement at the bottom of your resume.[1] This gives you an opportunity to make a final impression and add an original touch. It is a way to say, "Here is something personal and interesting about me that might help you, the employer." If you decide to write a personal statement, be sure it is a sincere reflection of you and not simply something that sounds good.

And, as with the entire resume, be sure it relates to your job target. Here are a couple of examples:

- "I enjoy being a part of a team where I can make a positive contribution by using my ability to remain calm and work efficiently under stressful conditions."
- "I get great satisfaction working with people from a variety of backgrounds who need assistance in resolving their health care problems."

If you decide to include a personal statement, review your reasons for choosing a career in health care along with what you believe are your best potential contributions to prospective employers. It is also a good idea to have someone else, such as your instructor, review your statement.

Step Eight: Leave out Personal Information

Don't include personal information such as your age, marital status, number of children, and health status. And never include false statements about your education or experience. If these are discovered later, they can be grounds for dismissal from your job.

Although it is important to have a Reference Sheet (list of references) available for potential employers who request it, it is not necessary to write a statement such as "References Available upon Request."

Step Nine: Plan the Layout

Each section of your resume, except the heading at the top and personal statement (optional) at the end, should be labeled: Objective, Education, Work History, and so on. Headings can be flush (aligned) with the left margin, with the content set to the right, as follows:

OBJECTIVE   XXXXXXXXXXXXXXXXXXXX
XXXXXXXXXXXXXXXXXXXX

EDUCATION   XXXXXXXXXXXXXXXXXXXX
XXXXXXXXXXXXXXXXXXXX

Alternatively, you can center your headings and list the information beneath and flush left.

OBJECTIVE
XXXXXXXXXXXXXXXXXXXXXXXXXXXXXX

XXXXXXXXXXXXXXXXXXXXXXXXXXXXXX

EDUCATION
XXXXXXXXXXXXXXXXXXXX

XXXXXXXXXXXXXXXXXXXXXXXX

XXXXXXXXXXXXXXXX

The information you list under the headings can be arranged in a variety of ways. The design should be based primarily on whether you need to use or save space on the page. The second consideration is personal preference. However you choose to lay out your resume, strive for a balanced, attractive look. Note the varied use of capitalization and boldface to draw attention to the job title in the following examples:

WORK HISTORY   Medical Transcriptionist
2001-Present
Hopeful Medical Center
Better Health, NJ

OR

MEDICAL TRANSCRIPTIONIST
2001-Present
Hopeful Medical Center
Better Health, NJ

OR

Medical Transcriptionist
2001-Present
Hopeful Medical Center
Better Health, NJ

Step Ten: Create an Attractive and Professional-Looking Document

Selecting and organizing content takes time and effort, so don't waste your efforts by failing to attend to the details of appearance. A poor appearance can land a resume in the wastebasket without even a review. The following tips will help you achieve a professional look:

- ☐ Leave enough white space so the page doesn't look crowded. Double-space between the sections.
- ☐ It is recommended that you limit your resume to one page. It is better to use two pages, however, than to crowd too much information onto one page. If you do use two pages, write "More" or "Continued" at the bottom of the first page and your name and contact information and "Page 2" or "Page Two" at the top of the second.
- ☐ Capitalize headings.
- ☐ Use bullets to set off listed items.
- ☐ Try using boldface for emphasis.
- ☐ Make sure your spelling and grammar are perfect.
- ☐ Leave at least a 1-inch margin on all sides.
- ☐ Use good-quality paper in white, ivory, or very light tan or gray.

Whether printing from the computer or using a copy machine, make sure the print is dark and clear. If you don't have access to a computer printer or a good copy machine, consider paying to have your resume printed. Although this limits your flexibility in customizing the resume for various employers, it will provide professional-quality copies.

See Box 10-3 for a resume checklist to ensure you have a comprehensive and high-quality resume that represents you well. Your basic resume can serve you throughout your health care career. Think of it as a living document on which you continually record your experiences and new skills.

See Figures 10-4, 10-5, and 10-6 for examples of completed resumes. Yours will look different, of course, but these will give you some ideas.

Go to page 286 to complete Prescription for Success 10-13

DISTRIBUTING YOUR RESUME

Make the best use of your printed resume by distributing it to people who have may have job openings—employers—and people who might know about jobs. Following are some suggestions to get you started:

☐ Employers who place help-wanted ads or post job openings on the Internet or elsewhere
☐ Employers who have unadvertised openings you have heard about from other sources
☐ Your networking contacts
☐ Friends and relatives
☐ Anyone who indicates that he or she knows someone who might be hiring
☐ Your school's career services department

Keep enough copies of your resume on hand to respond to unexpected opportunities. Take copies to interviews (even if you have sent a copy in advance), career fairs, and the human resource departments of health care facilities. Be sure to have plenty on hand if you decide to drop in on employers as described in Chapter 9. A well-prepared resume in many hands is an effective way to get the word out that you are a serious job candidate.

It is usually not recommended, however, that you send resumes to dozens of employers in the hope of locating one that has a job opening. One exception is when there are more job openings than applicants. This can occur when there is a shortage, such as the current nationwide shortage of registered nurses. When there is a shortage, you are more likely to receive responses when sending unsolicited resumes. A second exception is when you are moving to a new area. Sending a large number of resumes, along with a cover letter explaining that you are relocating, may be more economical and productive than calling many potential employers.

NEW DEVELOPMENTS IN RESUMES

The capacities of the computer to sort and organize data, along with the speed and convenience of the Internet, have resulted in new forms of resumes and ways for job searchers and employers to connect.

E-Resumes

You will need to modify your resume if you are sending it to an employer electronically, if it will be scanned, or if you are posting it on an Internet site. This is to ensure that it transmits and scans properly. You will note that some changes require you to do exactly the opposite of the directions given in the previous sections to create an attractive printed resume! But this doesn't mean destroying or not using your original version—it means creating an additional version.

Start by converting your resume to what is called "plain text." If you created your resume using MS Word (on either a PC or a Mac), use the "save as" command and choose the plain text format (the ending will be .txt). This format strips your document of all special formatting—things like bullets, boldface, and italics. The instructions embedded to create these "special effects" do not translate well electronically, and your resume can become scrambled or interspersed with odd-looking characters.

Once you have created a plain-text version, do the following[2]:

1. Proofread it for oddly wrapped lines, scrunched up words, and similar problems that can happen when text is converted.
2. Delete "continued" or "page 2" if these exist.
3. Use caps to emphasize words that otherwise would have been boldfaced or italicized—your name, for example.
4. Replace bullets with standard keyboard symbols such as *, +, --, or ~. (Bullets may have converted to little boxes or other odd characters.)

RUDY MARQUEZ
1909 Franklin Blvd.
Philadelphia, PA 19105
(610) 765-4321   MAmarquez@aol.com

OBJECTIVE   Position as a clinical medical assistant in an urgent care setting

QUALIFICATIONS

- 13 years experience as a certified medical assistant
- Current certifications in CPR and Basic Life Support
- Proven ability to communicate with patients and staff
- Proactive employee who anticipates office and physicians' needs
- Fluent in Spanish and Italian

WORK HISTORY   Medical Assistant   2005-present
Founders Medical Clinic   Philadelphia, PA
- Perform clinical and laboratory duties
- Assist physicians with exams, procedures, and surgeries
- Reorganized patient education program, including selection of updated brochures, videos
- Provide patient education and present healthy living workshops
- Train and supervise new medical assistants

Medical Assistant   1999-2005
North Side Clinic   Pittsburgh, PA
- Performed clinical and laboratory duties
- Developed system for monitoring and ordering clinic supplies that resulted in annual savings of over $25,000
- Received commendation for providing outstanding patient service

Medical Assistant   1997-1999
Dr. Alan Fleming   Erie, PA
- Assisted Dr. Fleming with procedures and minor office surgeries
- Prepared treatment and examining rooms
- Took vital signs and administered injections
- Performed routine laboratory tests
- Handled computerized recordkeeping tasks
- Assisted in researching and purchasing new office computer system

EDUCATION   Associate of Science in Medical Assisting   1997
Emerson College of Health Careers, Erie, PA

Recently Completed Workshops and Continuing Education Courses
- Health Care Beliefs of Minority Populations
- Medical Spanish
- New Requirements for Maintaining Patient Confidentiality

ORGANIZATIONS   American Association of Medical Assistants (AAMA)
Pennsylvania Association of Medical Assistants
Philadelphia Lions Club

Figure 10-4 Example of a chronological resume. This type of resume, which lists a detailed work history, is recommended for applicants who already have experience working in health care.

5. If you need to add spaces, use the space bar, not the tab key.
6. If you use quotation marks anywhere, these only convert if they are straight, not curly (curly quotation marks are also called "smart quotes"). Check your word-processing program to see how to do this.

Just as with the original version of your resume, it is critical that this version be free of errors. Once

sent or posted online, it is there for potentially millions of people to view.

Posting Your Resume on the Internet

There are many types of websites on which you can post your resume. Some are general employment sites, such as Monster. Others are specific to health

HEATHER DIETZ
10532 Cactus Road
Yuma, AZ 85360
(520) 321-7654   thedietz@linkup.com

OBJECTIVE

Entry-level position in health information management in which I can apply up-to-date knowledge and skills. I especially enjoy applying my organizational skills and working on challenging tasks that must be complete and accurate.

EDUCATION

Associate of Science in Health Information Technology   2009
Desert Medical College   Yuma, AZ

COMPUTER SKILLS

- Created electronic spreadsheet to track fund raising for Sage Elementary School PTA
- Taught self to efficiently use leading brand software programs in the following areas: word processing, database, spreadsheets, and accounting
- Set up and managed electronic accounting system for family-owned construction business
- Teach computer classes at Girl Scout summer day camp

ORGANIZATIONAL SKILLS

- Created system to monitor all church collections and fund-raising projects
- Initiated and developed computer career awareness program for Girl Scouts
- Secretary for college HIT student organization
- Completed HIT associate degree program with perfect class attendance while working part-time and managing family life

CLERICAL/ADMINISTRATIVE SKILLS

- 7 years bookkeeping experience
- Keyboarding speed of 78 wpm
- Excellent written communication skills

WORK HISTORY

Unpaid Internship at St. John's Medical Center, Yuma, AZ   2009
Medical Records Department

Bookkeeper   2003-2007
Buildwell Construction Company, Yuma, AZ

Bookkeeper   1998-2003
Perfect-Fit Cabinetry, Yuma, AZ

Secretary   1995-1998
Caldwell Insurance Company, Yuma, AZ

ORGANIZATIONS

Desert Medical College Health Information Technology Student Organization, Secretary
Sage Elementary School PTA, Treasurer
Faith Community Church, Member of Social Service Committee

Figure 10-5 Example of a functional resume. This type of resume, which lists skills that support a health care job, is recommended for applicants who have not worked in health care.

care. And still others are employer websites that allow—or even require—you to apply electronically for specific job openings. Deciding whether to place your resume on the Internet and which type of website to choose depends on your job target and the kind of employer you are seeking. Although many websites allow job searchers to post their resumes for free, they charge employers to place help-wanted ads online and to view the resumes in their databases.

Therefore larger organizations are the ones most likely to pay for this service. A physician's office or small clinic may not be able to justify the expense for its relatively small number of hires. Organizations with many employees, such as Kaiser Permanente or even a single hospital, may have their own websites and online application capabilities.

Spend some time considering whether to post your resume on the Internet. Although posting

EMILY COLLINS
8215 Mile High Drive
Denver, CO 80201
(303) 987-6543

OBJECTIVE Position as an Occupational Therapy Assistant working with clients who have physical disabilities

EDUCATION Associate of Science   Occupational Therapy Assistant   2010
Salud College   Denver, CO
Graduated with Honors
Passed national certification exam
Fieldwork completed at Central Rehabilitation Hospital

Certificate   Nursing Assistant   2005
San Juan Medical Center   Denver, CO

HEALTH CARE WORK EXPERIENCE
Nursing Assistant   2005-2008
GoodCare Nursing Home, Denver, CO
- Encouraged patients to achieve their maximum level of wellness, activity, and independence
- Demonstrated interest in the lives and well-being of patients
- Helped patients to perform prescribed physical exercises
- Organized and participated in activities with patients
- Assisted patients with basic hygiene and dressing

INTERPERSONAL SKILLS
- Provided daily care for parent with Alzheimer's disease for 18 months
- Answered telephone, directed calls, and took messages for busy sporting goods manufacturer
- Received Connor Memorial Award from Salud College for making positive contributions and assisting classmates

TEACHING SKILLS
- Teach swim classes to all ages at YMCA
- Conduct CPR instruction for the American Heart Association
- Organize holiday programs and outings for nursing home residents (volunteer)
- Planned and supervised craft and play activities for school-age children
- Tutored ESL students at Salud College

WORK HISTORY
Preschool Aide   2004-2005
Bright Light Preschool, Denver, CO

Swim Instructor (part-time)   2004-present
YMCA, Denver, CO

Receptionist   2000-2004
Sportrite Manufacturing Co., Denver, CO

ORGANIZATIONS
American Occupational Therapy Association
American Heart Association, Chair of Local Fundraising Committee

Figure 10-6   Example of a combination resume. This type of resume is recommended for applicants who have some experience working in health care but who also want to highlight other skills that support their target job.

on a large website makes your resume available to millions of viewers, you are also competing with millions of other job seekers. Experts suggest that posting your resume on a few carefully chosen sites is worth some of your time but is not as likely to help you find a job as methods such as networking and applying directly to specific employers. (This advice does not apply to employer websites with job postings and instructions for applying and sending your resume electronically.)

Deciding on which public websites to post your resume should receive careful consideration.

In general, experts recommend that you should not pay to have your resume distributed. Many of these "services" simply send out mass e-mails containing the resumes of anyone who pays them. The resumes may or may not match the jobs posted (if indeed, the targeted employers even have job openings), and it is reported that resumes are often sent without contact information, such as your name and telephone numbers, so employers cannot reach you even if they are interested in learning more about you. You must explore websites for yourself, but starting with the recommendations of well-known job-search experts will help you avoid unreliable websites. The following three sites are well-established and appear on all "recommended" lists:

1. Monster.com
2. HotJobs.com
3. CareerBuilder.com

In addition, check sites dedicated to health care or your particular occupation and the website of your professional organization. (See the information on health-specific websites in Chapter 9.)

The following suggestions can help you choose an appropriate website[3]:

☐ Do not use websites that won't allow you to review at least a sample of their job lists before you provide personal information or your resume.

☐ Read the privacy policy! Some websites sell or give your information to other businesses. Important: *Never* put your social security number on your resume.

☐ Check the wording. Do the lists provided include real jobs, or are they examples of what the website claims to be trying to fill?

☐ Check for currency. Are there dates on the jobs listed? Are they recent?

☐ Look for information about who sponsors the site. Do they have credentials and/or experience in the job-search industry?

☐ If you do not get any responses to your resume within 45 days, remove it and find another website on which to post it.

As a courtesy to those who are looking for applicants, remove your resume from all websites on which you have it posted once you become employed. Another consideration is that your new employer may see your resume online and wonder if you are still looking for a better deal.

INTRODUCING YOUR RESUME: COVER LETTERS

A cover letter should be sent along with your resume, whether it goes by conventional ("snail") mail or is sent electronically. The purpose of a cover letter is to provide a brief personal introduction. It should be short, informative, persuasive, and polite. The fact that you write a letter can be persuasive in itself. It shows that you took the time and made the effort to consider why and how you meet this particular employer's qualifications. You did more than simply put a resume in an envelope or send it electronically.

Cover letters can be customized for different circumstances. Before discussing the different types, let's look at a few how-tos common to all cover letters:

1. Use a proper business letter format. Figure 10-7 contains an example.
2. Be sure your spelling and grammar are error-free.
3. Direct your letter to a specific person whenever possible. Look for a name in the employment ad, ask your contact for the name of the appropriate person, or call the facility and ask. If you are writing in response to an unadvertised position, having a name on your correspondence is especially important. Letters without names can get misdirected or discarded. Busy facilities don't have time to determine to whom to direct your inquiry.
4. Write an introduction. State who you are, why you are writing, who referred you or what ad you are responding to, and what position you are applying for. Employers may have more than one position open, so don't assume they will know which job you are applying for.
5. Develop the body of the letter. Explain why the employer should interview you—that is, what you have to offer and how you can help him or her. Summarize your qualifications for the job. Do your best to match them with what you believe the employer is seeking. At the same time, don't simply repeat the same information that is on your resume.
6. Include a closing paragraph. Ask the employer to call you for an interview or state that you will call for an appointment.
7. If you are sending your cover letter electronically (in the body of an e-mail, for example), keep the format simple: don't use bolding, bullets, or other special features and avoid using tabs to indent text.

Letter for an Advertised Position

In Chapter 9, we discussed responding to employment ads in a way that demonstrates how you meet the employer's needs. Use language in your letter that mirrors the words used in the ad or job announcement. Review the examples in Figures 9-4 and 9-5; then take a look at Figure 10-8, which is an example of a complete cover letter.

	Your address 1234 Graduate Lane *and the date* Collegeville, CA 90123 June 6, 2010
Samantha Ernest, Office Manager Good Health Clinic 922 Wellness Avenue Cassidy, CA 91222	*Receiver's name, title, and address*
Dear Ms. Ernest:	*Salutation. Note use of colon.*
Introductory paragraph	*Identify yourself, why you are writing, and the source of your information.*
Body of letter	*Explain how you meet the employer's requirements. Provide examples.*
Closing paragraph	*Request an interview, state that you will call, etc. Offer thanks for employer's time and consideration.*
Sincerely,	*Closing*
Gwen Graduate	*Written Signature*
Gwen Graduate	*Typed name*

Figure 10-7   Format of a business letter. (*Adapted from Hacker D: A writer's reference, ed 5, Boston, 2003, Bedford/ St. Martin's and Yena D: Career directions, ed 3, Chicago, 1997, Irwin/Times Mirror.*)

 Go to page 286 to complete Prescription for Success 10-14

Letter for an Unadvertised Opening

You may learn about unadvertised job openings through your school or from your networking contacts. Mention your source of information in the introduction of your cover letter. (Be sure to obtain permission from the contact person before using his or her name!) Before writing the letter, learn as much as possible about the job. Sources of information include the person who told you about it, the employer's website, or an inquiry call to the facility. See Figure 10-9 for an example of this kind of letter.

Letter of Inquiry

There may be a facility where you would like to work, but you don't know if it has any job openings. Perhaps you have a friend who is happily employed there and has recommended it as a great place to work. Or it may have a reputation for excellent working conditions and educational and promotional opportunities. When you are not responding to a specific job opening, state your general qualifications that meet the current needs in health care. Explain why you are interested in working at the facility. Learn as much as possible about the facility so you can emphasize specific contributions you can make (Figure 10-10).

1234 Graduate Lane
Collegeville, CA 90123
June 6, 2010

Samantha Ernest, Office Manager
Good Health Clinic
922 Wellness Avenue
Cassidy, CA 91222

Dear Ms. Ernest:

I was excited to see your ad in the Cassidy Times on June 5 for a medical assistant. As a recent graduate of Medical Career College, I believe I can make a positive contribution to your health care team. In addition to submitting my resume for your review, I would like to point out how I believe I meet your needs for this position.

Your requirements:	How I Meet Them:
75% clerical duties	I enjoy and am proficient in front office duties. I received top grades in all my administrative classes. I understand the importance of efficiency, accuracy, and confidentiality when performing clerical functions in the medical office. I have very good written and oral communication skills.
25% clinical duties	I have up-to-date skills in all medical assisting back-office procedures.
Computer literate	I have basic computer literacy skills, can work in a Windows environment, and am proficient in Medical Manager, Word, and Excel.

I am an energetic, detail-oriented person with good interpersonal skills. I understand the need to maintain high-quality patient relations in today's health care environment and know I am capable of providing efficient, caring service.

Good Health Clinic has an excellent reputation in Cassidy and it would be a privilege to have the opportunity to discuss my qualifications with you in person. I will call next week to schedule an appointment or you can contact me at (760)123-4567. Thank you for your time and consideration.

Respectfully,

Gwen Graduate

Gwen Graduate

Figure 10-8   Example of a cover letter for an advertised position. Note how the writer responds to the specific qualifications the employer is seeking.

Go to page 286 to complete Prescription for Success 10-15

APPLICATIONS

Applications are commonly requested of job applicants, even if they have submitted a resume. Applications provide the employer with complete, standardized sources of information. Once you have been hired, the application is placed in your personnel file and can serve as a legal document and record of information about you and your previous employment.

Some applications contain important statements you are required to read and sign. For example, employers of home health care workers may protect themselves from **liability** if employees have an accident when they are driving to and from job assignments. Read all statements carefully before

5687 Success Avenue
Schoolville, MI 48755
September 10, 2010

Joseph Featherstone, Laboratory Supervisor
North Valley Medical Laboratory
4657 Flanders Road
Schoolville, MI 48757

Dear Mr. Featherstone:

Kim Lee, the academic director of the Laboratory Technician Program at High Tech Institute, told me that your facility has an opening for a laboratory technician. North Valley has an excell- ent reputation for performing high-quality work and providing learning opportunities for employees. As a recent graduate of High Tech, I am enthusiastic about starting my career in an environment in which I can make a positive contribution and at the same time, continue to acquire new skills.

I am dedicated to performing my work accurately and efficiently. High standards are important to me and I earned top grades in all my classes at High Tech. At the same time, I maintained near- perfect attendance and served as president of the student council.

My resume is enclosed for your review. Because a resume can only partly communicate my qualifications, I would appreciate the opportunity to meet with you personally. I will call you on Friday to arrange a time that is convenient for you. I can be contacted at (906) 123-4567.

Sincerely,

Sandy McDougal
Sandy McDougal

Figure 10-9   Example of a cover letter for an unadvertised position identified through professional networking.

signing. Applications and employment contracts may contain legal language and unfamiliar words. Don't hesitate to ask for an explanation of anything you don't understand.

After the work of constructing a resume, filling out an application may seem easy. But don't take it for granted. Take time to read the instructions, and fill it out as accurately and neatly as possible. This is especially important when applying for health care positions because neatness and accuracy are job requirements. Use this opportunity to demonstrate that you meet these requirements.

Success Tips for Filling out Job Applications

☐ Read the entire application before you begin to fill it in.
☐ Fill out all sections completely. Do not leave blanks or write in "See resume."

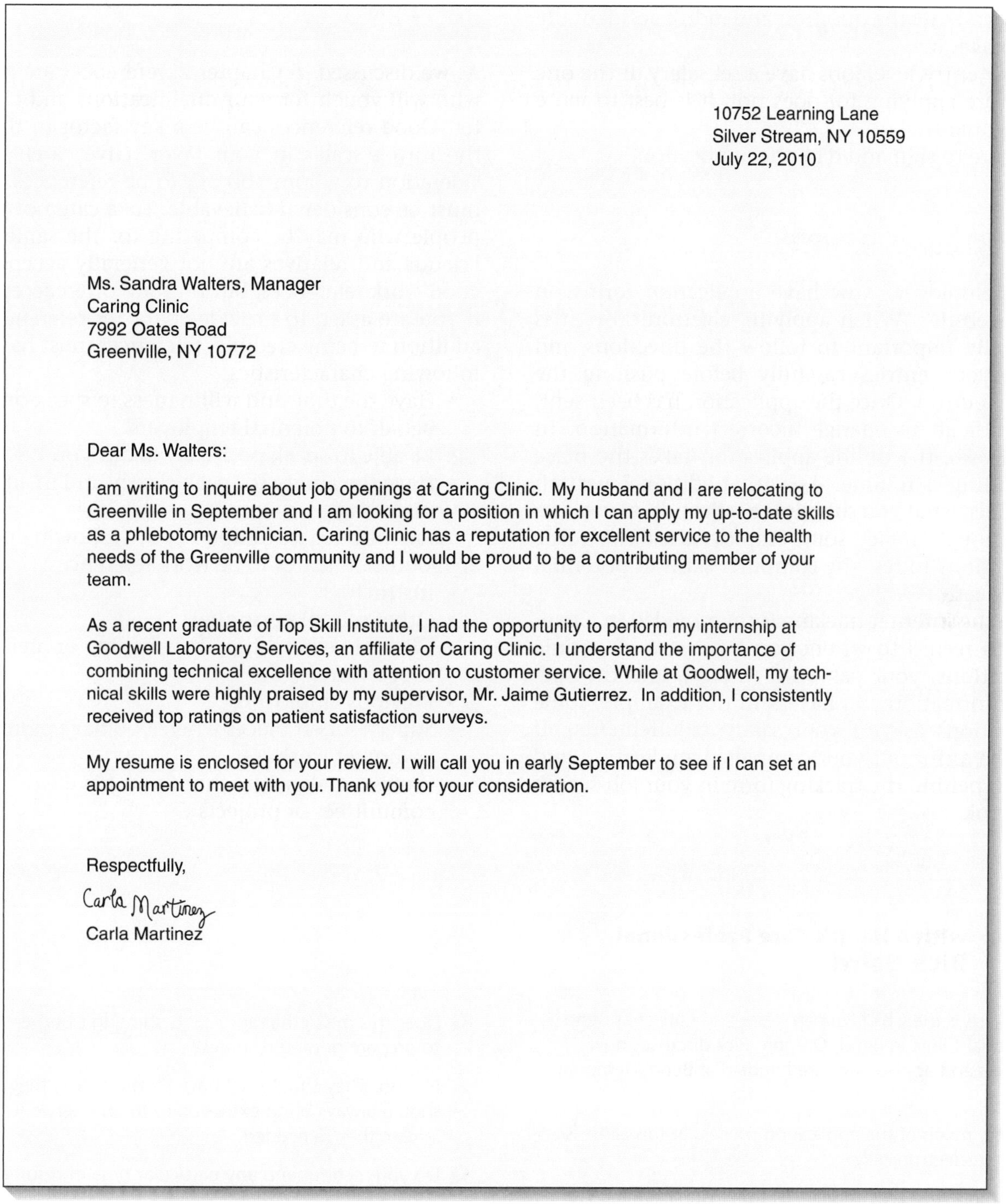

10752 Learning Lane
Silver Stream, NY 10559
July 22, 2010

Ms. Sandra Walters, Manager
Caring Clinic
7992 Oates Road
Greenville, NY 10772

Dear Ms. Walters:

I am writing to inquire about job openings at Caring Clinic. My husband and I are relocating to Greenville in September and I am looking for a position in which I can apply my up-to-date skills as a phlebotomy technician. Caring Clinic has a reputation for excellent service to the health needs of the Greenville community and I would be proud to be a contributing member of your team.

As a recent graduate of Top Skill Institute, I had the opportunity to perform my internship at Goodwell Laboratory Services, an affiliate of Caring Clinic. I understand the importance of combining technical excellence with attention to customer service. While at Goodwell, my technical skills were highly praised by my supervisor, Mr. Jaime Gutierrez. In addition, I consistently received top ratings on patient satisfaction surveys.

My resume is enclosed for your review. I will call you in early September to see if I can set an appointment to meet with you. Thank you for your consideration.

Respectfully,

Carla Martinez
Carla Martinez

Figure 10-10 Example of a cover letter used to inquire about possible job openings.

- [ ] Use black or blue pen, never pencil.
- [ ] Print neatly.
- [ ] Go to interviews prepared to fill out an application. Take complete information with you, including the following:
  - Social security number
  - Education, including dates and locations
  - Work history, including names of employers and dates of employment
  - Military service
  - References
- [ ] Proofread what you have written before submitting it.
- [ ] Be honest when answering questions. Giving false information can be grounds for dismissal if you are hired.
- [ ] For questions that don't apply to you, write "N/A" instead of leaving them blank. This way it is clear

that you saw the question and didn't accidentally skip over it.

☐ Many entry-level jobs have a set salary. If the one you are applying for does not, it is best to write "negotiable."

☐ Be sure to sign and date the application.

Electronic Applications

Many employers now have application forms on their websites. When applying electronically, it is especially important to follow the directions and check your entries carefully before pushing the "send" button. Once the application has been sent, it is difficult to change incorrect information. In some cases, the online application takes the place of sending a resume. As with traditional written materials, what you submit is a reflection of you as a professional. In fact, some employers use electronic applications to test the computer skills of potential employees.

Use the Internet tracking form provided in Chapter 9 to record to whom you have sent electronic applications, your password (if any), and the specific information you have sent (for example, some applications ask for your salary requirements). If possible, print out your completed application and place it behind the tracking form in your job-search notebook.

REFERENCE SHEETS

As we discussed in Chapter 2, references are people who will vouch for your qualifications and character. Good references can be a key factor in tipping the hiring scales in your favor. Give careful consideration to whom you ask to be references. They must be considered believable. Take care not to ask people who may be competing for the same jobs. Friends and relatives are not generally accepted as good work references, but they are often acceptable if you are asked to provide character references. In addition to being credible, references must have the following characteristics:

- Have the time and willingness to speak on your behalf to potential employers
- Be able to speak positively about you
- Have the ability to speak clearly and in an organized way

As mentioned in Chapter 2, the following people are good candidates to be work references:

- Instructors
- Other school personnel
- Clinical, externship, internship, or fieldwork supervisor(s)
- Previous employers
- Supervisors at places where you have performed volunteer work
- Professionals with whom you have worked on committees or projects

 with a Health Care Professional
Rick Baird

Rick Baird is the Chief Human Resources Officer at Bend Memorial Clinic in Bend, Oregon. Rick discusses how resumes and applications are handled at Bend Memorial Clinic.

Q How much of the application process at this clinic is done electronically?

A Actually, we accept only electronic applications. We also prefer that resumes be submitted electronically, either typed into the electronic application or sent as an attachment. There are a couple of reasons for this. One is that people who work here must have computer skills, so the application process requires that they demonstrate these skills. The second reason is so we can maintain an electronic database of applicants. If someone submits an application and resume today, we may not have a job that matches their skills. But an opening may come in a month. Then we can electronically review the resumes that we've scanned into our database and quickly identify potential candidates.

Q Does this mean that applicants shouldn't bother to prepare printed resumes?

A No, no. They should still have them. In fact, they should always bring extra copies to an interview, in case they're needed.

Q Do you recommend any particular type of resume?

A No, the standard resumes—chronological and functional—are still acceptable. One thing a resume should demonstrate is the applicant's computer skills. Its appearance is important, too—proper alignment, consistent fonts, that kind of thing. Resumes should also show that candidates have thought about where they want to go in their careers.

Q How do applicants access an application?

A They can go to our website. We list all current job openings on the site along with our general application. For applicants who don't have computers, we have one they can use in the human resources office.

Contact each person you want to serve as a reference. Do this before you begin your job search. Never give out a name and then ask the person for permission afterward. This can put the person on the spot and makes it difficult if he or she prefers not to be a reference. Inform your references about the types of jobs you are applying for and what qualifications are important. This will enable them to be prepared to answer the potential employer's questions.

Create a written list of at least three references. At a minimum, include their names, titles, telephone numbers, and e-mail addresses. You may also want to include their addresses. Ask them if they can be contacted at work. If not, provide recommended times to call. It is essential that the telephone numbers be current and accurate. If you list a work number and the person is no longer employed there, your credibility may be questioned. Potential employers don't have time to call you back or make numerous calls trying to locate your references. Make it easy for them. This makes it easier for them to hire you.

Organize your reference list in an easy-to-read format, and print it on the same kind of paper as your resume. Write "References for (your name)" at the top of the page. The reference sheet should not be mailed with your resume unless it is specifically requested. Take copies with you to interviews to give to potential employers who ask for it. If you are visiting a human resource department, take a copy with you, because many employment applications have a section for listing references.

Be sure to let your references know when you are hired. Thank them for their willingness to assist you. Keep them posted about your career progress. In the future, you may be in a position to help them, and that is what true networking is all about—mutual career support.

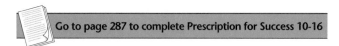
Go to page 287 to complete Prescription for Success 10-16

LETTERS OF RECOMMENDATION

Another type of reference is provided through letters of recommendation. These letters are usually written by supervisors or people in authority, such as instructors, who write statements about your work record, skills, and personal qualities. It is a good idea to request reference letters from employers throughout your career because they can serve as a record of endorsements and achievements over the years. As you leave each job (on good terms, it is hoped!), ask for a letter of recommendation from your supervisor.

Make copies of your letters of recommendation to place in your portfolio and/or to give to potential employers who request them. It is appropriate at interviews to mention that you have them available.

As with other references, be considerate. Ask only those people who you believe can write a positive letter. Also, try to give people enough time to compose a letter. Avoid giving a day's notice. Finally, let your references know what kind of job you are seeking so they can phrase their letters appropriately.

THE PORTFOLIO: SUPPORTING WHAT YOU SAY

Look over the items you have been collecting to put in your portfolio. (Review the suggestions given in Chapter 2.) Choose the ones that represent your best work and support the qualifications needed for your target jobs. Think about others you can include. For example, you might add a list of the courses you have taken if your educational program included classes not commonly offered in your program of study.

Organize your materials in a logical order, grouping related items together in sections. Place them in a binder or presentation folder using plastic protection sheets. It is not necessary to go to a lot of expense, but the folder should be well made and in a plain, conservative color. Prepare a title page labeled "Professional Portfolio" and include your name, address, and telephone number. If you have a large number of items, number the pages and prepare a table of contents.

You need to make only one portfolio if it is rather large; if it consists of only a few pages, make a few copies in case a potential employer asks you to leave it after the interview. Portfolios are not generally sent with your resume but are taken to interviews. You may mention to the interviewer that you have a portfolio. Don't simply hand it to the employer and expect him or her to read it (unless you are asked for it, of course). It is to be used during the interview to demonstrate your capabilities. For example, if you are asked about your knowledge of coding, you could show assignments in which you accurately coded a variety of diagnoses and procedures. Chapter 11 contains a section on using your portfolio at interviews.

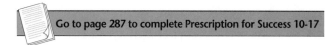
Go to page 287 to complete Prescription for Success 10-17

⇨ SUMMARY OF KEY IDEAS

1. Preparing high-quality written materials is a key part of the successful job search.
2. Your resume is a major method for advertising your qualifications.

3. The main purpose of a resume is to secure an interview.
4. Good cover letters can increase the effectiveness of your resume.
5. Written materials for health care jobs should reflect the job requirements of accuracy, neatness, and orderliness.
6. Good references are vital links to future employment.
7. A portfolio is a tool to support your qualifications.

Positive Self-Talk For This Chapter

1. My resume is a good representation of my skills and qualifications.
2. I write effective cover letters.
3. I fill out applications accurately and neatly.
4. My portfolio supports my claims and qualifications.

To Learn More

Career Builder

http://msn.careerbuilder.com

Click on the Career Builder's Resume Center for advice and examples of resumes.

Enelow W, Kursmark L: *Expert resumes for health care careers,* Indianapolis, 2004, JISTWorks.

Dozens of examples of resumes for health care positions.

Marino K: *Resumes for the health care professional,* ed 2, New York, 2000, John Wiley and Sons.

Dozens of examples of resumes for health care positions.

U.S. Department of Labor: Occupational Outlook Handbook

www.bls.gov/OCO

This is a source of detailed information about hundreds of careers, including typical job descriptions, educational requirements, and average salaries. It is updated every 2 years.

Online Writing Lab—Purdue University

http://owl.english.purdue.edu/owl

A very comprehensive source of help for all types of writing, including resumes and cover letters.

Quintessential Careers: "Researching Key Words in Employment Ads"

http://www.quintcareers.com/researching_resume_keywords.html

Riley Guide

www.rileyguide.com

The *Guide* has links to dozens of online resume-writing resources. All have been reviewed and evaluated for content and quality.

REFERENCES

1. Ellis D, Lankowitz S, Stupka E, Toft D: *Career planning,* ed 2, New York, 1997, Houghton Mifflin.
2. Ireland S: *How to format your resume for email:* http://susanireland.com/eresumeguide/email/index.html.
3. Dickel MR, Roehm F: *Guide to Internet job searching 2008-2009,* Columbus, Ohio, 2008, McGraw-Hill.

INTERNET ACTIVITIES

For active links to the websites needed to complete these activities, visit **http://evolve.elsevier/Haroun/career/.**

1. Locate two employment websites on which resumes can be posted. List the name and address of each website. Explain what you must do to post a resume (register, etc.).
2. Find three health care–employer websites that include electronic applications for job applicants. List the names of the employers and the website addresses.
3. Use key words such as "professional portfolio" and "employment portfolio" to find information about employment portfolios. Report on any suggestions you find useful for creating an effective portfolio or using a portfolio at interviews.
4. The Job Hunt website contains articles about protecting your privacy when posting your resume on the Internet. Read one of the articles and write a list of dos and don'ts for people who want to post their resumes.

Prescription for Success 10-1
First Impressions

1. Imagine yourself behind the employer's desk. You have placed an ad for a medical receptionist. You receive a large number of resumes, and among them you find the following:
   - Misspelled words

   - Pages lightly printed so that they are difficult to read

   - Lack of information about related training or experience

   - No telephone number for the applicant

   - No mention of what type of work the applicant wants

   - Paragraphs misaligned

2. Answer the following questions:
   What is your impression of these applicants?

   _____

   _____

   _____

   _____

   What does each of these errors say about the person who submitted the resume?

   _____

   _____

   _____

   _____

   Would you call any of them for an interview? Which one(s)? Why or why not?

   _____

   _____

   _____

   _____

   Are the errors in the resumes more significant because this is a job in health care? Explain why or why not.

   _____

   _____

   _____

Prescription for Success 10-2
Writing a Targeted Objective

1. Find an advertised position in your occupational area.
2. Underline the portions of the ad or posting that describe what the employer is looking for.
3. Write a targeted objective that responds specifically to the stated needs of the employer.

_____

_____

_____

Prescription for Success 10-3
Write Your Objective

Use the Resume Building Block #1 form to write a general objective to use on your resume.

Prescription for Success 10-4
Write Your Education Section

Use the Resume Building Block #2 form to complete the Education section of your resume. List all the schools you have attended, starting with the most recent one.

Prescription for Success 10-5
Write Your Professional Skills Section

If this section applies to you, complete the Resume Building Block #3 form.

Prescription for Success 10-6
Write Your Work History Section

Use the Resume Building Block #4 form to complete the Work History section of your resume, starting with the most recent job held.

Prescription for Success 10-7
Write Your Licenses and Certifications Section

If this section applies to you, complete the Resume Building Block #5 form.

Prescription for Success 10-8
Write Your Honors and Awards Section

If this section applies to you, complete the Resume Building Block #6 form.

Prescription for Success 10-9
Write Your Special Skills Section

If this section applies to you, complete the Resume Building Block #7 form.

Prescription for Success 10-10
Write Your Community Service and Volunteer Work Section

If this section applies to you, complete the Resume Building Block #8 form.

Prescription for Success 10-11
Write Your Organizations Section

If this section applies to you, complete the Resume Building Block #9 form.

Prescription for Success 10-12
Write Your Language Section

If this section applies to you, complete the Resume Building Block #10 form.

Prescription for Success 10-13
Write Your Resume!

Using the information from the Resume Building Block forms and what you have learned in this chapter, put together your resume. Have your instructor, someone in your career services department, or someone with good proofreading skills look it over for you. (A good hint for proofreading you can try is to read your resume backwards. That way, you don't anticipate the words and "correct" mistakes with your eyes.)

Prescription for Success 10-14
Respond to Some Advertised Positions

1. Find three ads or postings for health care jobs.
2. Write complete cover letters, in sendable form (containing all features mentioned in this chapter and having no errors), that respond to the requirements stated in each ad. (Attach the ads to your letters.)

_____

_____

_____

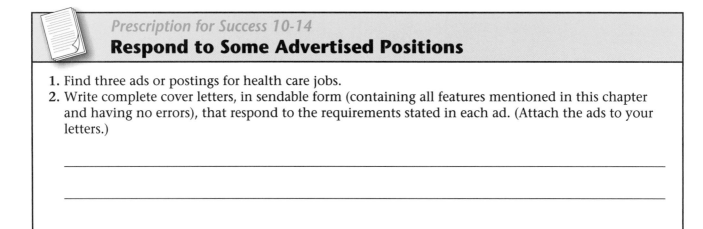

Prescription for Success 10-15
Inquire about the Possibilities

1. Select a facility where you might like to work.
2. Learn as much about it as possible. Sources of information include networking contacts, the Internet, acquaintances who work there, school personnel, and published information such as brochures and newspaper articles.
3. Write a complete inquiry cover letter in mailable form.

_____

_____

_____

Prescription for Success 10-16
Preparing Your Reference Sheet

Contact possible references, gather the data you need about each, and put together your reference sheet.

Prescription for Success 10-17
Preparing Your Portfolio

Using the items you have gathered and the information in this chapter, put together a portfolio that demonstrates your qualifications for the kind of job you want.

CHAPTER 11

The Interview

OBJECTIVES

The information and activities in this chapter can help you:

- Explain why the interview should be considered a "sales opportunity."
- Identify the needs of potential employers.
- Prepare to answer interview questions in ways that demonstrate what you can offer an employer.
- Demonstrate appearance and behavior that create a positive first impression.
- Communicate courteously and effectively.
- Use your portfolio to support your qualifications.
- Deal appropriately with difficult situations, including illegal questions.
- Distinguish between appropriate and inappropriate questions to ask at interviews.
- Make a gracious exit when the interview is over.

KEY TERMS AND CONCEPTS

Behavioral Interviews: Job applicants are asked to describe how they handled specific situations in the past.

Discriminate: Using unfounded bias as a reason for not hiring someone.

Illegal Questions: Requests for information that cannot be used to make a hiring decision about a candidate.

Interview: A meeting, usually in person, in which a job applicant and an employer or representative exchange information.

Mirroring: A communication technique in which you match your communication style to that of the other person for the purpose of increasing mutual understanding.

THE INTERVIEW—YOUR SALES OPPORTUNITY

"You don't have to be perfect. Just be the best for the job."

—Rick Baird

Finally! The words you have been hoping to hear: "When can you come in for an **interview**?" Your job-search efforts are paying off. But wait a minute! You begin to worry: "What if I can't think of anything to say?" "What if I don't have the skills they are looking for?" "What if they ask me about…?"

The purpose of this chapter is to help you put the "what ifs" to rest and see the interviewing process as an opportunity to present yourself at your best. In Chapter 3 we discussed the power of attitude and how, with practice, you can choose your reaction to any situation. Many applicants view interviews as opportunities to be rejected. But you have another choice. You can view an interview as an opportunity to determine an employer's needs and to show how you can meet them.

Think about it. Employers are busy people who don't have time to conduct interviews with people who are unlikely job candidates. You obviously meet the minimum qualifications. The interviewer wants to see whether you are a person who can back up your qualifications, communicate well, and contribute to the organization.

By learning what will be expected of you at an interview and practicing your presentation skills, you can attend each interview with confidence. A common reason for not being hired is lack of preparation for the interview. And this is a factor over which you, not the interviewer, has control.

The Customer's Needs

Good sales presentations are based on showing customers—employers—how they can benefit by buying a product—in this case, by hiring you. Recall from Chapter 1 that identifying the customer's needs is an important step for students who are beginning a program of career preparation. As we pointed out, it doesn't make sense to create a product that no one needs.

In the same way, if you attend an interview without knowing anything about what the employer is looking for, you put yourself at a disadvantage. This is because in order to be at your best during the interview, the following preparations must be completed in advance:
- Identify possible needs of the employer.
- Think of ways you might meet those needs as an employee.

- Anticipate what types of questions might be asked.
- Practice answering them.
- Create examples to demonstrate your qualifications.
- Prepare appropriate questions to ask.

All employers have general qualities they look for in applicants such as the ones identified in the SCANS report. And health care employers have expressed their needs through the National Healthcare Foundation Standards discussed in Chapter 1. In addition, individual employers have more specific requirements based on factors such as patient population, services offered, size of facility, budgets, and so on. It is important for you to learn as much as possible before attending the interview. Here is a checklist of possible sources of information:

☐ Direct contact by phone or in person: ask questions, request a job description, observe the facility
☐ Brochures produced by the organization
☐ People who work there, such as friends, classmates, or networking contacts
☐ The local newspaper: large facilities are sometimes the subject of news articles
☐ The employer's website
☐ Your school's career services department
☐ The Chamber of Commerce and other organizations that have information about large employers
☐ The local chapter of your professional organization
☐ Information gathered at career fairs and employer orientation meetings
☐ Employment ad if the position was advertised

If the facility is small, such as a one-physician office, you should know, at a minimum, the type of specialty practiced and the patient population served. When you are unable to learn very much before the interview, it is especially important that you listen carefully to the employer and ask good questions. How to do this is discussed later in this chapter.

 Go to page 306 to complete Prescription for Success 11-1

The Interviewer Is Human, Too

"Research into interviewing shows that the person conducting the interview is often more stressed than the candidate."

—Allan-James Associates

In addition to knowing the employment needs of the employer, consider the personal situation of the interviewer. Many applicants view the interviewer as a person of great confidence who has all the power in the hiring process. Applicants mistakenly see themselves as the underdogs in a game they have little chance of winning. In reality, interviewers may be experiencing a number of pressures:

- Concern about finding the right candidate who can perform the job as needed
- An extremely busy schedule
- Lack of interviewing skills
- A demanding supervisor who will hold them responsible for the performance of the person who is hired
- Concern about finding the time and resources to orient and train a new employee

Understanding the interviewer's point of view requires empathy—attempting to see the world through the eyes of others (see Chapter 8). This may not seem easy in a job interview when you are nervous and concentrating on presenting yourself well. But it is this very shift of focus—from yourself to the interviewer—that leads to a more successful interviewing experience. It is through this attempt to understand and then show how you can help solve the employer's problems that you best present yourself as the candidate for the job.

HEADS UP! KNOWING WHAT TO EXPECT

Some interviews are highly structured, meaning that each candidate is asked the same set of prepared questions. Others are more like a conversation, with topics and questions generated freely. Most interviews fall somewhere between these patterns, with interviewers preparing at least a few questions in advance. The style of the interview and types of questions most likely depends on the size of the organization. Large health care systems, hospitals, and clinics usually have dedicated personnel to conduct initial interviews. As human resource professionals, they have the time and expertise to study the latest hiring practices and develop their interviewing skills. They are most likely to conduct **behavioral interviews**, described later in this chapter. A physician who has a single practice is more likely to focus on what skills you have acquired through your education and experience—specific skills he needs, for example, in a clinical medical assistant or receptionist.

In any case, always base your answers on the needs of the health care industry in general and the specific needs of the employer. Your purpose is to demonstrate how *you* can contribute to *their* success.

Traditional Interview Questions

There are many "golden oldie" questions that interviewers have been using for years. Here are a few examples:

1. How would you describe yourself?
2. What are your long-range career objectives?
3. Why did you choose this career?
4. What makes you qualified for this position?
5. How well do you work with people?
6. What motivates you to go the extra mile on a job?
7. How do you define success?
8. Why should I hire you?

You can see that these questions are very open-ended. You can answer them in many ways, which actually can present a problem if your answers are too vague or not related to the job under consideration. In each case, what employers want to know is how your answer applies to *them*. For example, in explaining why you chose a career in health care, focus on what it is about you that relates to the job you are applying for. Be specific. Saying, "I've always been a people person" doesn't give much information. Saying, "I've been interested in health care since I was 11, when I spent time playing chess with my grandfather after he had his stroke. I noticed how he really perked up when he played, and I became fascinated by how the brain works better when stimulated with an enjoyable activity. This led me to explore a career in occupational therapy" is more specific and gives the interviewer more insight into who you are and what this means in terms of health care employment. When answering, "Why should I hire you?" mention specific skills and personal and professional qualities that will make a positive contribution to the physician's practice, the department's success, patient satisfaction, and so on.

Prepare for traditional interview questions by reviewing your inventories of skills and qualities, along with specific supporting examples, and then thinking about how you can incorporate them into your answers.

 Go to page 306 to complete Prescription for Success 11-2

Behavioral Interview Questions

Behavioral interviews have been part of the hiring process in many large organizations since the 1970s and are being increasingly used in the health care industry. In this type of interview, applicants are asked questions about their past performance—how they handled specific situations. Behavioral interviews are based on the premise that past performance is a good indicator of future performance.

Interviewers prepare in advance by listing the key qualifications for the jobs they post. Then they develop questions to help determine whether applicants possess the desired characteristics. Here is an example: suppose that getting along with others is very important. A question might be, "Describe a time when you had to work with someone with whom you found it difficult to get along." As you tell your story, the interviewer follows up with additional questions, such as "In what ways was this person difficult?" "What was it you needed to do together?" "What did you say to this person?" "Did you get the job done in spite of the difficulties?" "How did you feel about this situation?" "What did you learn from this?" There may be additional probing questions from the interviewer to get more detail as you tell your story and verify that this is an experience you really had. In the case of the difficult person, these might be, "How did these difficulties affect others, such as co-workers and customers?" "Did your supervisor become involved?" Table 11-1

contains examples of behavioral interview questions.

It has been shown that this kind of questioning about real events is more difficult for applicants to answer because they must be supported by facts. For this reason, behavioral interviewing has been found to be 55% predictive of future behavior on the job as compared with traditional interviewing, which is 10% predictive.[1]

Preparing to answer behavioral questions generally takes more preparation than for traditional questions. However, if you have been collecting examples of your skills and qualifications, as was first suggested in Chapter 2, you are already getting ready. The key is to anticipate the kinds of qualifications an employer wants and then search your inventory—and memory—for experiences you've had that illustrate that qualification. Examples can come from any area of your life. You may never have worked in health care. In fact, you may have limited work experience of any kind. But perhaps you have raised children. That experience may help you answer questions about making an unpopular

TABLE 11-1	Behavioral Interview Questions
Qualifications	**Sample Questions**
Interpersonal skills	Tell me about a time when someone disagreed with you about a major decision. What did you say or do? How was the decision ultimately made? Describe a situation in which you were able to use persuasion to successfully convince someone to consider your ideas.
Flexibility	Describe a situation in which you were required to conform to a work policy you really didn't agree with. What was the policy? Why didn't you agree? How did you feel about the situation? Give me an example of a job in which your working conditions frequently changed. How did you adapt to these changes? Tell me about a time when you had to reorganize your schedule in order to help a co-worker meet a deadline. How did you help? What was the result?
Communication	Give me a specific example that shows how you typically deal with conflict. Describe a time when you had to communicate something difficult to your supervisor. What was the situation? How did you plan your communication? What did you say? What was the result? Describe a situation in which you felt you didn't communicate well. How did you follow up? What did you learn?
Customer service skills	Tell me about a time when you had to deal with a very upset customer or patient. How did you handle the situation? What was the result? Give me a few examples of what you have said to customers or patients who have approached you for help. How did you decide the appropriate way to work with each one? Describe something you did to help an employer improve customer service.
Stress management	Describe a stressful situation in which you applied your coping skills. What specifically caused the stress? How were you feeling at the time? What techniques did you use? How was the situation resolved?
Problem solving	Describe a time when you anticipated a potential problem and developed preventive measures. How did you identify the problem? What were the signs? How did you determine ways to prevent it? How did others feel about your actions? What was the final result? Describe a time when you were asked or assigned to do a task you didn't feel qualified to handle. What did you do?
Integrity	Describe an incident in which you made a serious mistake. How did you handle this with your supervisor and/or co-workers? Tell me about a time when you had to make an unpopular decision. What were the circumstances? Why were others unhappy with the decision? Why did you believe you were making the right decision?

decision. These were likely based on good judgment, your values, even ethics and morality. Employers want to know you can make decisions that are guided by what is right rather than by what is popular. In addition to family life, there are other experiences you can draw from, such as the following:

- Clinical experience
- Previous work experience
- School: classes, labs, extra activities
- Community and service work

In a behavioral interview, it is essential to *listen carefully*. Not only must you understand the question, you need to understand *what it is the interviewer wants to know*—that is, what qualification is obviously important for this job, and how you can demonstrate that you have that qualification. Don't hesitate to ask for clarification if you don't understand the question.

It is totally acceptable to take a few moments to think about an answer. You undoubtedly have many experiences to draw from. However, if the question asks for an example you simply don't have—for example, "Tell me about a time when you had to fire a friend," and this has never happened to you—say so rather than trying to make up a story.

Many job-search experts recommend using the **STAR** approach when answering a behavioral question. It helps you organize your response and goes like this:

1. **S and T**: Choose and describe a **S**ituation or **T**ask that enables you to best demonstrate you have the qualification.
2. **A**: Explain the **A**ctions you took in dealing with the situation. Give enough detail to show your skills, but take care not to ramble or give unnecessary information.
3. **R**: Describe the **R**esults. Explain what happened, what you learned, and how the results made a difference. Give numbers and percentages when possible.

Being prepared in advance is especially important for behavioral interviews. Try to anticipate the qualifications the interviewer might be interested in. Some will probably be general, such as those listed in the SCANS skills. Others may be specific to the hiring facility or the job. It's a good idea to write your examples out in the form of stories so you'll have the details in mind if you need them. Some questions may ask you to describe failures and how you've handled them, so you might think of some examples. Reflect on what you learned from experiences that didn't turn out as you hoped they would.

Although it is advisable to have examples in mind and practice telling your "stories," take care not to try to memorize what to say. You need to think about what you are saying during the interview and not give a canned response that may not exactly apply.

 Go to page 307 to complete Prescription for Success 11-3

Situational Questions

Situational questions present situations and problems you might encounter on the job. You are asked to explain how you would respond and/or handle the problem. (See Box 11-1 for examples.) As with behavioral questions, you need to do some advance planning to be prepared to answer them:

- Learn as much as possible about the organization and the specific job. If possible, read the mission statement and goals of the organization.
- Recall your own values and mission statement. These may provide guidelines in answering questions that don't have easy answers but can be based on your sense of right and wrong.
- Review your personal inventory of skills and qualifications.

 Go to page 308 to complete Prescription for Success 11-4

Occupation-Specific Questions

Questions in this category explore your specific knowledge, skill mastery, willingness to learn new procedures, and the general content of your training.

BOX 11-1   Examples of Situational Questions

What would you do?
- You see a co-worker who does not have the authority to administer medications taking some from a locked cabinet.
- You disagree with your supervisor about how to handle a problem.
- You hear a co-worker discussing confidential patient information with her friend, who is not involved in the patient's care.
- You aren't sure how to prioritize your work, and no one is available to discuss it with you.
- You are working with an angry patient who insists on seeing the physician—who is not available—immediately.
- You have a problem to solve. What steps would you take?
- You offer ideas at staff meetings, but no one seems to take them seriously.

The type of question will vary, as in the following examples:
- ☐ Describe how to perform a specific procedure.
- ☐ Explain how to operate certain equipment.
- ☐ Describe appropriate action to take in a given situation that directly relates to this job.
- ☐ Suggest how to solve a health care problem.
- ☐ Explain how you plan to keep your skills updated.
- ☐ What do you know about…? (a theory, new procedure, etc.)
- ☐ Why do you want to work in pediatrics (dermatology, children's dentistry, etc.)?

Some employers give practical skill tests or ask you to physically demonstrate your knowledge. Examples of these tests include a keyboarding speed test, filing or record-keeping exercise, spelling test, calculation of drug dosages, or demonstration of a procedure. If you are asked to perform a practical test that is appropriate for your level of training, do so willingly. Use the request to show that you have confidence in your abilities and can handle stress. If the task is something you have not been trained to do but is required for the job, tell the interviewer you would welcome the opportunity to learn.

Go to page 309 to complete Prescription for Success 11-5

Work Preference Questions

You may be asked about your job preferences. Review your answers to Prescription for Success 9-2, "What Do I Want?" In addition, be prepared to answer questions such as the following:
- ☐ Do you want full-time or part-time work?
- ☐ What hours you are willing to work?
- ☐ What length of shift you prefer?
- ☐ What days and time of day you can work?

Remember to be realistic when applying for jobs. Don't waste employers' time—or your own—interviewing for jobs with conditions you already know are absolutely impossible for you to meet.

Go to page 310 to complete Prescription for Success 11-6

Personality Tests

In today's employment world, you may be asked to take a personality test as part of the interviewing process. Personality assessment tests are increasingly being used, especially in larger organizations. As many as 30% of all companies now use personality tests.[2] These tests consist of answering a series of questions on paper or on the computer and measure such qualities as persistence and whether a person is an extrovert or introvert (highly social or more private). Studies claim that better matches are found when applicants take these tests. This is because certain jobs require specific characteristics, and these are more reliably determined by tests than by interviews. Another claim is that individuals hired tend to be happier with their jobs because of this matching process.

The best advice for taking a personality test is to answer the questions honestly. The tests contain a variety of questions to assess each trait. If you answer as you think you should or if you randomly select answers, this can show up negatively. If you do not "pass" such a test, it is very possible you would not have enjoyed either the work or the setting. This has been one of the reported benefits of personality assessments: less turnover among employees who, with traditional hiring methods, end up deciding the job just isn't for them

Computerized Job Interviews

Yes, believe it or not, some employers are conducting interviews with the help of a computer. The advantage for the employer, in addition to saving time, is that every applicant is asked a prepared set of questions, often as many as 100. Most interview programs consist of answers to be checked. This enables the comparison of "apples with apples" when deciding who to interview in person. The advantage for you, the applicant, is you have more time to think about your answers and can, through the type of questions asked, learn a little about the organization before coming face-to-face with a human interviewer.

Answer the questions carefully and honestly. Computers are able to notice inconsistencies in your answers. Studies have shown that people are more likely to "tell" a computer information they would never reveal to another person.[3] If you are ever faced with a computerized interview, take care not to give unnecessary information that may harm your chance of getting hired. Also, be aware that most computer-assisted interviews must be completed in a certain length of time, so be sure you know how much time you have and keep track of it as you move through the questions.

Other uses of the computer in the hiring process include scenarios in which applicants explain what they would do in a given situation, skill tests, integrity tests, and personality tests. Some organizations administer computerized interviews and tests on their own computers at their facility; others make them available on the Internet and give applicants a password to gain access to testing websites.

PRACTICE: YOUR KEY TO SUCCESS

"Successful interviews usually depend on good preparation."

—*John D. Drake*

Of course you cannot anticipate the exact questions that interviewers will ask. What you can do is prepare yourself to answer a variety of questions. There are some things you can practice to improve your interviewing skills:

☐ Listening carefully
☐ Asking for clarification when necessary
☐ Thinking through your "inventory" of capabilities and characteristics that apply when answering questions
☐ Thinking of examples to back up your answers
☐ Projecting self-confidence

Preparation means practice—actually answering questions, aloud, under conditions as close to those of an actual interview as possible. The best way to practice is to role-play with someone who acts as the interviewer. This can be an instructor, classmate, mentor, networking contact, friend, or family member. Many schools require mock (pretend) interviews as part of professional development classes. Take advantage of these opportunities, and do your best to conduct yourself as if you were at a real interview. Videotaping or having an observer take notes can be helpful, even if it's a little nerve-wracking. It's better to make a few mistakes now so you can avoid them at interviews.

If you believe that you might be asked to demonstrate skills or react to a scenario, include them in your practice sessions. The career services personnel at your school may be familiar with the interviewing practices of facilities in your area and can give you additional information about what to expect and how to best prepare.

The goal of interview rehearsals is not to memorize answers you can repeat. It is to develop a level of comfort about the interviewing process and have facts fresh in your mind so you can call on them as needed and respond to questions intelligently and confidently.

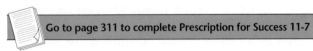
Go to page 311 to complete Prescription for Success 11-7

BE PREPARED: WHAT TO TAKE ALONG

Having everything you might need at the interview will help you feel organized and confident. It also demonstrates to employers that you are organized and think ahead, valuable qualities for health care professionals. Although your own list will be different, here are some suggestions for what to take along:

☐ Extra copies of your resume
☐ Your portfolio
☐ Copies of licenses, certifications, and other documentation
☐ Proof of immunizations and results of health tests
☐ Reference sheet
☐ Any documentation of skills and experience not included in your portfolio (or if you have chosen not to create a portfolio)
☐ Pens
☐ Small notepad
☐ Your list of questions (discussed later in this chapter)
☐ All information needed to fill out an application (see Chapter 10)
☐ Appointment calendar, planner, or electronic organizer
☐ Anything you have been requested to bring
☐ For your eyes only: extra pantyhose, breath mints, other "emergency supplies"

A small case or large handbag is a convenient way to carry your papers and supplies. It can be inexpensive, but it should be a conservative color, in good repair, and neatly organized so you can quickly find what you need.

FIRST IMPRESSIONS: MAKE THEM COUNT!

"The way in which we think of ourselves has everything to do with how our world sees us."

—*Arlene Raven*

Just 30 seconds! That's how long you have to make a lasting impression. The average person forms a strong opinion of another in less than 1 minute. This is why so much emphasis is placed on professional appearance both during the job search and later, on the job. Although it is possible to eventually reverse a negative first impression, it's a lot easier to make a good one in the first place. Employers are basing their opinions on this first meeting. They will be thinking, "If this is the best this person can do, what might I expect from them on the job?"

In Chapter 2 we discussed the messages that dress and grooming communicate. When you are applying for a job in health care, appropriate appearance can let the interviewer know that you:

• Understand the impact of your appearance on others (patients, other professionals)
• Know what is appropriate for the job
• Apply the principles of good hygiene
• Respect both yourself and the interviewer
• Take the interview seriously

There is no universal agreement about the proper clothing to wear when applying for health care jobs. Some schools encourage their students to wear a clean, pressed uniform. Other schools advise them to wear neat, everyday clothing that is not too casual. It is important to pay attention to the professional advice of the staff at your school. The best choices for clothing are generally conservative colors and simple styles. Figure 11-1 shows examples of professional appearance for interviews.

There are a few don'ts that apply wherever you live. Never wear jeans or clothing that is revealing or intended for sports and outdoor activities. Don't wear a hat or sunglasses during the interview. If you're not sure about what to wear, ask your instructor or someone in your school's career services department for help. If extra money for interview clothes is a problem, ask if your school has a clothes-lending program. Many cities have excellent thrift shops that sell nice clothes at reasonable prices. Some even specialize in helping people dress for job interviews.

You may arrive at an interview and discover that most people at the facility are dressed very casually. Don't worry. It is far better to be overdressed in this situation than underdressed. You can adjust your style later, after you get the job.

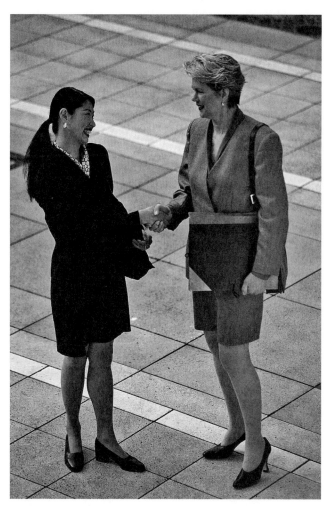

Figure 11-1 Your appearance makes an impression—make it a good one!

There are some additional guidelines that apply to all health care job applicants:

☐ **Be squeaky clean.** Take a bath or shower, wash your hair, scrub your fingernails, and use a deodorant or antiperspirant.

☐ **Save the fashion trends for later.** Hair and nails should be natural colors, tattoos covered up, and visible rings and studs from piercings removed. Limit earrings to one set. Women should apply makeup lightly for a natural, not painted, look.

☐ **Show that you know what is acceptable for the health care professional.** Avoid long fingernails, free-flowing hair, and dangling accessories that can be grabbed by patients or caught in machinery. Wear closed-toe shoes. Strive to be odor-free. For example, don't smoke on the way to the interview. Even the fragrances in perfumes and other personal products, intended to be pleasant, should not be worn because many patients find them disagreeable or have allergic reactions.

☐ Men who wear facial hair should groom it neatly.

 Go to page 311 to complete Prescription for Success 11-8

Your appearance may be perfect, but if you arrive late for an interview, it may not matter. Being late is a sure way to make a poor impression. Time management is an essential health care job skill, and you will have failed your first opportunity to demonstrate that you have mastered it. In addition, arriving late is a sign of rudeness and inconsideration for the interviewer's time. Making a few advance preparations will help to ensure that this doesn't happen to you:

☐ Write down the date and exact time of the appointment.

☐ Verify the address and ask for directions, if necessary.

☐ If the office is in a large building or complex, get additional instructions about how to find it.

☐ Inquire about parking, bus stops, or subway stops.

☐ If you are unsure of the location and it is not too far away, go there a couple of days before the interview to be sure you can find it.

☐ Allow extra time to arrive, and plan to be there about 10 minutes before the appointed time.

☐ If there is an emergency that can't be avoided (a flat tire or unexpected snow storm), call as soon as possible to offer an explanation and reschedule the interview.

Many job applicants don't realize that the interview actually starts before they sit down with the person asking the questions. That's right. From the first contact you made to inquire about a job opening or set the appointment, you have been making an impression. If you arrive for the interview and are rude to the receptionist, you may have already failed in your bid for the job. You cannot know what information is shared with the hiring authority. (Keep in mind, too, that these may be your future co-workers!)

Learn the name of the person who will be conducting the interview. Be sure you have the correct spelling (for the thank-you note, discussed in Chapter 12) and pronunciation. When you are introduced, the following actions express both courtesy and self-confidence:

1. Make and maintain eye contact.
2. Give a healthy (not limp or hesitant) handshake.
3. Express how glad you are to meet him or her and how much you appreciate the opportunity to be interviewed.
4. Don't sit down until you are offered a chair or the other person is seated.

 Go to page 311 to complete Prescription for Success 11-9

COURTESY DURING THE INTERVIEW

Maintaining eye contact (without staring, of course) while the other person is speaking indicates that you are interested in what he or she is saying. When you are speaking, it is natural to look away occasionally. Most of the time, however, you should look at the listener. This is a sign of openness and sincerity. (Review the guidelines for respectful communication in Chapter 8.) The following is a summary of behaviors to definitely avoid (even if the interviewer engages in them):

- Interrupting
- Cursing
- Using poor grammar (such as the word "ain't") or slang
- Gossiping, such as commenting on the weaknesses of other facilities, professionals, or your previous employer
- Telling off-color jokes
- Putting yourself down
- Chewing gum
- Appearing to snoop by looking at papers or other materials on the interviewer's desk, shelves, and so on
- Discussing personal problems

You don't want to come across as stiff or stuffy, but you do want to come across as professional. Try to be at ease and act natural while maintaining your best "company manners."

APPLY YOUR COMMUNICATION SKILLS

A successful job interview depends on the effective use of communication. An interview is essentially a conversation between two people who are trying to determine whether they fit each other's employment needs. As a job applicant, you must take responsibility for making sure that you understand the employer's needs, questions, and comments. At the same time, you have to express yourself clearly so that the interviewer understands you.

Active Listening

Understanding begins by listening actively. The importance of carefully listening to the interviewer cannot be overemphasized. So many times we become so caught up in thinking about what we're going to say next that we fail to fully hear, let alone actively listen, to the other person. This is especially true in an interview when we are nervous and worried about whether we will say the right thing. But this is the very situation in which we can most benefit from listening carefully so we can base what we say on what we hear.

Recall from Chapter 5 that active listening consists of paying attention, focusing on the speaker's words, and thinking about the meaning of what is said. This takes practice. When you participate in the mock interviews suggested earlier, do not look at the questions the person role-playing the interviewer is going to ask. Instead, focus on listening carefully to the questions and then formulating an appropriate response. Pausing to think and compose a good answer will be appreciated by interviewers. You are more likely to be evaluated on the quality of your answer, not on how quickly you gave it.

Mirroring

An effective communication technique for interviews is known as **mirroring**. This means you observe the communication style of the interviewer and then match it as closely as possible. This does not mean mimicking or appearing to make fun of the other person. It does mean adapting a style that will be most comfortable for the interviewer and help to build trust. Table 11-2 provides examples of mirroring.

Feedback

Whatever the style of the interviewer, use feedback when necessary to ensure that you understand the message. Feedback, as you recall from Chapter 8, is a communication technique used to check your understanding of the speaker's intended message. It is not necessary—or even desirable—to repeat everything the speaker says. It is annoying to

TABLE 11-2	Examples of Mirroring at the Job Interview	
If the Interviewer Is	**It Is Best To**	
Very businesslike. Direct and to the point.	Answer questions concisely, quickly getting to the point. Avoid long introductions, wordiness, and unnecessary detail.	
Warm and friendly. Conversational tone.	Reflect the interviewer's warmth without becoming too casual. Include human interest and details, when appropriate, in your answers.	
Seemingly unhurried. Spends time describing the job in detail.	Include details to support your answers and fully explain yourself (without giving unnecessary or unrelated information).	

speakers to have everything they say repeated, and you don't want to sound like a parrot. Using feedback unnecessarily will use up time better spent learning about the job and presenting your qualifications. Used when needed, however, feedback can help you understand the other person so you can respond appropriately and intelligently.

Organization

When speaking, do your best to present your ideas in an organized manner so they are easy for the listener to follow. This can be difficult when you are nervous, so take your time to think before you speak. Recall the STAR technique described earlier in this chapter. Sometimes we are uncomfortable with silence and feel that we have to talk to avoid it. But taking a few moments to consider what you are going to say will result in better answers. Saying something meaningful after a pause is more important than simply responding quickly.

 Go to page 311 to complete Prescription for Success 11-10

Nonverbal Communication: It Can Make You or Break You

"If you want a quality, act as if you already have it."

—*William James*

You can speak smoothly and answer questions correctly and yet fail in your communication efforts. What has gone wrong? Your actions have betrayed

 Q&A **with a Health Care Professional Rick Baird**

Rick Baird is the Chief Human Resources Officer at Bend Memorial Clinic in Bend, Oregon. Rick shares some interview tips for applicants.

Q What advice would you give applicants who are interviewing for a job at your clinic—or at any health care facility?

A First, I would say they should use sound common sense. I might add here that common sense is not always so common! What I mean is, applicants need to think about the impression they are giving the employer. If applicants are not at their best when they come in for an interview, what is the employer going to expect from them once they are on the job?

Q Can you be more specific?

A Sure. Good candidates for jobs in health care are friendly, concerned, and respectful. They show this in the way they interact with the interviewer. For example, they are on time, showing they respect the other person's schedule. Health care today is a high customer service environment, and we are looking for employees who take their work seriously. After all, we aren't selling shoes. Health *matters,* and that's what we're taking care of.

Q You mention appearance. Have the standards changed in today's health care facilities?

A To some degree, the answer is "yes." Social values drive business values, and, as we all know, styles and trends have changed. What we're looking for is "reasonable standards." For example, piercings and tattoos used to be job-blockers. But now they're more accepted if they aren't excessive or too outlandish.

Related to appearance is language. Communication and the impressions given to patients are really important, so inappropriate language is really not okay. Anything off-color or offensive—that kind of thing.

Q What kinds of questions should interviewees be prepared for?

A Patients today are considered to be *customers,* so I'm interested in knowing what an applicant can do that will help us make our patients satisfied with our service. What will they do to make our patients feel important? Those are questions I would ask. The bottom line is that I'm looking for people who want to help make this place better. And I want to know how they're going to do it.

We sometimes give behavioral interviews. This means we give applicants scenarios of typical work situations and ask how they would handle them. What we are looking for is caring and respect for others—their general approach to work. Sometimes we require a demonstration of a skill related to the job.

you. That's right: what you do communicates as much as—or even more than—what you say. As we discussed in Chapter 8, our movements, posture, gestures, and facial expressions usually reveal our true feelings. You can enthusiastically claim that you would love the challenge of working in a fast-paced, think-on-your-feet clinical environment. But if your face and body language reflect fear, anxiety, or subtle expressions of "yuck!," your verbal message will not ring true. Remember that more than half of the meaning of our messages is communicated nonverbally. This is why videotaping yourself is very helpful when practicing interviewing skills. You can observe your nonverbal language and catch inappropriate facial expressions and other behaviors that might betray your words.

The point is not to suggest that you should try to mask your true feelings and put on an act to impress interviewers. Rather, the purpose of this discussion is to encourage you to be aware of how important your actions are and what they say about you. If there are aspects of a job you know you can't or don't want to perform, this is the time to find out. Keep in mind that one of your goals in an interview

is to learn about the job and the organization so you can decide whether this is the place for you.

Developing a positive attitude about the interviewing process and having confidence in your own abilities will help ensure that your body language communicates appropriate positive messages. At the same time, developing the body language of a positive, confident person will help you become that person. Table 11-3 provides a number of ways to communicate self-confidence and, at the same time, respect for the other person. Figure 11-2 shows an example of body language that sends a positive message.

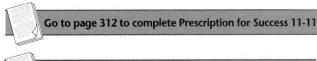

Go to page 312 to complete Prescription for Success 11-11

Go to page 312 to complete Prescription for Success 11-12

USING YOUR PORTFOLIO WISELY

Portfolios are gaining popularity among job seekers, including those in the health care field. They can be a very effective way to support your claims of

TABLE 11-3	Positive Body Language	
What You Do	**The Message You Send**
Stand up straight, with your head held up and shoulders back.	"I am a candidate worthy of your consideration."
Maintain eye contact.	"I am sincere in what I am saying."
Avoid nervous actions such as jiggling a leg or fidgeting with your hands.	"I want to be here."
Lean forward slightly toward the other person.	"I am interested in what you are saying."

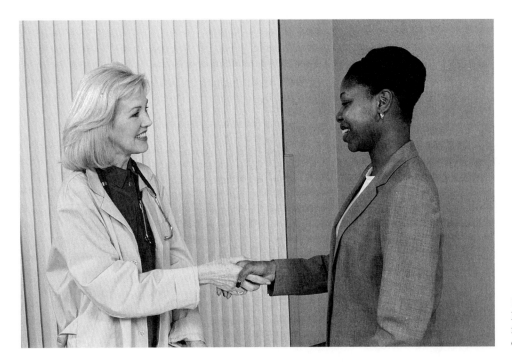

Figure 11-2 Use body language that communicates respect for the interviewer and confidence in yourself.

competence by providing evidence of your accomplishments and qualifications.

Not all employers are familiar with portfolios. Announcing at the beginning of interviews that you have brought one and asking interviewers if they would like to see it is not the most effective way of using it to your advantage. Remember that one of your main goals at the interview is to show how you meet the employer's needs. You won't know enough about these needs until you spend a little time listening. Then you may be able to use your portfolio constructively. The following interviewer questions and statements might be answered with material in your portfolio:

1. Asks a question about your skills and abilities
   "Can you…?"
   "Have you had experience…?"
2. States what skills are needed or provides a job description
   "This job requires…"
   "We need someone who can use medical terminology correctly and chart accurately."
3. Shares a problem or concern
   "One of our problems has been with ensuring accurate documentation…"
   "We have difficulties with…"
4. Isn't familiar with the contents of your training program
   "Did your program include…?"
   "What skills did you learn…?"
5. "Asks for verification of licenses, certifications, and so on
   "Have you passed the _____ exam?"
   "Are you a certified medical assistant?"
   "Are you licensed in this state?"

It isn't necessary—or even a good idea—to try to back up everything you say with your portfolio. In fact, if overused, a portfolio loses its effectiveness. And many questions are better answered with an oral explanation and/or example.

Become very familiar with your portfolio's contents so you can find items quickly. If necessary, create an easy-to-read table of contents. Frantically flipping through pages to find something will make you look (and feel) unprepared and disorganized. You will also waste valuable time, a very limited resource in most interviews.

Use your portfolio to give a brief summary presentation if you are given an opportunity at the end of the interview. For example, the interviewer might say, "Tell me why I should hire you," or ask, "What else should I know about you?" Use this presentation to quickly review your qualifications or to point out those that haven't been mentioned.

You may attend interviews where you don't use your portfolio at all. This is okay. It is always better—both during the job search and on the job—to

be overprepared. This prevents you from missing opportunities when they do present themselves.

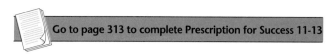

Go to page 313 to complete Prescription for Success 11-13

HANDLING STICKY INTERVIEW SITUATIONS

In spite of your best efforts, some interviews can be a little rocky. Remember, not every employer is skilled at interviewing. Consider this: you may have prepared and practiced more than the person conducting the interview! Table 11-4 contains difficult situations and suggestions for handling them gracefully. Keep in mind that the questions reveal something about the interviewer and possibly about the organization, so consider them when deciding if this is a place you want to work.

Dealing with Illegal Questions

It is illegal for employers to **discriminate** against an applicant on the basis of any of the following factors:
- Age (as long as the applicant is old enough to work legally)
- Arrests (without a conviction—being proven guilty)
- Ethnic background
- Financial status
- Marital status and children
- Physical condition (as long as the applicant can perform the job tasks)
- Race
- Religion
- Sexual orientation

Questions that require the applicant to reveal information about these factors are illegal. They are sometimes asked anyway. Some employers are ignorant of the laws. Or the interview becomes friendly and conversational, and personal information is shared. ("Oh, I went to Grady High School, too. What year did you graduate?") Employers may take the chance that applicants won't know the questions are illegal. And a few will ask because they know that most applicants will not take the time to report them for discrimination. It may not be obvious from the questions that answering them will, in fact, reveal information that cannot be considered when hiring. Take a look at the following examples:

Question	What It Can Reveal
What part of town do you live in?	Financial status
Do you own your home?	Financial status

Question	What It Can Reveal
Where are your parents from?	Ethnic background
Which holidays do you celebrate?	Religion
When did you graduate from high school?	Age

Illegal questions put you in a difficult situation, and there are no easy formulas for handling them. In deciding what to do, you need to ask yourself the following questions:

☐ Is the subject of the question of concern to me?
☐ Do I find the question offensive?
☐ Does the interviewer appear to be unaware that the question is illegal?
☐ What is my overall impression of the interviewer and the facility?
☐ Would I want to work here?
☐ How badly do I want this particular job?

☐ If this person is to be my immediate supervisor, is the question an indication that this is a person I don't really want to work with?
☐ What do I think the interviewer's real concern is? Is it valid?

Based on your answers, there are several ways you can respond to the interviewer.

1. Answer honestly.
2. Ask the interviewer to explain how the question relates to the job requirements.
3. Respond to the interviewer's apparent concern rather than to the question.
4. Ignore the question and talk about something else.
5. Refuse to answer.
6. Inform the interviewer that the question is illegal.
7. Excuse yourself from the interview and leave.
8. State that you plan to report the incident to the Civil Rights Commission or Equal Employment Opportunity Commission.

TABLE 11-4	Handling Difficult Interview Situations
If the Interviewer	**What You Can Do**
Keeps you waiting a long time.	If you are interested in the job, do not show annoyance or anger. It is best not to schedule interviews when you have a very limited amount of time. Remember, this person may be overworked, and that's exactly why there is a potential position for you! Keep in mind that health care work does not always proceed at our convenience. A patient with an emergency, for example, will certainly have priority over an interviewee.
Allows constant interruptions with phone calls and/or people coming in.	Again, do not show that you are irritated. This person may be very busy, disorganized, or simply having a difficult day. (This could be another good sign that this employer really needs your help.)
Does most of the talking and doesn't give you an opportunity to say much about yourself.	Listen carefully, and try to determine how your qualifications relate to what you are hearing. Being a good listener in itself may be the most important quality you can demonstrate.
Seems to simply make conversation. Doesn't discuss the job or ask you questions.	Try to move the discussion to the job by asking questions: "Can you tell me about what you are looking for in a candidate?" "What are the principal duties that this person would perform?" It is possible that this is a test to see your reaction, so take care to be courteous.
Tries to engage you in gossip about school, etc.	Say you don't really know about the person or other professionals, facilities, or situation and cannot comment. Ask a question about the job to redirect the conversation.
Allows long periods of silence.	This may be a test to see how you react under pressure. Don't feel that you have to speak, and do your best to remain comfortable. (Say to yourself, "This is just a test, and I'm doing fine.") If it goes on too long, you can ask: "Is there something you'd like me to tell you more about? Discuss further?"
Doesn't seem to understand your training or qualifications.	Explain as clearly as possible. Use your portfolio, as appropriate, to illustrate your skills.
Makes inappropriate comments about your appearance, gender, ethnicity, etc.	Depending on the nature of the comment and your interpretation of the situation, it may be best to excuse yourself from the interview. For example, comments of a sexual nature or racial slurs should not be tolerated. You should discuss this situation with your instructor or career services department for advice on how to proceed.
Is very friendly, chatty, and complimentary about you.	Why in the world, you ask, is this a problem? It may not be. But be careful not to get so comfortable that you share personal problems and other information that may disqualify you for the job.

TABLE 11-5	Addressing Employer Concerns	
Question	**Possible Concern**	**Possible Responses**
Do you have young children?	Your attendance and dependability	Explain your childcare arrangements, good attendance in school and on other jobs, and your understanding of the importance of good attendance.
Where do you live?	Reliable transportation and punctuality	Describe your transportation and previous good attendance.
Which religious holidays are you unable to work?	Scheduling problems	Explain that you are a team player and understand that all workdays must be covered. You are willing to cover when co-workers have a holiday you do not observe.

Employers do have the right—as well as the responsibility—to make sure that applicants can both physically and legally perform the job requirements. Sometimes there is only a small difference in wording between a legal and an illegal question, as in the following examples[4]:

Illegal	Legal
How old are you?	Are you over 18?
Where were you born?	Do you have the legal right to work in the United States?
What is your maiden name?	Would your work records be listed under another name?
Have you ever been arrested?	Have you ever been convicted of a crime?

Are you beginning to understand how employers can get confused and ask illegal questions? It is possible to be an excellent dentist or physical therapist but not an expert in the details of employment law. However you choose to respond to questions you believe are illegal, it is best to remain calm and courteous. You may decide you don't want to work there, but conduct yourself professionally at all times.

Many employment experts recommend that you respond to the employer's concerns rather than the questions. This requires that you determine what the concerns are. See Table 11-5 for examples.

One recommended strategy for handling common employer concerns is to bring them up before the interviewer does. This gives you the opportunity to present them in a positive light. Employers may be uncomfortable addressing certain issues and will simply drop you from the "possible hire" list. By taking the initiative, you gain the opportunity to defend your position and stay on the list. Table 11-6 contains suggestions for showing the employer the positive aspects of various employment "problems."

PERSONAL REFLECTION

1. Is there anything you think employers might see as an obstacle to hiring you?

_____

_____

_____

2. How can you turn the obstacle into a positive characteristic?

_____

_____

_____

STAY FOCUSED ON THE POSITIVE

"Employers are hiring based on attitude: "Give me a 'C' student with an 'A' attitude."
                        —*Melva Duran*

Interviews are a time to do your best to stay positive. They are not the place to bring up problems or what you believe you can't do or don't want to do. Be positive and future-oriented, and prepared to emphasize the following:
- What you can do
- How you can help
- Ways you can apply what you've learned

As mentioned before, you should never criticize a previous employer, instructor, or anyone else. Potential employers realize they may someday be your previous employer and don't want to be the subject of your comments to others in the

TABLE 11-6	Point Out the Positives	
The Problem	**The Bright Side**
You're very young, with little work experience.	You are energetic, eager to learn, "trainable," and looking for long-term employment. ("One of the advantages of being young is….")
You have a criminal record.*	You have learned from your mistakes and are eager to have an opportunity to serve others.
You're over age 40.	You are experienced, have good work habits, and are patient.
You've had many jobs, none for very long.	You have a variety of experiences, are flexible, can adjust to the working environment, and have now found a career to which you want to dedicate your efforts.

*Note: Some states do not allow individuals who have been convicted of specific crimes to work in certain health care occupations. In some cases, these individuals are not even allowed to take certification exams.

profession. It is also possible that the interviewer is a friend of the person you are criticizing!

Keep in mind that every interview is a sales presentation. A sales presentation is not the time to point out the product's faults. You want to emphasize the positive aspects of your skills and character, not your weaknesses. However, if you sincerely feel that you are not qualified for a job (and this is an important consideration in health care), you should never pretend that you are. Lacking needed skills is not a negative reflection on you as a person. It simply means that this job is not appropriate for you. Other jobs will be. In fact, there may be many reasons why jobs and applicants do not match. After all, that's the whole purpose of job interviews—for you and the employer to make that determination.

Discussion of personal problems should always be avoided. You are there to help solve the employer's problems, not find solutions to your own. Employers are looking for independent problem solvers. Bringing your own problems to the interview will not give them a good impression of your capabilities in this area. (There are exceptions. For example, if you are responsible for a disabled family member and need some consideration regarding your work schedule, it would be appropriate to mention this at the interview.)

Focusing on your own needs is negatively received by employers. Giving the impression that you are more concerned with what you can get from the job than what you can give is a sure way to get nothing at all. The following questions send the message "What's in it for me?" and should be avoided until you know you are actually being considered for the job:

- How much does the job pay?
- What are the other benefits?
- How many paid holidays will I get?
- Is Friday a casual day?

- Can I leave early if I finish my work?
- When will I get a raise?

It is acceptable to inquire about the work schedule, duties, and other expectations. The time to negotiate specific conditions, including your salary, is after you have been offered the job. (This is discussed in Chapter 12.)

IT'S YOUR INTERVIEW, TOO

Interviews are not only for the benefit of employers. You have the right, and the responsibility, to evaluate the opportunities presented by the jobs you are applying for. This may seem to contradict what we discussed in the previous section, but it doesn't. In fact, well-stated questions about the job communicate motivation and interest.

When you are in class, it is generally true that "there are no stupid questions." However, at a job interview, the quality of your questions does count. There is a difference between questions that should be avoided and ones that demonstrate that you:

- Have a sincere interest in the job
- Want to understand the employer's needs
- Understand the nature of health care work
- Have thought about your career goal
- Want information that will enable you to do your best

What you ask will depend on the job, the interviewer, and how much you already know about the job and the organization. It is a good idea to prepare in advance a list of general questions, along with a few that are specific to the job and the facility. This will help you remember what you want to ask. As we pointed out earlier, it is easy to forget when we feel under pressure, as may happen in the interview situation. Not everyone is skilled at "thinking in the seat," especially when it feels like the hot seat!

Here are a few suggested questions to get you started:

1. How could I best contribute to the success of this facility?
2. What are the most important qualities needed to succeed in this position?
3. What is the mission of this organization or facility?
4. What are the major problems faced by this organization or facility?
5. How is the organization structured? Who would I be reporting to?
6. What values are most important?
7. I want to continue learning and updating my skills. What opportunities would I have to do this?
8. How will I be evaluated and learn what I need to improve?
9. Are there opportunities for advancement for employees who work hard and perform well?

It is perfectly acceptable to ask questions throughout the interview where they fit in. This will be more natural and lead to a smoother interview than asking a long list at the end. You don't have to wait until you are invited to ask them.

 Go to page 313 to complete Prescription for Success 11-14

In addition to asking questions, observe the facility and the people who work there. Does this "feel" like a place you would want to work? Is it clean? Organized? Does it appear that safety precautions are followed? What is the pace? Are the people who work there courteous and helpful? How do they interact with patients and with each other? If your interview is with the person who would be your supervisor, do you think you would get along? Do you believe you would fit in?

It may not be possible for you to see anything other than the interviewer's office. In fact, at a large facility your first interview may take place in the personnel office. You won't see the area where you would work. If this is the case, you will want to ask for a tour if you are offered a job. (More about this will be covered in Chapter 12.)

LEAVING GRACIOUSLY

The end of the interview provides you an opportunity to make a final impression, so make it a good one. It is important to be sensitive to any signals the interviewer gives that it is time to wrap up. Failure to do so shows a lack of consideration for his or her time, and this is definitely not the parting message you want to leave. Some interviewers will make it

obvious the interview is almost over by doing the following:

- Telling you directly
- Asking whether you have any "final" questions
- Telling you that everything has been covered

Less obvious signs include looking at his or her watch, clock, appointment book, or papers on the desk; pushing his or her chair back; or saying that the interviewer has "taken enough of your time." Show respect for the interviewer's time by moving along with the final steps of the interview:

1. Ask any final questions (limit these to a couple of the most important ones that haven't been answered).
2. Make a brief wrap-up statement.
3. Thank the interviewer for his or her time.
4. Inquire about what comes next.

If you are interested in the job, say so in the wrap-up statement. Tell the interviewer why you believe you can make a contribution; what impressed you about the organization; why you believe your qualifications fit the position; and so on. Express your enthusiasm about working there and state that you hope you are chosen for the position.

Whether you want the job or not, always thank the interviewer for his or her time. This applies even if the interview did not go well. Health care professionals and personnel staff are extremely busy. Let them know how much you appreciate being given the opportunity to present your qualifications.

Finally, if you aren't told about the next step in the application process, don't hesitate to ask. Inquire about when the hiring decision will be made. Find out if there is anything you need to send. If asked, give the interviewer your reference sheet. Be sure to get the interviewer's last name and correct title. An easy way to do this is to ask for his or her business card. And be sure that he or she has your telephone number and any other information needed to contact you. Then smile, give a firm handshake, and leave as confidently as you entered, regardless of how you believe the interview went.

 Go to page 314 to complete Prescription for Success 11-15

SOME FINAL THOUGHTS

"You wouldn't be nervous if you didn't care."
—Robert Lock

You may be feeling a little—maybe very—overwhelmed at this point. "How can I remember all this and act natural and maintain eye contact and give good examples and...?" It is a lot, and that's why it is so important to spend time learning about

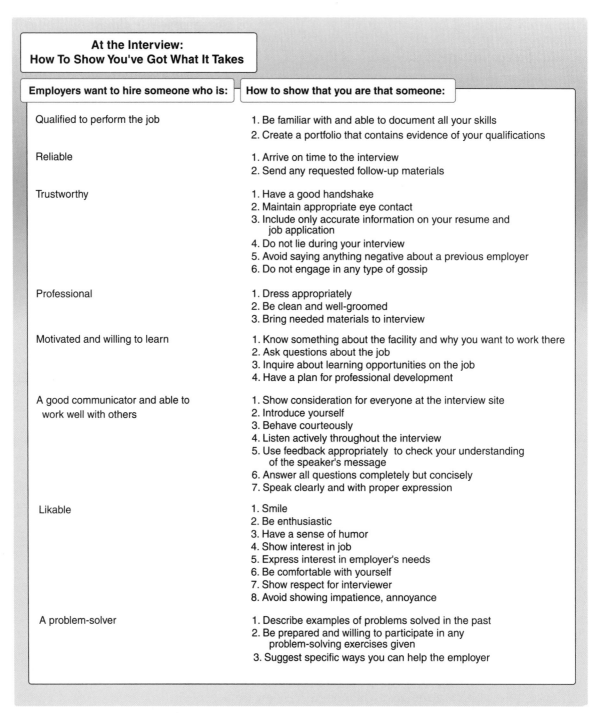

At the Interview:
How To Show You've Got What It Takes

Employers want to hire someone who is:	How to show that you are that someone:
Qualified to perform the job	1. Be familiar with and able to document all your skills 2. Create a portfolio that contains evidence of your qualifications
Reliable	1. Arrive on time to the interview 2. Send any requested follow-up materials
Trustworthy	1. Have a good handshake 2. Maintain appropriate eye contact 3. Include only accurate information on your resume and job application 4. Do not lie during your interview 5. Avoid saying anything negative about a previous employer 6. Do not engage in any type of gossip
Professional	1. Dress appropriately 2. Be clean and well-groomed 3. Bring needed materials to interview
Motivated and willing to learn	1. Know something about the facility and why you want to work there 2. Ask questions about the job 3. Inquire about learning opportunities on the job 4. Have a plan for professional development
A good communicator and able to work well with others	1. Show consideration for everyone at the interview site 2. Introduce yourself 3. Behave courteously 4. Listen actively throughout the interview 5. Use feedback appropriately to check your understanding of the speaker's message 6. Answer all questions completely but concisely 7. Speak clearly and with proper expression
Likable	1. Smile 2. Be enthusiastic 3. Have a sense of humor 4. Show interest in job 5. Express interest in employer's needs 6. Be comfortable with yourself 7. Show respect for interviewer 8. Avoid showing impatience, annoyance
A problem-solver	1. Describe examples of problems solved in the past 2. Be prepared and willing to participate in any problem-solving exercises given 3. Suggest specific ways you can help the employer

Figure 11-3   The interview is your sales opportunity.

the interviewing process, preparing, and practicing. Take every opportunity to role-play. Make your practice sessions as realistic as possible. Figure 11-3 contains a summary list of positive interview behaviors.

When you inventoried your skills, were you surprised at how much you can do now that you would never have attempted before you started your educational program? You learned these skills by studying and practicing them—over and over. If you have been working on developing these skills, this is your chance to use them for job success. You are almost certainly more qualified for the job search than you realize. And using your skills to get a job will reinforce your ability to use them once you are on the job.

A final note: It's okay to be nervous. It can even be a good thing, because it means you are not taking this experience for granted. Interviewers know you are nervous, and it tells them that this job is important to you and that you care about the outcome. This is a positive message to communicate.

PERSONAL REFLECTION

1. What is my biggest concern about inter-viewing?

_____

_____

_____

2. What can I do to best prepare for inter-viewing?

_____

_____

_____

⇨ SUMMARY OF KEY IDEAS

1. An interview is a sales opportunity, so consider the customer's—the employer's—needs.
2. Advance preparation is the key to a successful interview.
3. Practice will help you present your qualifications effectively.
4. First impressions are critical.
5. It's natural to be nervous.

Positive Self-Talk for This Chapter

1. I am well prepared for interviews.
2. I present myself and my qualifications effectively.
3. I answer questions clearly and confidently.
4. I make a positive impression.

To Learn More

About.com

http://jobsearch.about.com/cs/interviews/a/aceinterview.htm

Read about all aspects of interviewing, including behavioral interviews, proper interview behavior, and suggestions for dress.

Quintessential Careers

www.quintcareers.com/intvres.html

Gain access to dozens of articles and links to websites with information about interviewing, including examples of questions.

REFERENCES

1. Hansen K: Behavioral interviewing strategies for job-seekers. www.quintcareers.com/behavioral_interviewing.html (Accessed 2/27/09)
2. Cha AE: "Employers relying on personality tests to screen applicants." The Washington Post. March 27, 2005. Page A01. http://www.washingtonpost.com/ac2/wp-dyn/A4010-2005Mar26?language=printer (Accessed 3/1/09)
3. Graber S: The everything online job search book, Holbrook, Mass, 2000, Adams Media.
4. Lock RD: Job search: career planning guide, Book II, ed 3, Pacific Grove, Calif, 1996, Brooks/Cole.

INTERNET ACTIVITIES

For active links to the websites needed to complete these activities, visit **http://evolve.elsevier.com/Haroun/career/.**

1. The Monster website has a section with links to helpful articles on interviewing. Choose two articles to read. Create a list of the 10 tips you find most useful.
2. Quintessential Careers has links to dozens of websites dealing with job interviews. Browse sites of interest, and summarize what you learn.
3. The *Riley Guide* contains links to advice from job-search professionals about handling improper questions at an interview ("Handling Questionable Questions"). After reading the advice offered, describe how you would handle a question whose answer would reveal your age.

Prescription for Success 11-1
Be Prepared

1. Select a facility where you might want to work.
2. Use the resources suggested in this chapter to learn as much as possible.

What type of work do they do? _____

What is their patient population or client base? _____

What is the size of the staff?_____

What are the duties and responsibilities of the job(s) for which you might apply?

_____

_____

_____

_____

_____

What is the mission of the organization? How does the organization describe its core values?

_____

_____

_____

_____

_____

Prescription for Success 11-2
Answering Traditional Interview Questions

1. Think of five traditional questions you might be asked in an interview.

1. _____

2. _____

3. _____

4. _____

5. _____

Prescription for Success 11-2—(Continued)

2. Choose a specific job and facility (real or imaginary) and prepare an appropriate response for each question.

1. _____

_____

2. _____

_____

3. _____

_____

4. _____

_____

5. _____

3. Say your answers aloud.
4. Continue to practice the exercise aloud until you can answer the questions smoothly, but without sounding "canned" or phony. You may not be asked these same questions, but this exercise will give you practice thinking quickly and creating targeted answers.

Prescription for Success 11-3
Answering Behavioral Interview Questions

1. Think of five behavioral questions you might be asked in an interview.

1. _____

2. _____

3. _____

4. _____

5. _____

2. Choose a specific job and facility (real or imaginary) and prepare an appropriate response for each question.

1. _____

_____

Continued

Prescription for Success 11-3—(Continued)

   2. _____

   _____

   3. _____

   _____

   4. _____

   _____

   5. _____

   _____

3. Say your answers aloud.
4. Continue to practice the exercise aloud until you can answer the questions smoothly, but without sounding "canned" or phony. You may not be asked these same questions, but this exercise will give you practice thinking quickly and creating targeted answers.

Prescription for Success 11-4
Answering Situational Interview Questions

1. Think of five situational questions you might be asked in an interview.

   1. _____

   2. _____

   3. _____

   4. _____

   5. _____

2. Choose a specific job and facility (real or imaginary) and prepare an appropriate response for each question.

   1. _____

   _____

   2. _____

   _____

Prescription for Success 11-4—(Continued)

3. _____
   _____

4. _____
   _____

5. _____
   _____

3. Say your answers aloud.
4. Continue to practice the exercise aloud until you can answer the questions smoothly, but without sounding "canned" or phony. You may not be asked these same questions, but this exercise will give you practice thinking quickly and creating targeted answers.

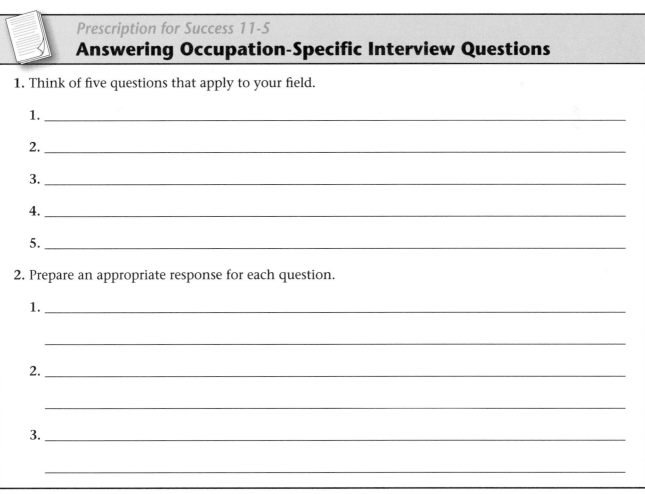

Prescription for Success 11-5
Answering Occupation-Specific Interview Questions

1. Think of five questions that apply to your field.

1. _____

2. _____

3. _____

4. _____

5. _____

2. Prepare an appropriate response for each question.

1. _____
   _____

2. _____
   _____

3. _____
   _____

Continued

Prescription for Success 11-5—(Continued)

4. _____

_____

5. _____

_____

3. Say your answers aloud.
4. Continue to practice the exercise aloud until you can answer the questions smoothly, and with confidence, but without sounding "canned" or phony.

Prescription for Success 11-6
Answering Questions about Your Work Preference

1. Think of five questions an employer in your occupational area might ask.

1. _____

2. _____

3. _____

4. _____

5. _____

2. Prepare an appropriate response for each question.

1. _____

_____

2. _____

_____

3. _____

_____

4. _____

_____

5. _____

_____

Prescription for Success 11-7
Dress Rehearsal

1. Choose someone to help you practice interviewing. Give him or her a list of questions to ask you in random order. (Better yet, find someone with interviewing experience and have this person surprise you with questions.)
2. If possible, videotape or record the session or have a third person observe.
3. Discuss how you did with your partner and the observer.
4. Create a plan to address anything you need to work on.

_____

_____

_____

_____

_____

Prescription for Success 11-8
Planning the Look

1. Select an appropriate outfit for interviewing, including shoes. Make sure everything is clean, pressed, and ready to go on short notice.
2. If in doubt, ask your instructor, mentor, or career services staff for advice about what to wear to interviews.

Prescription for Success 11-9
Practice until It Comes Naturally

1. In front of a mirror, practice your smile and posture.
2. With a partner, practice your handshake.
3. Rehearse the meeting until you feel comfortable with these actions: approach, smile, handshake, sitting down, maintaining positive posture.

Prescription for Success 11-10
Apply Your Communication Skills

Apply your communication skills at every opportunity: active listening, mirroring, and feedback. These are not just interviewing skills. Making an effort to use them consistently will benefit every aspect of your relationships with others.

Prescription for Success 11-11
Tune in to Nonverbal Messages

1. Observe the behavior of other people throughout the day. Can you find examples that communicate cooperativeness? Self-confidence? Respect for others?
2. Describe some of the behaviors you observe that communicate positive messages.

_____

_____

_____

_____

_____

Prescription for Success 11-12
Would You Hire This Person?

1. Check your posture and smile in a full-length mirror. Do you look confident? Approachable? Like a person you would choose to work with?
2. Explain why or why not.

_____

_____

_____

3. Is there anything you think you should change?

_____

_____

_____

4. If yes, what is your plan for improvement?

_____

_____

_____

_____

_____

Prescription for Success 11-13
Portfolio Practice

1. Think of five questions a potential employer might ask in which you could use your portfolio to support your answer.

    1. _____
    _____

    2. _____
    _____

    3. _____
    _____

    4. _____
    _____

    5. _____
    _____

2. Role-play with a partner. Have him or her play the part of the employer and choose questions to ask you at random. Answer each question, using your portfolio to document your answer.

Prescription for Success 11-14
What Do You Want to Know?

Make up at least five questions you could ask at an interview. The purpose of your questions should be to help you find out whether the job and organization are a match for your work preferences and qualifications.

1. _____

2. _____

3. _____

4. _____

5. _____

Wrapping It up

1. Create several short summaries that express your interest in various jobs and statements about why you should be hired.
2. Practice your statements aloud, along with a "thank you" and questions about follow-up.
   (**Note:** The purpose of this exercise is not to prepare a canned summary but to practice giving a good summary.)

_____

_____

_____

_____

_____

_____

_____

_____

_____

_____

_____

_____

_____

_____

_____

_____

_____

_____

_____

_____

_____

_____

After the Interview

OBJECTIVES

The information and activities in this chapter can help you:
- Learn from every interview you attend.
- Write appropriate thank-you letters to interviewers.
- Explain when and how to call and inquire about hiring decisions.
- Develop appropriate criteria for determining whether to accept a job offer.
- Calculate the total value of a compensation package.
- Accept or turn down job offers properly.
- Describe how to deal with and learn from the experience if you are not selected for a job.

KEY TERMS AND CONCEPTS

Benefits: Items of value provided by employers in addition to salary. They include insurance, tuition reimbursement, paid days off, and a uniform allowance.

Compensation: The payment an employer gives for work done. It includes wages and other benefits.

401(k) Retirement Plan: A retirement plan offered by some employers. It gives you an opportunity to save and invest for your retirement.

REWARD YOURSELF

"Celebrate all successes on the job search journey."

Attending an interview is a success, whether or not you are hired for a particular job. You have qualifications that were worthy of the interviewer's time, you prepared well, and you met the challenge of presenting yourself one-on-one to a potential employer. Take a moment to reward yourself for completing this important step.

MAXIMIZE THE INTERVIEW EXPERIENCE

"Nothing is a waste of time if you use the experience wisely."

—Auguste Rodin

Making the most of every interview means that you view each one as an experience that provides opportunities to improve your presentation skills and to learn more about the health care world. This knowledge can help you in future interviews and work-related situations such as performance evaluations. When you leave the interviewer's office, your reaction may be "Whew! That's over!" and the last thing you want to do is spend more time thinking about it. This is especially true if you feel the interview didn't go well. But this is precisely when you need to spend some time thinking about and evaluating the experience and your performance. Using an interview evaluation sheet will help you focus on the important factors that determine the success of an interview and create a plan for improvement. Make copies of the form provided in Prescription for Success 12-1, and keep a record of your interviews in your job-search notebook.

Go to page 327 to complete Prescription for Success 12-1

You might want to discuss your self-evaluation with someone you trust. Sometimes we are too hard on ourselves and need a second point of view to help us see the real situation. Review the interview with your instructor, career services personnel, or mentor. You may have friends and family members who can provide insight and support. Create an improvement plan and practice so you'll feel more confident at the next interview.

When seeking help or discussing interviews with others, it is best not to make negative remarks about the interviewer or the facility. This serves no purpose, unless you are seeking advice about whether to accept a job you have doubts about. A friend may have a friend who works there, and your words, said "in confidence," may be passed along to the wrong party.

You may believe you will receive a job offer. You very well might. But don't cancel or turn down other interviews until you are formally hired. You may have done a superb job and the facility plans to hire you. Then the next day, your soon-to-be supervisor is informed of a facility-wide hiring freeze. You don't want to be left out in the cold with no other options. You may even find something better before they make the offer. Stay actively involved in the search until you have a job.

THANK YOU LETTER

Whether the interview went like a dream or a nightmare, send a thank-you note. This courtesy is something many job seekers don't do. Yet it is a simple action that can set you apart from the others. Suppose the employer interviewed nine people in 2 days, in addition to carrying on a normal workload. Tired? Very likely. Able to remember each candidate clearly and recall who said what? Maybe. But why take the chance of being lost in the crowd?

If you know for sure that you don't want the job, send a thank-you note anyway. Keep it simple, say something positive about the interview, and express your appreciation for the time taken to meet with you. Do not say that you are not interested in the job. Figure 12-1 is an example of this kind of note.

Why, you might ask, would you write if you don't want to work there? There are at least three good reasons:

1. The employer may know someone else who is hiring. Impressed by your follow-up, he or she recommends you.
2. An opening for a job that you do want becomes available at this facility. You are remembered for your thoughtfulness.
3. At this time, when courtesy and consideration for others are disappearing, it is the right thing to do.

Go to page 330 to complete Prescription for Success 12-2

Thank You–Plus Letter

If you want the job (see the next section for how-tos on making that decision), then take the time to write a thank-you–plus letter. The "plus" refers to

1642 Windhill Way
San Antonio, TX 78220
October 18, 2010

Nancy Henderson, Office Manager
Craigmore Pediatric Clinic
4979 Coffee Road
San Antonio, TX 78229

Dear Ms. Henderson:

Thank you so much for the time you spent with me yesterday. You have a busy schedule, and I appreciate the time you took to describe the opening for a medical assistant at Craigmore Pediatric. The Clinic enjoys a good reputation in San Antonio for the services it provides children in the community, and it was a pleasure to learn more about it.

Sincerely,

Karen Gonzalez

Karen Gonzalez

Figure 12-1   A simple thank-you letter.

a paragraph or two in which you do at least one of the following:

- Briefly summarize your qualifications in relation to the job as it was discussed in the interview
- Point out specifically how you can make a positive contribution—again, based on details you learned

Let the employer know you want the job and hope to be the candidate selected. Include your full name and telephone number. Figure 12-2 shows an example of a thank-you–plus letter.

Thank-you notes should be sent no later than the day after the interview. Consider keeping a box of cards in the car and writing the note immediately after you leave the interview. Interviewers will be impressed when they receive your note the very next day.

For some jobs, such as administrative positions, e-mailing a thank-you note may be acceptable because it demonstrates computer proficiency. Take the same care you would with a written letter: include a salutation, write complete sentences, use correct grammar, spell all words correctly, and use a proper closing. (Review Figure 10-7, which shows the proper format for a business letter.)

1642 Windhill Way
San Antonio, TX 78220
October 18, 2010

Nancy Henderson, Office Manager
Craigmore Pediatric Clinic
4979 Coffee Road
San Antonio, TX 78229

Dear Ms. Henderson:

Thank you so much for the time you spent with me yesterday. You have a busy schedule, and I appreciate the time you took to describe the opening for a medical assistant at Craigmore Pediatric. The Clinic enjoys a good reputation in San Antonio for the services it provides children in the community, and it was a pleasure to learn more about it.

After visiting your facility and meeting the health professionals who work there, I sincerely believe I could make a positive contribution to your facility. My ability to communicate in both English and Spanish would allow me to work with patients from various cultural backgrounds. My previous experience working in a day care facility gave me a love for and understanding of children that enables me to work effectively with them. Finally, my organizational skills and knowledge of current insurance requirements would be of benefit in helping to develop the new billing system you described.

I am interested in this position and enthusiastic about working at Craigmore Pediatric. Please let me know if you need anything further from me. I can be reached at (210) 123-4567. I look forward to hearing from you.

Sincerely,

Karen Gonzalez

Karen Gonzalez

Figure 12-2 Thank-you–plus letter.

Go to page 330 to complete Prescription for Success 12-3

ALERT YOUR REFERENCES

If you left a reference sheet with the interviewer, call your references as soon as possible to tell them they may receive a call. Of course, they already know that you have given their names out as references. (You did ask them, right?) Give them the job title, nature of the work, and type of facility. Add anything you learned about the type of candidate the employer is seeking. This gives your references an opportunity to stress those features that best support your bid for the job. Help them to help you by keeping them informed.

WHEN TO CALL BACK

Following up after an interview is a kind of balancing act: you don't want to be considered a pest by calling too soon and too frequently. On the other hand, you took the time to attend the interview and have a right to be informed when the hiring decision is made.

The best strategy is to wait until the day after you were told a decision would be made. Call and identify yourself and inquire about the decision. If none has been made, ask when you might expect to hear. Use your best telephone manners. This is still part of the interview, and courtesy counts. Never express impatience about a delay. You want to show interest, but you don't want to pressure the employer for a decision he or she is not ready to make. Sometimes the interviewer is deciding between two candidates and the decision may be influenced by your follow-up.

IS THIS THE JOB FOR YOU?

Jobs are usually not offered on the spot during the first interview. If this does happen to you, it is a good idea to ask when a decision is needed and say that you are very interested (if you are) but need a little time to make a decision. There are exceptions, of course. You may have performed your clinical work at this site and know for sure that this is the place for you. In this case, the interview may be a formality and it makes sense to accept the position immediately.

Interviewers will usually give you a time range during which a hiring decision will be made. You, too, need to make a decision: if this position is offered, will you accept it? Many factors will influence your decision. In Chapter 9, we discussed how the job market is affected by various economic and governmental conditions. When the unemployment rate is high, you probably can't be as choosy about the job you take. In fact, you may have very few choices, because there will be more candidates competing for a limited number of positions. You can be more selective when the unemployment rate is low. Of course, your location and specific occupation will influence the number of opportunities available to you. Some parts of the country are highly desirable places to live, and competition is intense. And some occupations will be in either high or low demand, depending on current health care trends. Box 12-1 contains questions to help you select an appropriate job.

Although you should consider these questions carefully, remember that the job that is "exactly what you want" probably doesn't exist. Finding

---

BOX 12-1 Questions to Guide the Job-Selection Process

Here are some questions to guide your thinking about the specific job and facility in which you would be working:

1. Do the job duties match my skills and interests?
2. How closely do the job and facility match my work preferences?
3. Does the facility appear to follow safe and ethical practices?
4. Do I agree with the mission and values of the organization?
5. Can I make a positive contribution?
6. Who are the clients or patients? Will I enjoy working with them?
7. How well do I think I would fit in?
8. Are there opportunities to learn?
9. Will there be opportunities for advancement?
10. Can I commit to the required schedule?
11. Is the management style compatible with my work style?
12. How did the facility "feel"?

---

the right job for you is a matter of finding a close match on the most important elements. You are starting a new career, and there are certain factors that will help your long-term success. Working with someone who is interested in teaching you, for example, may be a better choice than choosing a slightly higher-paying position that offers no opportunities for acquiring new skills. Many health care facilities make it a practice to promote from within. If there is a facility where you want to work, consider taking a job that gets you in the door.

DISCUSSING SALARY: WHEN AND HOW

Most career experts recommend that you not discuss salary with a potential employer until you have been offered the job. In many cases, this won't be an issue because salaries are predetermined and not negotiable. Some occupations, such as nursing, have labor unions, and the employer cannot change agreed-on salaries for specific positions.

Doing your research before you attend an interview may provide you with this information. If a range of salary is given for a position, the amount offered to you will most likely depend on the experience you bring to the job. Recent graduates tend to start at the low end of a range, earning more as they gain experience.

CONSIDERING AN OFFER

A job offer may be extended in a telephone call, at a second or even third interview, or in a letter. Even if you feel quite sure that this is the right job, you still need to be sure that you have all the information needed to make a final decision. It is essential that you understand the following:

☐ The **exact duties** you will be required to perform. If you haven't seen a written job description, ask for it now. If there is no written description, ask for a detailed oral explanation if this wasn't done in the interview.

☐ **Start date.** Be sure you are clear about the exact date and time you are to report for work.

☐ The **days and hours** you will work. Ask about the likelihood of required overtime and any change of hours or days that might take place in the future.

☐ Your **salary.** Earnings are expressed in various ways: hourly, weekly, biweekly, monthly, or annual rates. If you are quoted a rate that you aren't familiar with, you might want to convert it to one you know. For example, if you are accustomed to thinking in terms of amount per hour but are given a monthly salary, you may want to calculate the hourly equivalent (Figure 12-3).

☐ **Orientation and/or training given.** This is especially important for recent graduates. Learning the customs and practices of the facility can make a big difference in your success. Letting the employer know that you are interested in learning as much as possible about the facility and the job communicates the message that you are motivated and interested in being prepared to do your best.

You may have received all this information in the interview(s). Don't hesitate, however, to ask about anything you don't fully understand. It is far better to take the time now rather than to discover later that the job or working conditions were not what you expected. If you didn't have an opportunity to see any more than the interviewer's office, be sure to ask for a complete tour of the facility before deciding whether to accept the job.

UNDERSTANDING BENEFITS

Benefits can represent a significant portion of your **compensation.** Health insurance, for example, can cost hundreds of dollars per month for a family of four. If full family coverage is offered by the employer, this may be worth thousands of dollars each year. Find out if you must pay part of the cost of the premiums and what type of coverage is provided. Health insurance for individuals (or families) is often more expensive than the group rates available through an employer. And many individuals find it difficult to qualify on their own. Health insurance is becoming an increasingly important benefit to consider

---

Calculating How Much You Will Earn

Basic Facts: Based on a 40-hour week: 1 year = 12 months = 52 weeks = 2080 work hours

If you are paid every 2 weeks, you will receive 26 paychecks per year.

Conversions Based on Annual Salary of $24,000.00

Monthly = $24,000/12 = $2000.00
Biweekly = $24,000/26 = $923.07
Weekly = $24,000/52 = $461.54
Hourly = $24,000/2080 = $11.54

Conversions Based on Hourly Rate of $11.00

Weekly = $11 x 40 = $440.00
Biweekly = $11 x 80 = $880.00
Monthly = $11 x 2080/12 = $1906.67
Annually = $11 x 2080 = $22,880.00

Figure 12-3 Calculating your pay: converting hourly, monthly, and annual wages.

when choosing where to work. There are other types of insurance, too, that can add value to the benefits package, including dental, vision, life, and disability.

If you are planning to continue your education, tuition benefits might be important to you. Some employers cover all or part of educational expenses if the studies are related to your work and you receive a grade of C or better. Time off to take classes and workshops is an additional advantage. This benefit is especially helpful for health care professionals who are required to earn continuing education units on a regular basis. Related professional expenses that some employers cover are the dues for professional organizations and required uniforms.

Other benefits to consider when calculating your overall compensation include the number of paid vacation, holiday, and personal days offered and whether there is a retirement plan such as a **401(k) retirement plan**. With this plan, you choose an amount to be deducted from your earnings each pay period. You pay no taxes on this money until you withdraw it anytime after you reach age 59½. The money is invested, often in mutual funds. Some employers match a certain percentage of the money you save, which is like giving you an additional, tax-free salary.

When considering the compensation offered by an employer, think in terms of the total package. One job may offer a higher hourly rate but require you to pay part of your health insurance premium. You may end up financially ahead by accepting the lower salary. On the other hand, if you are included on your spouse's group insurance plan, this might not be significant. Salary alone should not be the determining factor when deciding whether a job "pays enough."

Let's look at an example. Suppose you are offered Job A, which pays $24,000 and includes medical insurance, for which the employer pays $2700. The total value of this package, then, is $26,700. Another employer offers you Job B at $27,000 in salary with no insurance benefits. You need insurance and plan to pay for it yourself with the extra salary you will earn. Assuming that everything else about the two jobs is equal, with which one would you come out ahead financially? Almost certainly Job A. Let's see why.

1. You will pay taxes on wages of $24,000 rather than $27,000. (Health insurance benefits are not taxed.)
2. The $2700 for medical insurance is the cost for a member of a group plan. If you buy insurance as an individual, it may cost you even more. (And you may have to qualify medically, which makes it more difficult to get.)

Job A		
$24,000 – $7200 (standard tax deduction and single exemption)	=	$16,800 (taxable income)
$16,800 × 15% tax rate	=	$2520 (taxes)
$24,000 – $2520	=	**$21,480** (amount of money you keep)

Job B		
$27,000 – $7200	=	$19,800 (taxable income)
$19,800 × 15%	=	$2970 (taxes)
$27,000 – $2970	=	$24,030
$24,030 – $2700 (amount spent on health insurance)	=	**$21,330** (amount of money you keep)

The lesson here is to collect information and consider all aspects of the compensation plan. Although this was just an example, it shows how important it is to do the math. If you are unsure about how to do these calculations, ask for help. Your long-term financial health depends on it.

ACCEPTING AN OFFER

When you accept a job, express your appreciation and enthusiasm. In addition to responding orally, write a letter of acceptance. The letter should include a summary of what you understand to be the terms of employment. Figure 12-4 provides a sample letter.

When speaking with the employer, inquire about any necessary follow-up activities. It is also a good idea to disclose any future commitments or other factors that will affect your work. For example, if your son is scheduled for surgery next month and you know you will need to take several days off to take care of him, let the employer know this during the hiring process. It is a sign of integrity to make important disclosures before the hiring is completed. There may be little risk of losing the job by revealing reasonable, unavoidable future commitments. If the employer does refuse to accommodate you, it is better to learn now that this job lacks flexibility regarding family needs. You may want to reconsider your acceptance. (Be aware, however, that employers cannot grant repeated requests for days off because of family responsibilities. Their first responsibility must be to the patients they serve.)

1642 Windhill Way
San Antonio, TX 78220
October 18, 2010

Nancy Henderson, Office Manager
Craigmore Pediatric Clinic
4979 Coffee Road
San Antonio, TX 78229

Dear Ms. Henderson:

I was very pleased to receive your telephone call this morning advising me that I have been chosen to fill the medical assistant position at Craigmore Pediatric. This letter confirms my response to accept your offer. I am very excited about joining your organization and look forward to reporting for work at 9:00 a.m. on November 8, 2010.

Thank you for placing your confidence in me. I will do my best to merit your support.

Sincerely,

Karen Gonzalez
Karen Gonzalez

Figure 12-4 A sample letter of acceptance.

You may want this job but need to negotiate some conditions. For example, suppose the work hours are 8:00 AM to 5:00 PM. You have a 3-year-old child who cannot be left at day care before 7:45 AM, and it takes at least 25 minutes to drive to work. It is better to ask if you can work from 8:30 AM to 5:30 PM than to take the position and arrive late every day.

Many problems on the job can be avoided by discussing them openly in advance. (Again, you must also consider the employer's needs. Accommodations like this are not always possible if they disrupt the facility's schedule and patient flow.) And sometimes, having a "Plan B" will save the day—in this case, having someone reliable who can take your child to day care.

Go to page 330 to complete Prescription for Success 12-4

WHAT TO EXPECT

Once you are hired, employers can ask questions that were unacceptable during the hiring process. Information that cannot be used to make hiring decisions is often necessary to complete personnel requirements. Examples include the following[1]:

1. Provide proof of your age (to ensure you are of legal age to work).
2. Provide verification that you can legally work in the United States.
3. Identify your race (for affirmative action statistics, if applicable in your state).
4. Supply a photograph (for identification).
5. State your marital status and number and ages of your children (for insurance).
6. Give the name and address of a relative (for notification in case of emergency).
7. Provide your Social Security number (for tax purposes).

There may be mandatory health tests and immunizations. In addition, some employers require drug tests and background checks for all employees.

If you are asked to sign an employment contract, read it carefully first. As with all other employment issues, ask about anything you don't understand. Also, be sure to ask for a copy of anything you sign.

TURNING DOWN A JOB OFFER

After careful consideration, you may decide not to accept a job offer. It is not necessary to explain your reasons to the employer. Do express your appreciation and thanks for the opportunity, and do send a thank-you note. In addition to being an expression of courtesy, this leaves a positive impression on all employers. You may want to work at this facility in the future. Figure 12-5 is a sample refusal letter.

Go to page 331 to complete Prescription for Success 12-5

IF YOU DON'T GET THE JOB

"Failure is a delay, but not a defeat. It is a temporary detour, not a dead-end street."
—*William Arthur Ward*

It can be difficult when you are not selected for a job you really want. There are many reasons

---

BOX 12-2   Why Job Applicants Fail to Get Hired

1. Failure to sell themselves by clearly presenting their skills and qualifications
2. Too much interest in what's in it for them rather than what they can give
3. Unprofessional behavior or lack of courtesy
4. Lack of enthusiasm and interest in the job
5. Poor appearance
6. Poor communication skills
7. Unrealistic job expectations
8. Negative or critical attitude
9. Arrived late, brought children or the person who provided transportation, or other demonstrations of poor organizational skills

---

why applicants don't get hired. Some you can't change and must simply accept, such as the following:

- There was another applicant with more experience or skills that more closely met the employer's current needs.
- An employee in the organization decided to apply for the job.
- The employer believed that someone else was a better "match" for the organization in terms of work style, preferences, and so on.
- Budget cuts or other unexpected events prevented anyone from being hired at this time.

On the other hand, you may have lost this opportunity for reasons you can change. How do you know? First, do an honest review of your postinterview evaluation, school record, and resume. Are you presenting yourself in the best possible way? Second, look over the list in Box 12-2. Health care employers and career services personnel name these as major reasons why job applicants fail to get hired. Do you recognize anything that might apply to you?

You must be honest with yourself and commit to improving your attitude and/or job-search skills. If necessary, seek advice from your instructor, career services personnel, or mentor. Work on creating a winning attitude that will help you develop the interviewing skills it takes to get hired. Seek support from friends and family members if you are feeling down. They can help you keep your perspective and boost your self-confidence if it's a little low.

Although you may not feel enthusiastic about writing a note to an employer who chooses another applicant, consider this: you may have come in a close second. The next opening may be

1642 Windhill Way
San Antonio, TX 78220
October 18, 2010

Nancy Henderson, Office Manager
Craigmore Pediatric Clinic
4979 Coffee Road
San Antonio, TX 78229

Dear Ms. Henderson:

Thank you so much for your telephone call this morning advising me that I have been chosen
to fill the medical assistant position at Craigmore Pediatric. I told you I would give you a
response within one day. After much careful consideration, I have decided to decline the offer
at this time.

This was not an easy decision to make, and I hope it does not exclude me from future consideration at Craigmore Pediatric. I am sincerely grateful for your time and consideration.

Sincerely,

Karen Gonzalez
Karen Gonzalez

Figure 12-5   A sample letter of refusal.

yours! So take a few moments and demonstrate your high level of professionalism by thanking the employer and letting him or her know that you are still interested in working for the organization (Figure 12-6).

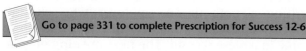

Go to page 331 to complete Prescription for Success 12-6

If you don't get hired after attending an interview that you think went well, ask for assistance from an instructor or career services personnel. You may be able to get good feedback. Or perhaps this person can call the employer on your behalf to find out how you might improve your presentation or to see if you appeared to lack needed skills. Employers are sometimes more willing to share reasons with school personnel so they can better assist their

1642 Windhill Way
San Antonio, TX 78220
October 18, 2010

Nancy Henderson, Office Manager
Craigmore Pediatric Clinic
4979 Coffee Road
San Antonio, TX 78229

Dear Ms. Henderson:

Thank you for letting me know that you have chosen another candidate for the medical assistant position at Craigmore Pediatric. I am still very interested in working at Craigmore and hope you will consider me for future openings. I believe I can make a real contribution.

I am sincerely grateful for your time and consideration. I was treated professionally by everyone at Craigmore and have great respect for your organization.

Sincerely,

Karen Gonzalez
Karen Gonzalez

Figure 12-6   A sample letter of response when you are not offered the position.

students. Be willing to listen to any constructive criticism offered and to make any needed changes.

PERSONAL REFLECTION

If you don't get a job you want, what can you learn from this experience?

_____

_____

_____

_____

_____

_____

_____

SUMMARY OF KEY IDEAS

1. Make it a point to learn something from every interview you attend.
2. Write thank-you notes to everyone who interviews you.
3. Consider all aspects of the job when deciding whether it is the one for you.
4. Learn to accept defeat gracefully.

Positive Self-Talk for This Chapter

1. I am performing better at each interview I attend.
2. I am a considerate person and follow up all interviews with a thank-you note.
3. I can gracefully handle being either selected or rejected for a job.

To Learn More

About.Com

> http://jobsearch.about.com/od/interviewsnetworking/a/intfollowup.htm
> "Job Interview Follow-Up"

Quintessential Careers

> "Job Interview Follow-Up Do's and Don'ts"
> www.quintcareers.com/interview_follow-up-dos-donts.html
> "The Art of the Follow-Up after Job Interviews"
> www.quintcareers.com/job_interview_follow-up.html
> "Job Interview and Thank You Letters"
> www.quintcareers.com/sample_thank-you_letters.html

REFERENCE

1. Lock RD: Job search, ed 3, Pacific Grove, Calif, 1996, Brooks/Cole.

INTERNET ACTIVITIES

1. Use the search phrase "job interview follow up" and write a summary of suggestions for increasing your chance of being hired.
2. Review sample letters at the Quintessential Careers website. Print copies of those you believe might be helpful models to use after your interviews.

Prescription for Success 12-1
How Did I Do? Postinterview Self-Evaluation

Name of Organization

_____

Interviewer's Name

_____

Job Title

_____

Date of Interview

_____

_____ I arrived on time.

If not, what can I do to make sure I'm not late for future interviews? _____

_____

_____

_____

_____ I displayed good nonverbal communication skills.

_____ Smiled

_____ Maintained good eye contact

_____ Waited to be seated

_____ Shook hands properly

If not, what do I need to improve?

_____

_____

_____

_____ I presented my qualifications effectively.

_____ Used examples to support my skills and qualities

_____ Used my portfolio effectively

Continued

Prescription for Success 12–1 (Continued)

_____ Accurately answered questions that tested my knowledge

_____ Performed hands-on skills correctly

If not, how can I improve my presentation skills? _____

_____

_____

_____

Are there subjects and skills I need to review? _____

_____

_____

_____

_____ I was prepared to answer the interviewer's questions.

_____ I understood the meaning of the questions.

_____ I was able to compose my thoughts and organize good responses.

_____ I had prepared for the types of questions that were asked.

If not, what steps can I take to prepare to handle interview questions more effectively?

_____

_____

_____

_____ I asked good questions.

_____ I was able to think of them as the interview progressed.

_____ I fit them in appropriately.

_____ I had appropriate questions prepared in advance.

If not, how can I be better prepared to ask what I need to know? _____

_____

_____

_____

Prescription for Success 12–1 (Continued)

What things seemed to make a positive impression on the interviewer?

_____

_____

_____

What things seemed to make a negative impression?

_____

_____

_____

What would I do differently if I could do it over?

_____

_____

_____

What things, on the part of the interviewer, made a positive impression on me?

_____

_____

_____

What things, on the part of the interviewer, made a negative impression on me?

_____

_____

_____

What did I learn from this experience?

_____

_____

_____

Continued

Prescription for Success 12–1 (Continued)

What questions, or kinds of questions, did the interviewer ask?

_____

_____

_____

_____

_____

_____

_____

_____

_____

_____

_____

Adapted from Drake JD: *The perfect interview: how to get the job you really want,* ed 2, New York, 1997, AMACOM.

Prescription for Success 12-2
Thank You

1. Imagine a job for which you interviewed and that you will probably not accept if offered.
2. Write an appropriate thank-you note.

Prescription for Success 12-3
Thank You-Plus

1. Imagine that you have interviewed for a job you would most likely accept if offered.
2. Write a thank-you–plus letter, including a description of what you can contribute.

Prescription for Success 12-4
I'll Take It!

Write a letter of acceptance for a job in your field.

Prescription for Success 12-5
No, Thank You

Write a sample refusal letter.

Prescription for Success 12-6
Thank You, Anyway

Write a follow-up letter for a position that you wanted but for which you weren't chosen.

CHAPTER 13

Success on the Job

OBJECTIVES

The information and activities in this chapter can help you:

- Choose positive actions to help you succeed at a new job.
- Make a good impression when starting a job.
- Apply your study skills to learning a new job.
- Create a personal workplace guide for quick and easy reference.
- Describe the qualifications that will increase your value as a health care professional.
- Develop—and maintain—a positive relationship with your supervisor.
- List five laws and one regulatory agency that protect the rights of employees.
- Develop effective ways to deal with difficult situations at work.
- Know when to use a grievance procedure.

KEY TERMS AND CONCEPTS

Approval Agency: An organization that sets standards for health care facilities.

Blood-Borne Pathogens: Microorganisms (germs) that cause disease and are transmitted from one person to another by means of the blood.

Burnout: A state of physical and emotional exhaustion related to conditions on the job.

Charting: Recording patient data in written or computerized form to document all aspects of diagnosis and care.

Code of Ethics: Standards of conduct created by professional organizations to guide the conduct of members of the profession.

Coding: Numbers (codes) that correspond to specific diagnoses and health care procedures. The three major sets of codes are the Current Procedural Terminology (CPT), the Health Common Procedure Coding System (HCPCS), and the International Classification of Diseases, Ninth Revision, Clinical Modification (ICD-9-CM).

Compliance Reports: Reports submitted to approval agencies to demonstrate that their standards are being followed.

Courtesy: More than saying "please" and "thank you," courtesy means treating others with kindness, consideration, and respect.

Cross-Training: Learning to perform tasks in addition to those traditionally assigned to a given occupation.

Employee Manual: A written document that contains policies, rules, and guidelines for employees.

Grievances: In the workplace, circumstances believed to be unjust and/or harmful to an employee and grounds for filing a formal complaint.

Integrity: The state of conducting oneself honestly, sincerely, and in a manner guided by high moral principles.

Morale: Group feelings of confidence, enthusiasm, and willingness to work hard to achieve goals.

Reasoning: Organizing facts so they make sense and/or help you draw correct conclusions.

Scope of Practice: Duties you are legally allowed to perform in a specific occupation. They are established and monitored by governmental or professional regulatory bodies.

Standard Precautions: Specific practices and procedures to prevent the spread of infection.

Toxic: Poisonous.

Work Ethic: A positive approach to work, including the willingness to do your best each day.

HIT THE GROUND RUNNING

Starting your first job in health care represents the achievement of a major goal. Enjoy the satisfaction of your success. At the same time, be aware that how you perform during the first months on the job will influence your future career success.

The first few weeks at work can be busy and stressful. There will be a lot to learn and many adjustments to make. Sometimes it may seem as if getting through each day is a major accomplishment. Be patient with yourself. Do your best, but remember that it takes time to learn a new job and to develop a level of comfort. There are three actions you can take to help you get a good start:
1. Shift your focus.
2. Make a good first impression.
3. Learn all you can about the job.

Action 1: Shift Your Focus

As a student, your main career-related concern was getting through school: mastering new material, learning new skills, completing assignments, and performing well on tests and evaluations. Your principal responsibility was to yourself, perhaps to a family and a job, and to your personal progress. As a health care professional, you must now shift your attention to the goals and needs of others: your employer, patients, and co-workers. You are now accountable to people who are depending on what you do and how well you do it.

Important components of professionalism in health care are the ability to understand and the willingness to attend to the needs of others. Being a professional includes possessing the ability to determine what is most appropriate and necessary to provide high-quality service. This is true whether you work in direct patient care or in services that support the health care delivery system, such as medical billing.

Demonstrate Empathy

Empathy, described in Chapter 8, means trying to see the world through the eyes of others. Health care is a people business, and understanding the feelings and experiences of others—patients, supervisors, and co-workers—is essential. Empathy means remaining professional while caring about the other person. Patients who have experienced an illness or injury sometimes feel as if they have lost control of their lives. The empathy expressed by caregivers and other support personnel can be a critical component of their recovery. Empathy is also important in relationships with supervisors and co-workers. Mutual understanding promotes effective working relationships.

Each of us will interpret a given set of circumstances differently. This interpretation is shaped by factors such as cultural background, education, religious beliefs, and previous experiences, which lead us to make certain assumptions about the world. Difficulties and misunderstandings arise because most of us take our assumptions for granted and don't see them as only *one* possibility out of many. Our view makes sense to us and provides us with a basis for dealing with life. We believe our way to be the right way, and it may not occur to us to question it. But the fact is, what is obvious to us is not necessarily obvious to others.

It takes awareness and effort to see beyond our own assumptions, but that's what is necessary to be empathetic. Let's review the following suggestions from Chapter 8 for developing empathy:
- Listen carefully to what the other person is saying. You must know his or her view before you can begin to understand, and you can't know unless you listen.
- Don't judge what you hear. You are gathering information to help you understand the other person, not to decide if he or she is right or wrong.
- Ask questions or give feedback to ensure that you have received the other person's message as it was intended.

An important point to keep in mind is that it's not necessary to agree with the beliefs of others. You must simply be aware of them and how they influence the perceptions and actions of others. In some cases, providing appropriate care requires that you try to persuade others to change ideas that may be harmful to their health. For example, many patients demand they be given antibiotics for colds and flu. They don't understand that these common illnesses are caused by viruses that cannot be killed by antibiotics. The overprescribing of these drugs has caused many bacteria (which antibiotics are intended to treat) to mutate and become resistant. In cases like this, being empathetic does not mean accepting the beliefs of the patients. It does mean respecting the individuals and understanding that what they want is relief from their symptoms. Through this understanding, you increase your chances of convincing them that they can benefit from your knowledge.

Action 2: Make a Good First Impression

Each time you meet someone new or perform a task for the first time, you have an opportunity to make a first impression. The saying "You have only one chance to make a first impression" is worth thinking about. Why is it so important? Because people tend to make judgments about others very quickly and often on the basis of very little information. In the employment setting, information from first contacts may be used by others to form opinions about the level of your professionalism and competence, as well as about the quality of the entire facility. You represent the organization for which you work.

As a recent graduate, you may not be 100% confident of your abilities. You may feel a little anxious about your performance. Keep in mind that no one expects you to know everything. However, there are two key factors under your control that influence first impressions: appearance and courtesy.

Most people are strongly influenced by visual impressions. If you look as though you know what you're doing, you are likely to be perceived that way. In Chapter 2 we discussed appropriate appearance for the health care professional. To review quickly, we said that the desired manner of dressing and grooming is as follows:

1. Conservative—out of consideration for patients
2. Clean—for the safety and consideration of others
3. Safe —for the benefit of self and others
4. Healthy—to provide a good example of wellness

The discussion about appearance in Chapter 11 applies to the workplace as well as to the interview. You will probably find there are variations in the dress and grooming considered appropriate. Some facilities are more formal than others, and what is appropriate in one is unacceptable in another. Follow the directions you receive during your interview or orientation. Read the written dress code. And remember, for a new employee it is better to be more rather than less conservative.

Much more than simply using good manners, **courtesy** refers to being considerate and helpful. It means respecting the feelings of others and showing appreciation for the help you receive when you are new on the job. You are establishing relationships with co-workers, and courtesy will go a long way toward providing a good foundation for these important relationships.

PERSONAL REFLECTION

Describe a time when someone made a negative impression on you when you first met. Did your impression change after you got to know the person? Why and how? Did it take a long time to change?

_____

_____

_____

_____

Action 3: Learn All You Can about Your Job

The first few weeks at a new job can seem overwhelming. Your educational program provided you with occupational knowledge and skills. But there will be a lot more to learn when you start your first job—any new job, in fact—because each facility has its own policies, rules, and procedures. Add to this the need to know the proper operation of equipment, location of supplies, and correct way to fill out forms, and you have a full course to master: Job 101.

The good news is you have what it takes to pass this course with flying colors. If you approach it with a "can do" attitude and apply the same skills that helped you succeed in school, you can learn and master your job systematically and effectively. Chapter 1 pointed out that "school skills" have valuable applications on the job. Let's see how you can use some of them now to succeed in your new environment.

Using Your Note-Taking Skills

Your supervisor and co-workers will be important sources of useful information. Just as you took notes in class, you can profit from taking notes on the job. These notes can serve as both learning aids and reference materials. Some note-taking situations will be formal, such as structured orientation sessions and employee training programs. Informal situations in which note-taking is useful include receiving explanations and demonstrations from your supervisor and fellow employees. You can gain a lot from taking notes, including the following:

- It allows you to concentrate on what is being presented.
- It reinforces what you hear, through the act of writing it down.
- It creates a record of information to study later.
- It allows you to put together a reference so you won't have to ask the same questions again.
- It demonstrates to your employer and co-workers that you care about your work and are detail-oriented.

Taking and using notes involves three different ways of learning: listening, writing, and reading. This variety will reinforce your learning and help you master the new information you need for your job.

Remember that a key factor in effective note-taking is careful listening. This applies, of course, to all communication, whether you are taking notes or not. Take full advantage of workplace learning opportunities by clearing your mind of other thoughts, focusing on what the speaker is saying, and asking questions to clarify anything you don't understand.

As you did in class, use an organizing scheme when taking notes: write down the key ideas, steps in a procedure, and/or important facts. Spend a few minutes after work editing your notes, if necessary, and reviewing the important points. Taking a few minutes each day to review them and "rehearse" your job duties will give you confidence and make your time on the job more productive. You might want to review the section on note-taking in Chapter 5.

Asking Questions

The potentially negative consequences of workplace errors make the ability to ask appropriate questions an essential professional skill. This applies to all types of health care employment situations, such as the following:

- Direct patient care in which the physical safety of both you and the patient is at risk
- Use of equipment, chemicals, and other materials that can be hazardous if handled incorrectly
- Administrative responsibilities in which errors can jeopardize the facility's standing with a regulatory agency
- Coding and billing tasks in which errors can cause rejection of payment by insurance companies, Medicare, and other agencies

Knowing when to ask questions is important. Whenever possible, use resources, observe, and think through situations to find the answer for yourself. If you cannot find the answer, there isn't time to do research, or the situation is urgent, don't hesitate to ask an appropriate person—someone who has the training and experience to know the answer or where to find it. In situations that are not urgent, choose a convenient time for the other person. It is also important not to ask questions about patients in the presence of anyone else, including other patients. Remember that the patient's right to privacy is protected by law. (Patient confidentiality is discussed in more detail later in this chapter.)

Creating a Workplace Reference Guide

When starting a new job, it can be helpful to create a workplace reference guide. If you started a personal reference guide, as recommended in Chapter 7, you can add an on-the-job section. What should you include? The following are some items you might find useful:

- ☐ Materials given to you during orientation or training sessions
- ☐ Notes taken during training sessions
- ☐ The name and telephone number of the person to contact if you must be absent
- ☐ Schedules: holidays, vacation, meetings, and weekly schedules if they vary
- ☐ Facility staff directories and important phone numbers
- ☐ Maps and floor plans if you work in a large facility
- ☐ Notes from meetings attended
- ☐ Printed instructions and other how-to information
- ☐ Instructions about what to do in case of an emergency
- ☐ Procedures to follow during inclement weather
- ☐ Organizational charts and chains of command (who supervises whom)

You can organize your guide in several ways. If you work mostly at a desk or in one location, a standard-sized three-ring binder is a convenient place to store information. For jobs that involve moving around, such as in a hospital, a pocket-sized reference system you can carry with you works well. For example, you can write important information on index cards, punch a hole in the corner of each card, and hook the cards together with a metal ring. Or carry a small notebook. You might want to use a personal digital assistant (PDA). Having everything in one place will be a big help when things get busy and you want to find something quickly.

Using Your Reading Skills

Reading is not limited to classroom-based learning. Printed materials are the source of important job-related information. The following examples highlight a few of the most common ones:

- **Employee manuals.** These contain policies and rules regarding employee conduct, holidays and vacations, the grievance procedure (discussed later in this chapter), and other topics related to the employer-employee relationship. Unfortunately, many people don't take the time to study the employee manual. Although it may not be very exciting reading, it contains facts to help prevent problems and misunderstandings that cause the kind of excitement you don't want to happen on the job. If you don't receive an employee manual your first day on the job, request one.

- **Policy and procedure handbooks.** Facilities create manuals to provide standard instructions for routinely performed tasks. Although it may not be necessary for you to read the entire manual, you should study the sections that apply to your job. Pay special attention to procedures to follow in emergency situations. Knowing where to find this information quickly when needed has the potential to save lives. It is your responsibility to read and study workplace manuals and handbooks. You may not be tested on them, but you cannot use the defense that you "didn't know" if the information was in a manual you should have read.

- **Regulatory and approval agency standards.** Health care facilities are regulated by a variety of government and private agencies. Following the standards and rules set by these agencies is critical in determining the success—even the survival—of a facility. For example, reimbursement for Medicare patients requires the strict observance of certain guidelines. It is important that you know and understand all requirements that affect your job. Important regulatory agencies include the Occupational Safety and Health Administration (OSHA), which oversees worker safety; the Clinical Laboratory Improvement Amendments (CLIA), which regulates all laboratory testing on humans; and The Joint Commission, which evaluates the quality and safety of care for more than 15,000 health care organizations.

- **Instructions and technical manuals.** Techniques and equipment for today's jobs are more complex than ever. Being able to read and follow instructions (often called *documentation,* especially when applied to computer software) is an important job skill. Examples include instructions for using equipment, performing laboratory tests, mailing special packages, and using computer programs. The proper use of equipment and supplies is essential in health care because their misuse can result in serious consequences, including injury to the professional and/or patient.

- **Professional publications.** These include general health care newsletters and journals and those that apply to your specialty. They help you keep up-to-date in your field, which is essential in

health care. (See the section entitled "Continue to Learn," later in this chapter.)

When reading technical material, apply the following techniques for effective reading, suggested in Chapter 5:

1. Preview the material quickly.
2. Ask yourself questions about the material and look for the answers as you read each section.
3. Mark anything you don't understand.
4. Periodically review the material.

Remember that repetition over time is the best way to learn. You can see the power of repetition in action by observing experienced professionals at work. Their self-confidence and ability to perform duties smoothly and effectively develop over time. Acquiring and applying knowledge is based on the same principle.

Using Your Observation Skills

There are important things you need to know about the workplace that no one will think to tell you. They are not written down anywhere and may not even be discussed. Everyone simply takes them for granted. These are the factors that make up the organizational culture, discussed in Chapter 8. Recall that this culture consists of the customs and expectations of an organization and includes the following:

- **Level of formality:** Does Dr. Patricia Abrams want the staff to call her "Dr. Abrams" or "Dr. Pat"?
- **Amount of at-work socializing among employees:** Does everyone go out to lunch to celebrate birthdays and holidays, or do individuals who have become friends at work plan these events on their own time?
- **Organizational values:** What are the most valued employee characteristics?
- **Management styles:** Are employees closely supervised or given lots of freedom?
- **Methods of communication:** Does your supervisor prefer all requests in writing?
- **Daily customs:** Who goes to lunch first?

You can learn the organizational culture and discover how to fit in as a new employee by observing carefully and asking questions. "Knowing the ropes" can influence your job performance. It usually takes time to understand the organizational culture, but it is well worth the effort.

You may notice that some of the procedures and methods used at your workplace are different from those you learned in school. As we discussed in Chapter 7, there is often a variety of correct ways to perform a given procedure. Some experienced professionals develop preferences or acceptable (in terms of safety and effectiveness) shortcuts. Your facility may have specific reasons for using a different method. Use the method that is most comfortable for you *and* meets facility requirements. Never suggest that another employee is wrong because he or she is not doing something the way you learned it in school. The only exception is if you believe a law or safety measure is being violated. Under these circumstances, it is usually best to speak first with your co-worker. Then, if necessary, speak with your supervisor. And never feel pressured, because you are new, to perform a task in a way you know to be unsafe.

Taking the Time to Learn

Taking the time to learn your job well will pay off in the future. Applying your study skills at work will increase your confidence and decrease your frustration. At the same time, you'll be building a foundation for progressing in your career and assuming increased responsibilities. For those who wish to climb the career ladder in their occupational area, this foundation will provide a solid base for advanced formal studies.

Go to page 351 to complete Prescription for Success 13-1

DEVELOPING YOUR WORKPLACE COMPETENCIES

In Chapter 1 we introduced lists of competencies that employers value in their employees, including items from the SCANS report and standards from the National Consortium on Health Science and Technology Education. What better way to learn about achieving success on the job than going directly to the source of information—the employers themselves? The following sections discuss a number of these competencies and how you can apply them to your job in health care.

Believe in Your Self-Worth

> *"Positive feelings about oneself are essential to enhancing the life force in self and others."*
> —*Mattie Collins*

Believing in your self-worth means that you value yourself and your actions. You consider both to be important and deserving of respect. This enables you to recognize that you and your work truly make a difference. These beliefs provide the foundation for all other career competencies, because they generate the self-confidence necessary to ask questions, learn new skills, and build positive relationships with others.

Go to page 351 to complete Prescription for Success 13-2

Demonstrate Integrity and Honesty

Integrity means having sound moral principles and being sincere and honest. Let's look at some examples of workplace behavior that demonstrate integrity.

☐ **Admit when you make a mistake.** Covering up errors in the health care environment can have serious consequences. For example, if lab results are reported for the wrong patient, a false diagnosis can cause ineffective—or even harmful—treatment to be prescribed.

☐ **Conduct yourself ethically.** This means conforming to established standards for moral and correct behavior. In addition to ethical standards that apply to society as a whole, each health care profession has a **Code of Ethics** that serves as a guide for proper conduct. Box 13-1 contains a Code of Ethics developed for medical assistants by the American Association of Medical Assistants (AAMA). (Note: The American Medical Technologists organization also has a code for medical assistants.) You should become familiar with the code for your profession.

BOX 13-1 **American Association of Medical Assistants Code of Ethics**

The Code of Ethics of the American Association of Medical Assistants (AAMA) shall set forth principles of ethical and moral conduct as they relate to the medical profession and the particular practice of medical assisting.

Members of AAMA dedicated to the conscientious pursuit of their profession, and thus desiring to merit the high regard of the entire medical profession and the respect of the general public which they serve, do pledge themselves to strive always to:

A. render service with full respect for the dignity of humanity

B. respect confidential information obtained through employment unless legally authorized or required by responsible performance of duty to divulge such information

C. uphold the honor and high principles of the profession and accept its disciplines

D. seek to continually improve the knowledge and skills of medical assistants for the benefit of patients and professional colleagues

E. participate in additional service activities aimed toward improving the health and well-being of the community

---

Copyright by the American Association of Medical Assistants Inc.

☐ **Develop a strong work ethic.** This means taking a positive approach to work. It means that you take your work seriously, are responsible, and give each task you perform your best effort.

☐ **Be loyal to your employer.** As long as you are being paid by an employer, it is your obligation to demonstrate loyalty. Examples of ways to show loyalty include the following:

• Dedicating your time on the job exclusively to work. Personal tasks and telephone calls should be limited to the lunch hour or break time.

• Not using your employer's computer to send personal e-mails or to surf the Internet at any time. This is becoming a growing problem for employers. Remember, anything that occurs online can be traced back to you.

• Never taking anything that belongs to the employer. Even small items, such as pens, add up when every employee thinks, "This is so small it won't make any difference." Taking something, however small or inexpensive, is theft. Don't contribute to the rising cost of health care by increasing your employer's expenses.

• Not speaking badly about your employer. Speaking badly serves no purpose other than lowering employee **morale.** If overheard by patients, it can create doubts in their minds about the quality of care they are receiving. Seek solutions by discussing legitimate concerns directly with your supervisor.

• Not complaining about your job, working conditions, and so on. Again, this does nothing to resolve the problem. Seek positive solutions through action or by speaking with someone who has the power to address the issue.

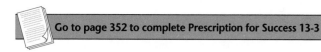

Go to page 352 to complete Prescription for Success 13-3

Respect Confidentiality

As a health care professional, you have an ethical and legal responsibility to respect patient confidentiality. As mentioned in Chapters 1 and 8, this includes both oral and written communications. You must be willing to monitor your work habits and conversation to make sure this important patient right is constantly guarded. Confidentiality must be safeguarded for both the patient's sake and yours. Serious or habitual disregard of this principle can be a cause for dismissal of health care personnel, as well as fines and disciplinary action against the facility.

The necessity to maintain patient confidentiality has increased in recent years as a result of federal legislation, known as HIPAA, passed in 1996. These letters stand for the Health Insurance Portability and Accountability Act. The following are a few of the major provisions in this act:

1. Make it easier for employees to maintain health insurance coverage when they change jobs
2. Adopt national standards for electronic health care transactions
3. Protect the privacy of every patient's health information

All health care facilities have developed policies and procedures to ensure that medical privacy is maintained. It is essential that you learn and strictly follow these policies to prevent problems for yourself and for your employer. The following suggestions, although not comprehensive, can help you avoid unintentional "leaks" of private information during a busy workday:

• Never discuss patient issues with anyone other than health care professionals who are directly involved in the care of the patient, and confine discussion to matters pertaining to this care.

• Limit allowable discussion to locations where you won't be overheard.

• When speaking with patients about personal matters, do so in a voice that they but not anyone else can hear.

• Take care when speaking to and about patients on the telephone so that you are not overheard by others in the area.

• Leave patient-related matters at the workplace. Although it is natural to want to share your work with family and friends, any reference to patients and "interesting cases" is illegal.

• Clear computer screens containing patient records when you leave the computer.

• Don't leave paperwork or files containing patient information on reception counters and other areas where they can be viewed by unauthorized individuals.

• Do not discuss any information with anyone, even a patient's spouse or relative, without the written permission of the patient.

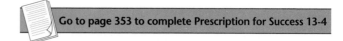

Go to page 353 to complete Prescription for Success 13-4

In addition to patient confidentiality, health care professionals have an obligation to protect the privacy of the facility where they work. Engaging in conversation about problems at work is a common employee activity. But airing what you consider to be the facility's "dirty laundry" does nothing to help the situation. In fact, it can have the opposite effect by damaging its reputation and undermining patient confidence. Problems must be addressed at the source if positive changes are to be made.

A final note regarding privacy is to respect your own. This means that personal problems don't belong at work and should not be discussed there. It is not the responsibility of co-workers to listen to and spend time advising you about personal affairs. Remember that your focus should be on work activities.

Be Responsible

Employees who are responsible and can be depended on to do what is expected—and then some—are worth their weight in gold. Today's health care environment puts many demands on employers. For example, they must provide high-quality services for patients, meet administrative deadlines, comply with a variety of regulations, and control operating costs. This is why it is essential that your employers be able to depend on you. Acting responsibly means that your actions include the following:

- ☐ **Complete all tasks.** This includes returning equipment and supplies to their proper places for the next person who needs them.
- ☐ **Strive for accuracy.** Examples of the many health care tasks in which accuracy is critical include patient **charting**, medical **coding** and billing, filling out **compliance reports** and lab reports, preparing sterile fields, and providing patient education.
- ☐ **Help out when needed, even when it's not your job.** The unexpected must be anticipated in health care. Co-workers are sometimes absent, emergencies occur, and situations can quickly change from routine to urgent. A career in health care requires that you be willing to do what it takes to get the job done.
- ☐ **Be on time.** This includes arriving at work on time every day, returning promptly from lunch and breaks, and getting to meetings and appointments on time. One of the major complaints of patients is having to wait. They feel that their time is not respected. Sometimes this cannot be helped, but avoid being the cause yourself. Absences should occur only for real emergencies. Have backup plans for transportation and childcare.
- ☐ **Follow through with everything you are directed or have offered to do.** If you cannot perform a task or need assistance, let your supervisor know so the task can be reassigned or help recruited. Don't allow work to go undone because you couldn't get to it yourself.

 Go to page 354 to complete Prescription for Success 13-5

Work Effectively with Others

Getting along with others is one of the most talked-about, yet taken-for-granted workplace skills. Failure to work well with others is a major cause of employee dismissal because it reduces the health care facility's capability to provide high-quality service. Applying the people skills discussed in Chapter 8 and earlier in this chapter will help you establish positive relationships with co-workers. How well you develop your people skills will greatly influence your future.

High-quality health care requires the cooperation of many specialized individuals. And new types of professionals, in response to medical advances and increasingly complex delivery systems, continue to join the team. Whatever your particular occupation, you will be working with a variety of people who will bring different personalities, work styles, personal goals, and skill levels to the job. Your challenge will be to work in harmony with them all because each one is equally important to successful care delivery.

Working with Your Supervisor

How well you get along with your supervisor can make the difference between looking forward to each workday or dreading the thought of showing up (Figure 13-1). The nature of this relationship influences promotions, raises, and the quality of work assignments. Indeed, it is a critical factor in determining both job success and worklife quality. But many people don't take the time or make the effort to get to know this important person. Using the information in this section will help you avoid missing what can be a career-enhancing opportunity.

Just as instructors have their own teaching and classroom management styles, described in Chapter 8, supervisors are characterized by a variety of management styles. These are shaped by the supervisor's personality, beliefs about management, personal experiences, and the organizational culture in which they work. Table 13-1 contains examples of different management styles. Your supervisor may demonstrate more than one of the styles listed. Keep in mind that there is no one right way to manage in all situations. Each has advantages and disadvantages. Certain styles are more appropriate than others in specific situations and work settings. The following are a few examples:

- Being friendly with employees is not positive if it results in too much downtime spent socializing. There is also the danger that some employees will believe there is favoritism if the supervisor is more friendly—or perceived to be—to some employees than to others.

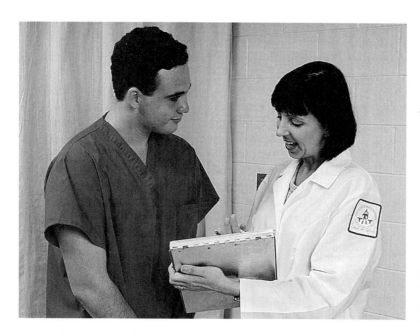

Figure 13-1 Developing a good relationship with your supervisor is an important part of career success—and work satisfaction. *(From Gerdin J: Health careers today, ed 4, St Louis, 2007, Mosby.)*

TABLE 13-1	Common Management Styles
Management Style	**Examples of Supervisor's Actions**
Micromanages	Closely monitors your work. Frequently checks on you and wants regular progress reports.
Believes employees work best on their own	Doesn't appear to pay much attention to your work unless something goes wrong.
Likes a friendly work environment	Conversation is warm and friendly. Interested in your family and other aspects of your personal life. Birthday and holidays are celebrated at the workplace.
Maintains a businesslike environment	Keeps most conversation work-related. Co-workers who become friends engage in social activities outside the workplace.
Disorganized or too busy to keep order	Loses reports you've turned in. Forgets scheduled meetings. Doesn't give you promised follow-up in a timely way. (Caution: Don't assume that because your supervisor is disorganized, he or she will tolerate *your* disorganization and accept actions such as completing assignments late.)
Values and practices order	Rarely misses deadlines and expects you to meet them, too, correctly and efficiently. Keeps lists, calendars, and orderly files.
Communicates directly	Lets you know how you are doing. Offers suggestions and criticism as needed. You know where you stand.
Communicates indirectly (or not at all)	Doesn't want to hurt your feelings. Avoids confrontations. May not tell you if you are doing something incorrectly or not to his or her liking. (Caution: May complain about you behind your back, thus depriving you of the opportunity to learn and resolve the problem.)
Believes it is the supervisor's responsibility to make most decisions	Employees are not consulted about policy changes, future plans, etc.
Believes that better decisions result when employees participate in making them	Employees are asked for their opinions. Some decisions are made as a group. (Caution: Group decision making can bog down the group and result in little being accomplished.)

- There are brilliant people who seem to be very disorganized. They may have numerous projects going and don't feel they have the time to tidy up. Don't lose the chance to learn from them because you have judged them negatively for their disorderliness.

- Inviting employee input and encouraging creativity is beneficial in some work settings. But in others, such as the emergency room, it is not appropriate. Here, employees must work as directed. Procedures must be strictly followed. Lives depend on doing work the right way—and quickly.

Your work style may not match the management style of your supervisor. This is not uncommon. Mature employees see these differences as challenges rather than obstacles. A number of constructive ways to work effectively with your supervisor in spite of differences include the following:

1. Keep communication open. One of the worst things you can do is avoid someone with whom you disagree or have difficulty. Cutting off contact is likely to increase distance and decrease understanding.

2. Follow the chain of command. This means speaking with your supervisor before going to the next level with concerns and complaints. If you are having problems with your supervisor, talk with him or her first. It is all too common for employees to bad-mouth their supervisors and discuss problems with everyone except the one person who can actually do something to resolve them: the supervisor. In fact, complaining usually results in everything but resolution. It may actually create new problems: lowered morale among co-workers who hear your complaints, lost work time, decrease in the quality of service to patients, and worsened relations with the supervisor who hears about the grumbling through the grapevine. Failure to follow the proper order can even result in dismissal.

3. Be empathetic. Your supervisor may have pressures and problems that explain his or her actions.

4. Ask questions to learn your supervisor's priorities and find out what is most important. If the following questions weren't answered in the job interview, ask them now:
   • What is the mission of this organization and/or department?
   • What are your expectations of me?
   • What do you most value in an employee?
   • How can I best contribute to the success of the organization and/or facility?
   • How often would you like me to report to you?
   • What is the best time to report to you, ask questions, and receive progress reports about my work?

5. Let your supervisor know how you work best. This can be a positive conversation: "I really want to be able to do my best work for the radiology department. I find that when my work is constantly being checked, I get nervous and tend to make more errors. Could we work out another way to monitor my progress that still meets the needs of the department?"

6. Ask for clarification if you are unclear about your job duties or exactly what is expected of you.

7. Realize the bottom line is this: you must work with your supervisor, and this means adapting to his or her style. Do your best to make the situation positive. Focus on learning as much as possible from both the supervisor and the situation.

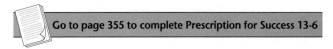

Go to page 355 to complete Prescription for Success 13-6

Think about What You Are Doing

Work in health care requires continual thinking. Nothing can be taken for granted. You must constantly pay attention to make sure that your actions make sense. Suppose that Mr. Cardenas, who doesn't understand English well, is scheduled for a lab test that requires him to follow certain procedures the day before. It wouldn't make sense for the medical assistant to give him a written instruction sheet in English. He will need directions in Spanish to ensure he is properly prepared for the test.

Health care professionals must keep their minds in gear, continually observing and thinking as they perform their duties. Your daily work can never be performed automatically. You must continually ask yourself questions, think about the significance of what you see, and use this information to determine the most appropriate action to take. As a health care professional, you cannot cruise along in neutral. Your work is too important, and the potential consequences of failing to be alert and thinking are too serious.

Solve Problems Effectively

The problem-solving method introduced in Chapter 7 is an essential workplace tool. To review quickly, it consists of the following six steps:

1. Define the problem.
2. Gather information.
3. Brainstorm alternative solutions.
4. Consider possible results and consequences.
5. Choose a solution and act on it.
6. Evaluate the results and revise as needed.

Good problem-solving skills involve both **reasoning** and creativity. Start by examining what you believe to be the problem. Try to see it from different angles. Mentally walk around the problem, looking at it from all sides. Are you defining the problem in terms of the symptoms rather than the problem itself? (Recall the case of Kathy in Chapter 7. She believed her problem to be low grades in pharmacology when it turned out to be her lack of math skills.)

Use brainstorming to come up with possible solutions. This means thinking of as many ideas as possible, from the sensible to the crazy. Seeing new possibilities requires you to think creatively because problems are often solved by using an original approach.

Although creativity generates ideas, reasoning helps you to put the ideas together in ways that work. It also helps you test potential outcomes mentally. Use it to check "What would happen if…" scenarios for the possibilities you have brainstormed. Reasoning helps you ask the right questions, such as the following:

- Based on what I know, could this solution work? Why or why not?
- Do all the pieces fit together?
- Does it make sense?

Effective solutions are the result of using creativity to generate new ideas and applying reasoning to test them. Creativity is the artist and reasoning is the critic.

Before you approach your supervisor with a problem, think it through. Do your best to come up with solutions to suggest. This demonstrates your initiative and willingness to take an active part in the problem-solving process. With experience, you will better know when to ask questions and when to choose and implement solutions on your own.

Continue to Learn

The need to learn is important in all fields today, but it is especially so in health care. This field is in a state of continual change brought about by medical discoveries, transformations in the delivery system and methods of payment, government regulations, and technologic innovations. Outdated knowledge and skills can be useless. You've got to keep up to remain effective. There are many ways to do this, including the following:

- ☐ Attend the meetings and learning activities sponsored by your professional organization.
- ☐ Read journals and publications devoted to your field, as well as books and articles about the general field of health care.
- ☐ Take courses at local schools and colleges.
- ☐ Observe and ask questions at work.
- ☐ Request information from organizations, such as the American Heart Association, that publish free educational literature. Most also have informative websites.
- ☐ Join newsgroups on the Internet, as described in Chapter 9.
- ☐ Use the Internet to explore topics of interest. (Be sure to check the reliability of Internet sources, as explained in Chapter 5.)

- ☐ Check the availability of resources at your workplace: library, reference books, journals, people with expertise and special interests.

Some employers pay for professional journal subscriptions, classes, and workshops, so ask about the policy where you work.

Go to page 356 to complete Prescription for Success 13-7

Practice Cost Control

Cost control is a major concern in health care today (Figure 13-2). The United States spends more of its total income on health care than any other nation. Unfortunately, this doesn't always result in better overall outcomes. There are several countries, for example, in which people live longer and have a lower infant mortality rate (number of babies who die within the first year of life).

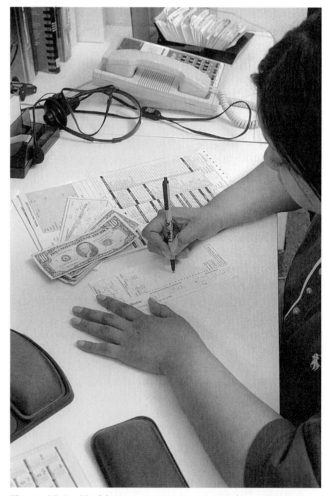

Figure 13-2 Health care costs are increasing faster than any other area of our lives. You can make a major contribution to the success of today's health care system by working to control expenses.

How can you help control costs? There are a number of ways. They may seem insignificant, but if practiced by everyone, they can make a difference.

☐ Work carefully and thoughtfully so tasks don't have to be repeated by you or anyone else. When you are being paid, time is a resource with monetary value.

☐ Don't waste supplies. Use what is needed and no more.

☐ Learn how to use supplies correctly. For example, follow the instructions when using lab test kits.

☐ Take care of equipment. Follow directions, use it carefully, practice preventive maintenance, and report any problems promptly.

☐ Never take supplies or use services for your personal use. A few "short" long-distance calls for personal business or runs through the copy machine add up quickly.

☐ Use work time for work. Your salary is a major employer expense.

Manage Yourself

Managing your personal habits effectively enables you to serve others better. How does this work? We discussed the following major components of self-management in Chapter 3:

- Attitude
- Personal organization
- Time management
- Stress reduction techniques

Failure to maintain control in these areas can negatively affect your work in a number of ways, as shown in the following examples:

- Arriving late can disrupt the schedules of patients and co-workers.
- Running out of energy before the workday is over can delay the completion of important tasks.
- Repeatedly calling in sick because of stress-related illnesses forces co-workers to fill in for you, disrupts schedules, and/or leaves tasks undone.
- Failure to prioritize tasks can result in missing important deadlines.
- Feeling tired can reduce your ability to concentrate and complete work assignments accurately.

As you can see, your personal habits are no longer just personal—they affect other people, too. Efficient use of time, for example, is especially critical in today's busy offices and clinics. The inability to maintain schedules and complete tasks in a timely way can be a serious liability on the job. By choosing a career in health care, you have made a commitment to serve others, and you owe it to your profession to offer your best efforts. And this requires good self-management.

This does not mean, however, that your life should be entirely devoted to work. In fact, just the opposite is true. You need to take time out to attend to your own needs. The key is to achieve a balance between your needs and those of others in your life: patients, employer, co-workers, family members, and friends. If you continually ignore your own needs, you can deplete your physical, mental, and emotional resources. The result will be that you have nothing left to give others.

Maintaining this balance between self, family, and work requires prioritizing and practicing good organizational and time-management skills. There will always be more to do than there is time and energy to do it. We all must make choices, and these should be based on our values. Your mission statement, described in Chapter 3, should guide these choices. For example, if spending time with your children is important to you, and you have only 2 free hours in the evening, you might choose to play games with the children instead of watching television. If your weekends are filled with housework and errands, you might look for ways your children can help with the chores and then plan a fun activity together as a family.

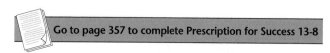
Go to page 357 to complete Prescription for Success 13-8

At the workplace, self-management means the ability to work without constant supervision. Supervisors don't have time to continually monitor their employees. You can increase your value as an employee by identifying what needs to be done and following through on tasks. Working without being reminded and told what to do will help you achieve a reputation as an excellent employee. In the event you complete your work and have extra time, look for something else to do or ask for an additional assignment. There is no such thing as "free time" on the job, and you owe it to your employer to stay busy and productive.

It is more likely you will experience the opposite problem: too much to do in too little time. In this case, learn to prioritize tasks according to the needs of your employer so the essential ones always get completed. If you are unsure about priorities, ask your supervisor for direction.

Adapt to Changing Conditions

Change is to be expected in health care environments. Adapting to change—and doing so willingly and agreeably—is an essential job skill. We have mentioned the continuing changes in health care. Other factors that require flexibility include responding to patient emergencies and ensuring that all responsibilities are covered when employees are absent. Here are a few everyday examples that demonstrate the need for flexibility:

- A dental assistant learning to assist the dentist with new laser equipment that has replaced traditional drills
- A medical insurance biller keeping informed and using revised reporting methods required for Medicare reimbursement
- An emergency medical technician agreeing to change her work schedule to cover for a fellow worker who is ill
- The members of a clinic staff learning to work with a new supervisor and under new policies that accompanied an ownership change
- A nurse developing relationships with new co-workers after the hospital reorganizes departments and staff to create a team approach to patient care
- A lab technician applying new OSHA requirements to the handling of chemicals and biologic waste
- A medical assistant learning new medical office management software

Change can be viewed as an opportunity to learn and avoid boredom on the job—or as an inconvenience that requires you to "grin and bear it." The approach you choose will influence how much satisfaction you gain from your work. Be aware that the words "That's not my job," if heard by your employer, can be fatal in the workplace. (Exception: performing tasks you are not trained or legally allowed to perform.)

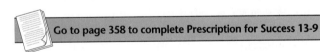

Go to page 358 to complete Prescription for Success 13-9

Be Willing to Cross-Train

Learning tasks that are usually—or used to be—performed by professionals outside your specific occupational area is known as **cross-training.** Job duties are not separated as distinctly by occupation as they once were. Certain tasks that were once performed only by nurses, for example, are now performed by other professionals. The movement toward the expansion of responsibilities has been encouraged by one of the major goals driving health care today: increasing the quality of patient care while controlling costs.

Learning additional skills adds to your value as an employee. In some cases, it will even determine your success in securing the job you want. Having opportunities to learn new skills on the job should

be viewed as a benefit, not an imposition. Take advantage of them. You are learning new skills that will enhance your career, and you're being paid at the same time!

One word of caution: check the **scope of practice** for your professional level. Some skills require you to be licensed or certified before you can legally perform them. Be sure that you know and stay within your legal limits.

Go to page 359 to complete Prescription for Success 13-10

Serve as a Role Model for Wellness

Personal habits are now recognized as having a major impact on health. In a dual effort to help people live healthier lives and avoid the expense of preventable medical problems, health care providers are placing more emphasis on promoting wellness. This is in contrast to the traditional focus on treating disease and injury. A growing number of patients want to take a more active role in the management of their health. Part of your work may involve teaching patients, as appropriate for your profession, about the practice of preventive and good wellness habits.

As a health care professional, you can encourage this positive trend by promoting the benefits of healthy living. Serve as an example of healthy lifestyle choices, as discussed in Chapter 2. Are you a good "advertisement" for the industry you represent? This applies to your life in the community outside the health care facility, too.

Avoiding Burnout

Burnout is a work-related condition in which a person experiences physical and emotional exhaustion. People experiencing burnout often have a feeling of hopelessness. They believe their efforts have no purpose.

Burnout is a growing problem among health care professionals because of the responsibilities of working with people who are ill, heavy workloads, and the increasing emphasis on efficiency and cost control. Signs of burnout include extreme fatigue, irritability, frequent illnesses, and a feeling of discouragement. Several conditions can lead to burnout, including the following:

- Continual job stress caused by factors such as constantly changing schedules, lack of feedback about work performance, and lack of recognition for accomplishments
- More tasks assigned than can be accomplished during work hours
- Long work hours and inadequate time for rest

BOX 13-2 — Suggestions for Avoiding Burnout on the Job

- Develop organizational and time management techniques that work for you to avoid feeling constantly rushed and to make time for rest and recreation. (Review Chapter 3 for suggestions.)
- Practice the stress management techniques described in Chapter 3.
- Get enough sleep. Increasing your efficiency during waking hours can make up for the extra time spent sleeping and resting.
- Make sure you are clear about your job tasks. Ask for a written job description if you don't have one. Talk with your supervisor about his or her expectations.
- Don't try to do everything yourself. Ask others for help when appropriate and needed. This includes family members and co-workers.
- Know your own limits. Don't take on more than you can manage physically and mentally.
- Develop and schedule time for interests outside of work, such as hobbies, social activities, and spiritual growth.
- Seek satisfaction within yourself. Don't depend on recognition from others. Reward yourself for your achievements.

- A feeling of never getting caught up on tasks
- Continual pressure to meet tight deadlines and complete demanding assignments

Consistent use of good self-management techniques provides protection against burnout. Box 13-2 contains a list of suggestions for avoiding burnout.

YOUR LEGAL RIGHTS

It may seem, as an employee, that you have an endless list of "shoulds" and "must dos." In fact, there are safeguards to protect your rights on the job. These range from laws to prevent discrimination to agencies charged with ensuring your physical safety. You should be aware of the major employment laws described in the following sections. Ask your employer for information about company policies, and check the library and/or the Internet for further resources.

Family Medical Leave Act

The Family Medical Leave Act (FMLA) is an act of federal legislation that was passed in 1993 to make it easier for employees to take time off to attend to health and family matters. There are certain eligibility requirements that include the following:

- ☐ You must be a public employee or work for an employer who has at least 50 employees.
- ☐ You must have worked for at least 12 months and at least 1250 hours during the 12 months immediately before the leave is to be taken.

The purpose of the leave must be (1) to take care of serious personal health problems or those of a spouse, parent, or child, or for the birth or adoption of a child; or (2) to take care of a family member who is in the Armed Forces and undergoing medical treatment or therapy or is on temporary disability because of a serious injury or illness.

Employees who take a leave under the act must be given their previous job or the equivalent at the same pay on their return. The employer is not required to pay the employee during the leave, but benefits such as medical insurance must stay in effect.

Equal Pay Act

The Equal Pay Act was passed in 1963 as an amendment to the Fair Labor Standards Act, the federal regulation of wages, hours, and working conditions. Its purpose is to protect workers from pay discrimination based on gender. Although the act protects both men and women, it is women who have traditionally been prohibited from performing certain jobs and have been paid less than men for doing the same work. Therefore most equal pay complaints are filed by women.

For a successful claim, the jobs in question must be proven to be equal. This means showing they are similar in skill, effort, and responsibility. Also, claims of unequal pay can only apply to employees in the same workplace. In other words, a medical assistant can't file a claim because the physician at another office pays a higher wage to medical assistants. She could, however, file a claim if a male medical assistant in the same office is paid more for performing similar work. The Equal Pay Act covers all categories of employees, including executives and managers.

Civil Rights Act of 1964

The Civil Rights Act is important legislation that was passed to protect the rights and opportunities of all Americans. Title VII of the act prohibits the denial of employment opportunities on the basis of race, color, religion, sex, or national origin. Once hired, employees cannot be treated differently based on these factors.

Sexual harassment is classified as a form of discrimination and is therefore illegal under Title VII.

It refers to unwelcome and unwanted sexual attention. Sexual harassment can take many forms, ranging in severity from telling dirty jokes to rape. It does not prohibit mutually agreed-on behavior between employees such as flirting and dating. (These behaviors are not recommended, however, because workplace romances that go sour can become workplace nightmares for the people involved.)

An important point to keep in mind is that the victim of sexual harassment does not have to be directly involved. Consider the example of two hospital employees who have become friends and regularly share jokes of a sexual nature. They find them amusing and stress-reducing. A third person, who works in the same department, finds them extremely offensive. She asks them to stop, but they consider her to be prissy and unreasonable. The third person may have a legitimate claim of sexual harassment.

Some people find any reference to sexual matters offensive, so it is best to play it safe by avoiding any speech or behavior that is sexual in nature. This is especially important when you are new on the job. It takes time to get to know people and the organizational culture. People respond differently, and it is best to avoid anything that might be misinterpreted. For example, remarks you intend as compliments, such as references to any part of the body, may be misinterpreted. You are in the beginning stages of establishing your reputation as a health care professional. Do everything possible to get a good start and avoid any behavior that might be interpreted as harassment.

At the same time, you need to know what to do if you are the victim. Most experts recommend that the first step of defense should be to speak directly with the harasser and request an immediate stop to the behavior you find objectionable. It is best not to let it go, hoping the problem will go away, because this can send the message that the person's actions are acceptable. As a result, the actions are likely to continue and may even get worse.

When speaking with the harasser, focus on the objectionable behavior. State exactly what you find unacceptable and tell him or her to stop. Keep a dated, written record of all events connected with the incident(s), including when you spoke to the harasser. If the behavior continues, report it to the appropriate person. This may be your supervisor or a specific person who has been appointed to deal with discrimination issues at your organization. Follow the proper procedures for filing a complaint. It is best to seek a resolution within the organization. If the problem is not resolved, however, a complaint can be filed with the Equal Employment Opportunity Commission. This must be done within 180 days of the incident.

Americans with Disabilities Act

The Americans with Disabilities Act (ADA) protects the right of disabled workers to secure and maintain employment. A disability can be either physical or mental. The act requires employers to make "reasonable accommodations" for disabled employees who have the necessary qualifications to perform the job. A reasonable accommodation refers to both the financial impact on the employer and how the modifications affect the ability of the organization to function. Examples of reasonable accommodations are to provide a specially designed desk and chair for an employee with a back injury or an adaptive computer keyboard for an administrative worker who has the use of only one hand. Ramps, wheelchair access to work areas, and phone equipment for the hearing impaired are other examples of accommodations that might be considered reasonable under the act.

Federal Age Discrimination Act

Passed in 1967, the Federal Age Discrimination Act protects workers over the age of 40 from discrimination in the workplace. Employers who have more than 20 employees are subject to this act. The following actions are prohibited if they occur because of an employee's age:

- Refusal to hire
- Dismissal
- Layoff
- Denial of a promotion
- Limits placed on wages and other benefits

Complaints about possible age discrimination that are not resolved at the workplace can be filed with the Equal Employment Opportunity Commission.

Occupational Safety and Health Act

OSHA, passed in 1970, requires employers to provide safe workplaces. The act is very comprehensive and contains a wide variety of provisions to protect workers by doing the following:

☐ Ensuring that equipment is safe and in good operating order.

☐ Keeping the environment free of **toxic** and potentially harmful wastes, chemicals, and other materials.

☐ Providing employees with training about the safe handling of chemicals, equipment, and other materials that are potentially hazardous when used improperly.

☐ Offering hepatitis B vaccines free of charge to employees who are at risk for contracting the disease. (Hepatitis B is a serious disease of the liver that can be transmitted through contact with the blood and other body fluids of an infected person.)

☐ Requiring that **Standard Precautions** be followed in the handling of blood and other body fluids. (Standard Precautions are specific practices and procedures to prevent the spread of infection.)

☐ Providing protective equipment, such as gloves and protective eyewear, to employees who are exposed to **blood-borne pathogens.**

☐ Disposing of medical waste properly.

☐ Having Material Safety Data Sheets (MSDSs) for all products used in the workplace. These sheets list every ingredient, as well as precautions and clean-up instructions in case of spills.

Although OSHA requirements are intended to protect workers, they also carry a burden of responsibility for employees. You will be required to follow certain OSHA policies and procedures on the job. It is essential that you become familiar with the ones that relate to your occupational duties because failure to comply can have serious consequences for both you and the facility where you work.

FOCUS ON THE GOAL

In spite of your best efforts, difficulties may arise on the job. These can range from the annoying to the intolerable. The ability to handle them effectively is a major job and life skill. Some problems can be handled with your own resources. Others require the assistance of others to resolve.

In Chapter 2 we introduced Stephen Covey's advice to "Begin with the end in mind." Slightly modifying this sentence gives us words to keep in mind when we are faced with a serious problem at work: "Act with the end in mind." This means that you approach problems with the intention of finding solutions to enhance rather than jeopardize your career. Choose actions that are appropriate for the situation and that will build your professional reputation. Some situations must simply be tolerated. For example, simple patience may be required when working with people who have annoying habits. Actions such as refusing to work with them and/or complaining to others behind their backs may hurt you professionally. On the other hand, resigning from a workplace in which illegal actions are taking place—and not being corrected—may be the most appropriate action. Your professional goals should guide your actions.

Dedicate your efforts to finding solutions to difficult situations. It's easy to wear yourself out by worrying or complaining about a problem, leaving you with little energy for actually dealing with it. Be clear about the resolutions you hope to achieve and look for ways to achieve them.

If you have a mentor, he or she may be a good source of advice for dealing with workplace issues. Talking them over with someone experienced in the field can help you gain perspective and see potential solutions that may not have occurred to you. Take care, however, to protect the confidentiality of the facility if your mentor does not work there.

The following are some examples of workplace problems that occur in health care settings:

1. *You are asked to perform duties that fall outside your scope of practice, tasks for which you were not trained, or tasks that are illegal.*

   Fortunately, this problem is rare. Unfortunately, when it does happen, it places the health care professional in a difficult situation. The best advice in these cases is "don't." Even if you are pressured by your supervisor or are assured that it is okay and "everyone does it," this is too big a risk to take. Once lost, your professional trustworthiness is very difficult to re-earn. Furthermore, illegal acts can result in fines and/or imprisonment.

2. *You find it difficult to get along with your supervisor.*

   Begin by taking an honest look at your own behavior to see whether there is something you are doing—or not doing—to contribute to the problem. Speak privately and frankly with your supervisor about how important your job is to you. Tell him or her that you want to have a good working relationship. Ask if there is anything you need to do to improve your performance.

   Identify your supervisor's priorities and communication style. Use mirroring, the technique discussed in Chapter 11, to match your communication styles. Not all supervisors have good communication skills. Listen carefully, and use feedback to increase the quality of communication and the likelihood of mutual understanding.

   Make an effort to find out what is important to your supervisor. Take a look at Table 13-1 to see descriptions of common management styles. Do your actions conflict with his or her management style? Does the management style conflict with your preferred way of working? Do you have different assumptions about the right way to do the work? This can lead to major misunderstandings in which each of you seems uncooperative and difficult to the other. We must become aware of the assumptions and expectations of the other person before we can attempt to get along with them.

When trying to communicate with your supervisor, keep in mind that your purpose is to promote mutual understanding and get the information needed to perform your job effectively. It is not to prove you are right or to tell your supervisor off, actions that will most likely make the situation worse. Look for ways to relieve your stress without venting your frustration at your supervisor.

3. *Low employee morale. Your co-workers are unhappy and complain a lot. You'd like to get along with everyone and be part of the group, but the conversation and atmosphere are getting you down.*

This can be a tough situation because it's unlikely you can change the opinion of the group. And being a newcomer, you want to fit in, but not at the expense of joining in the complaint sessions. Complaints that are justified are resolved through action, not endless discussion that wastes time, drains energy, and generally leads nowhere. Apply your communication and problem-solving skills to try to find solutions. And do your best to avoid participating in complaint sessions. It's a negative note on which to start a new career.

4. *There's too much to do and you can't finish all your work.*

Start by reviewing your work habits. Are you taking too much time to complete each task? Are there some tasks that you are still learning? Are you practicing good time management skills? You may be able to draw on the experience of your supervisor and/or co-workers to help you increase your efficiency. Talk with your supervisor about prioritizing your work. If you can't complete everything, which tasks are the most critical? What help is available? The time crunch is a growing problem in health care as professionals are being required to do more work in less time. Learning to maximize your efficiency will serve you well.

Work can be very satisfying in spite of problems like these. At best, problems provide opportunities for professional growth. Some situations, however, cannot be resolved or require compromises that you are not willing to make. You may choose to leave and seek employment elsewhere, a topic that is discussed in Chapter 14. In the meantime, it is critical that you do everything possible to maintain your professionalism and build a good reputation as a competent and cooperative employee.

Go to page 359 to complete Prescription for Success 13-11

Grievance Procedure

A grievance procedure is a written policy that gives employees a formalized, structured method to resolve workplace issues, or **grievances,** that they do not believe have been satisfactorily resolved by the supervisor. Common grievances concern fair treatment, discrimination, and disciplinary actions. For example, if an employee believes she did not receive a promotion because her supervisor favors another employee, she should first speak with her supervisor. If she is dissatisfied with the explanation or believes that company policy regarding promotions was not followed, she can speak with her supervisor's manager. If after seeking resolution by following the chain of command she still believes she has been treated unfairly regarding the promotion, she can file a grievance.

Organizations develop their own procedures, which consist of specific steps to take to file a grievance. This procedure is usually described in the employee handbook or in a policy and procedure manual. If you belong to a labor union, ask your representative how to file a grievance. It is important to follow the directions and meet any deadlines outlined in the policy. Grievances should be filed only when all of the following conditions are met:

1. You have made a sincere attempt to handle the issue, starting with speaking to your supervisor about the problem.
2. The issue is serious.
3. You are willing to follow a formal process.

Used appropriately, the grievance procedure can be an effective and fair means of resolving employee issues in an organization.

SEEK SATISFACTION IN YOUR WORK

Many of your waking hours are spent at the workplace. If you are to live a high-quality life, it makes sense that your work be a source of satisfaction. This doesn't mean finding the "perfect job." In fact, it is unlikely such a thing exists. It does mean approaching work with a positive attitude and focusing on those aspects that give you the opportunity to do the following:

- Perform meaningful work
- Make a positive contribution to the well-being of others
- Work in an interesting environment
- Continue to learn

Satisfaction is self-perpetuating. This means that health care professionals who project a positive attitude and like their work are likely to create satisfaction in those who receive their services. Performance levels and efficiency are also raised, further increasing the professional's sense of satisfaction.

Q&A with a Health Care Professional Bernie Stults, Registered Nurse

Bernie has 42 years of experience as a registered nurse in hospitals and clinics. Bernie discusses tips for career success.

Q What advice would you give graduates who are starting their first job in health care?

A The basics are still very important for success on the job. Things like professional appearance. In the last 10 years or so, trends like tattoos have become a problem because some older patients find them objectionable. They don't understand they are just a fashion statement and no longer have the negative connotations they had years ago. Another style that's a problem is low-cut blouses and tops on female employees. These are seen just about everyplace these days, but they just aren't appropriate on the job in health care.

Q Along with appearance, what other recommendations would you offer?

A It's important to show an interest in the job. New employees should want to learn, and they can do this by asking questions—and then following up. By this I mean writing the information down and making an effort to learn and remember it. We had a new hire recently who would ask questions and

then fail to pay attention. She ended up doing the work her way, which unfortunately wasn't always correct.

Q There are instances in which recent graduates believe their current training actually makes them more qualified than experienced health care workers. Have you run into this problem?

A Yes. This know-it-all attitude is a problem with quite a few graduates. What they don't realize is that much of their learning will be based on years of experience on the job. They need to do their best to perform efficiently and correctly while also being willing to learn.

Q What other advice do you consider essential for success in health care?

A In a few words: be prepared to meet the needs of others. And I don't just mean your patients. I used to work in the ER. When there was a seriously injured accident victim, for example, I was not only helping the patient, but dealing with the family members, friends, and working with other hospital personnel. There were lots of things to consider, and they all dealt with people. Regardless of the situation, good social skills are really a must.

A win-win situation is created in which everyone benefits.

To keep yourself on the right track, ask yourself the following questions as you work:

- Who is benefiting from the tasks I am performing now?
- What contributions am I making to the well-being of others?
- What can I learn today?
- Are there positive aspects of my work that I am overlooking?

 Go to page 360 to complete Prescription for Success 13-12

 ## SUMMARY OF KEY IDEAS

1. Your first job sets the groundwork for your future career success.
2. Your study skills are also useful employment skills.
3. Mastering workplace competencies leads to workplace success.
4. Learning to work well with your supervisor is worth the effort.
5. Employees have rights that are protected by law.

Positive Self-Talk for This Chapter

1. I will be a confident and competent health care professional.
2. I have the skills to handle various kinds of workplace problems.
3. I work well with others.
4. My health care career is off to a good start.
5. My job will bring me great satisfaction.

To Learn More

About.com: Workplace Survival and Success
http://careerplanning.about.com/od/workplacesurvival/Workplace_Survival_and_Success.htm
This page contains links to dozens of short articles that include topics such as getting along with your boss and co-workers, office etiquette, and personal issues at work.

Covey SR: *The 7 habits of highly effective people,* New York, 1990, Fireside.
This popular book lists seven principles that help individuals live effective lives. These can be applied for success in the workplace.

Flight M: *Law, liability, and ethics for medical office professionals,* ed 4, Clifton Park, NY, 2004, Cengage Delmar Learning.

This book presents legal and ethical matters for health care professionals in an interesting and easy-to-read format. Actual cases are used as examples.

Mind Tools

www.mindtools.com

The "tools" include skills that contribute to workplace success including time management, problem solving, and stress management.

INTERNET ACTIVITIES

For active links to the websites needed to complete these activities, visit **http://evolve.elsevier.com/ Haroun/career/**.

1. Many specific OSHA regulations apply to workers in health care facilities. Explore the OSHA website and choose a topic related to your future career, such as blood-borne pathogens or needlestick prevention. Write a short report about the extent of the problem and OSHA's recommendations for the protection of workers.

2. Concern about medical privacy has increased significantly with the passage of HIPAA and the creation of federal privacy standards that took effect on April 14, 2003. The U.S. Department of Health and Human Services has created fact sheets on patient privacy that are available online. Read the fact sheets for consumers, and list the five provisions designed to protect patient health information.

3. Health care providers have created guidelines to help employees follow HIPAA regulations. The guidelines for the Department of Radiology at Massachusetts General Hospital are available online. Read the guidelines, and list 10 that you believe apply to the tasks you will be performing in your future occupation.

4. Mind Tools has information on job success topics such as stress and time management, problem solving, and practical creativity. Choose a topic to explore, and write a plan for incorporating suggestions you find useful into your daily life.

5. The Professional Personnel Development Center at Pennsylvania State University has a short module available online with information about communicating with supervisors. Study the material provided, and then complete the four student activities.

Prescription for Success 13-1
Applying Your Study Skills

Think of three "study skills" not discussed in this chapter that might help you succeed in your job.

1. _____

2. _____

3. _____

Prescription for Success 13-2
Recognize Your Value

1. List five things you like about yourself.

1. _____

2. _____

3. _____

4. _____

5. _____

2. List five accomplishments that give you pride.

1. _____

2. _____

3. _____

4. _____

5. _____

3. List five things you believe will make you a good employee.

1. _____

2. _____

3. _____

4. _____

5. _____

Prescription for Success 13-3
The Code as Your Guide

1. If you don't already have one, obtain a copy of the code of ethics for your profession.
2. Read the code and describe how it addresses the following issues:
   A. Integrity

   _____

   _____

   _____

   B. Human dignity

   _____

   _____

   _____

   C. Loyalty

   _____

   _____

   _____

   D. Honesty and sincerity

   _____

   _____

   _____

   E. Responsibility to patients

   _____

   _____

   _____

   F. Lifelong learning

   _____

   _____

   _____

Prescription for Success 13–3 (Continued)

G. Community service

_____

_____

_____

Prescription for Success 13-4
Focus on Confidentiality

1. Does the code of ethics for your profession include a statement about patient confidentiality?
2. List at least five techniques you can use in your work to guard patient confidentiality.

1. _____

_____

_____

2. _____

_____

_____

3. _____

_____

_____

4. _____

_____

_____

5. _____

_____

_____

_____

Prescription for Success 13-5
Consider the Consequences

A medical assistant who works in a busy pediatric office fails to autoclave the instruments as directed. As a result, the physician cannot perform minor elective surgery scheduled for a young patient. Discuss the possible impact on the following:

1. Patient _____

_____

_____

_____

_____

_____

2. Parents _____

_____

_____

_____

_____

_____

3. Physician _____

_____

_____

_____

_____

_____

4. Medical assistant _____

_____

_____

_____

_____

_____

Prescription for Success 13-6
Management Styles

1. What types of supervisors have you worked for in the past?

_____

_____

_____

_____

_____

_____

_____

2. How did you get along?

_____

_____

_____

_____

_____

_____

_____

3. Did you learn any strategies that you can apply at future jobs?

_____

_____

_____

_____

_____

_____

_____

Prescription for Success 13-7
What's Available?

1. Does your professional organization have a local chapter?

_____

_____

2. What types of learning activities does it sponsor?

_____

_____

3. What are names of journals available in your field?

_____

_____

_____

_____

Where are they available?

_____ Subscription

_____ Part of professional membership

_____ Library

_____ Health care facility

4. What types of continuing education classes are available in your occupational area?

_____

_____

5. Choose a topic of interest in health care, and conduct an Internet search for information. What kind of information is available?

_____

_____

_____

_____

Prescription for Success 13–7 (Continued)

Who are the sponsors?

_____

_____

_____

_____

How reliable do you believe the information to be? Why?

_____

_____

_____

_____

Prescription for Success 13-8
Are You Ready?

1. What are your backup plans for transportation, childcare, and/or any personal responsibilities that could interfere with your job?

_____

_____

_____

2. What organizational strategies have you developed to help balance your professional and personal lives?

_____

_____

_____

3. Do any of your self-management skills need improvement? If so, what can you do to improve them?

_____

_____

_____

Prescription for Success 13-9
Knowing Ahead Gives You the Edge

Research your occupation to see how it has changed over the last 20 years. Sources of information include interviewing someone who has worked in the field for several years, your professional organization, the Internet, and your instructors.

1. Does your occupation require more training than it did in the past?

_____

_____

_____

2. Describe any duties and responsibilities that have been added and/or deleted.

_____

_____

_____

_____

3. Have licensing or certification requirements been added or changed?

_____

_____

_____

_____

4. What changes are anticipated for the future?

_____

_____

_____

_____

5. How can you start preparing to be ready for these changes?

_____

_____

_____

_____

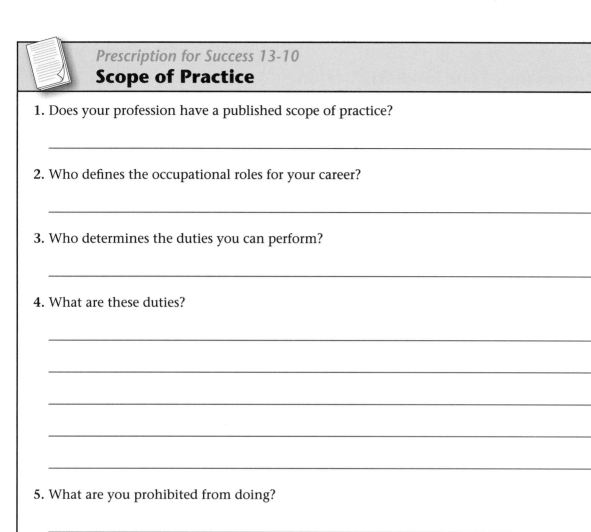

Prescription for Success 13-10
Scope of Practice

1. Does your profession have a published scope of practice?

_____

2. Who defines the occupational roles for your career?

_____

3. Who determines the duties you can perform?

_____

4. What are these duties?

_____

_____

_____

_____

5. What are you prohibited from doing?

_____

_____

_____

Prescription for Success 13-11
Handling the Tough Ones

Suppose you are newly hired and have been trying your best to complete what you understand to be your assignments. However, you received only a 1-hour orientation to the job and are not completely clear about your duties, the policies at the facility, and exactly what you are expected to do. You haven't been able to locate all the supplies and resources you need and aren't sure how to operate the computer system. Your supervisor is always rushed. You now have 15 minutes to talk with him. What would you say?

Prescription for Success 13-12
Increasing Your Job Satisfaction

1. What were your reasons for choosing a career in health care?

_____

_____

_____

_____

_____

2. In what ways do you think you will receive satisfaction from your work?

_____

_____

_____

_____

_____

3. How will you measure your success and satisfaction at work?

_____

_____

_____

_____

_____

4. What can you do to make your work fulfilling?

_____

_____

_____

_____

_____

Navigating Your Career

OBJECTIVES

The information and activities in this chapter can help you:

- List ways to gain maximum benefit from performance reviews.
- Describe the continuing education requirements for your career, if applicable, and list ways to earn them.
- Explain why it is important to maintain your professional network throughout your career.
- Explain how to increase your chances of earning a promotion.
- List the characteristics of an effective supervisor.
- Use self-questioning and a decision matrix to choose the right job.
- Describe the proper actions to take when leaving a job voluntarily.
- Explain how to survive and learn from the experience of being fired from a job.
- List ways to add variety to your work and keep it interesting.

KEY TERMS AND CONCEPTS

Decision Matrix: A table you create to help you compare and rate alternatives.

Downsizing: Reducing the number of employees.

Entrepreneur: Someone who starts and operates a business.

Job Shadow: To spend time with a professional during typical workdays to observe the kinds of tasks performed, the environment in which the work takes place, and so on.

Step-Up Programs: Educational programs in which credits and/or experience earned for one occupational level can be applied for credit when studying for a higher level.

STAYING ON COURSE

"Only he who keeps his eye fixed on the far horizon will find his right road."
                        —Dag Hammarskjöld

You're on your way! You have launched your health care career and should be enjoying the results of your efforts. But maintaining a successful career is like traveling successfully by ship. Without plotting and paying attention to your course, you can end up drifting aimlessly. Even worse, inattention can result in collisions that can sink your ship.

PERFORMANCE REVIEWS

Many people think that performance reviews (work evaluations) are the responsibility of supervisors. This is not true. In fact, you should be conducting regular self-evaluations to monitor your progress and keep yourself on course. Review your performance periodically using your job description and your employer's evaluation form as guides. Figure 14-1 is a sample evaluation form. Honest self-evaluations are like an internal quality control system. They can alert you to the need to seek help from your supervisor and ask questions about your job. You may discover that some of your skills need improvement, and you may look for resources and information to learn more.

Self-awareness empowers you to be proactive and in control. You don't wait for others to suggest needed improvements, but rather you continually review your performance and set your own goals. At the same time, you should be documenting your achievements on the job.

Your supervisor is, of course, a valuable source of information and feedback about your progress. Take the initiative to maximize the value of your formal performance evaluations. More than one-sided progress reports, these meetings should be an opportunity for you to review your supervisor's expectations and determine whether you are meeting them. Take advantage of your meeting to ask questions such as the following:

1. Which tasks am I performing well?
2. Which tasks need improvement?
3. Do you have suggestions for improvements?
4. Can you recommend sources that might help me?
5. How can I increase my value to the team (department, facility)?

Don't hesitate to request information. If you are unsure about certain job duties, rules, policies, or procedures, use this opportunity to ask. If you receive a low rating in some area and don't understand why, ask for an explanation and examples that demonstrate how you do not meet the criteria or performed poorly. In the case of low ratings, you can offer explanations, but don't make excuses. If you believe you have a good reason for performance on which you were rated poorly or believe there has been a misunderstanding, it is perfectly acceptable to give an explanation. For example, if it turns out you were given incorrect instructions about how to perform a procedure, let your supervisor know and ask for help.

Help your supervisor to help you. In the spirit of developing a positive relationship and increasing your value to the facility, tell your supervisor how he or she can assist you. Examples include providing additional information about the job, explaining rules, giving you regular feedback about your work, or directing you to sources of additional training and information. Work with your supervisor to set professional goals for yourself. In some organizations, setting and reviewing goals are the main part of the performance review.

Withhold criticism and complaints during the review. This is not the appropriate time to present your list of complaints about the workplace. You will come across as defensive. Do not become angry. Use your energy to learn as much as possible in the current situation. Suggestions from your perspective can best be presented at another time.

Formal performance evaluations, when approached as opportunities rather than something to be endured, can be constructive experiences. Combine them with self-evaluations to help keep your career on course.

 Go to page 378 to complete Prescription for Success 14-1

KEEPING CURRENT

In Chapter 13 we discussed the importance of staying current in your field and how you can count on continual changes and advances in health care (Figure 14-2). In some professions, earning a certain number of continuing education units (CEUs) or participating in continuing professional education (CPE) is mandatory for renewing your license or certification. The required numbers are set by licensing boards, state regulatory agencies, and/or professional organizations. It is important for you to know exactly what is required for your profession. There

Wellness Plus Physicians Group
Employee Performance Review

Name: _____   Position: _____

Hire Date: _____   Date of Last
                                                    Performance
Supervisor: _____   Evaluation: _____

Rating Scale: 1 = Excellent   2 = Very Good   3 = Satisfactory   4 = Needs some improvement   5 = Needs much improvement

A. Quality of work performed   Comments:
   Rating   1   2   3   4   5

B. Use of judgment   Comments:
   Rating   1   2   3   4   5

C. Dependability   Comments:
   Rating   1   2   3   4   5

D. Cooperation with others   Comments:
   Rating   1   2   3   4   5

E. Appearance and hygiene   Comments:
   Rating   1   2   3   4   5

F. Attendance and punctuality   Comments:
   Rating   1   2   3   4   5

G. Time management   Comments:
   Rating   1   2   3   4   5

H. Proper use of equipment   Comments:
   and supplies
   Rating   1   2   3   4   5

I. Ability to work independently   Comments:
   Rating   1   2   3   4   5

(1)

Figure 14-1 Sample performance review.   *Continued*

**Wellness Plus Physicians Group
Employee Performance Review**

Rating Scale: 1 = Excellent   2 = Very Good   3 = Satisfactory   4 = Needs some improvement   5 = Needs much improvement

J. Communication skills
    Rating   1   2   3   4   5

Comments:

K. Willingness to take direction
   and suggestions
    Rating   1   2   3   4   5

Comments:

L. Ability to adapt to change
    Rating   1   2   3   4   5

Comments:

Employee's greatest strengths: _____
_____

Progress in meeting goals from last review: _____
_____

New goals for improvement: _____
_____

Plan for achieving goals: _____
_____

Overall evaluation of this employee: _____
_____

Reviewed by: _____

Date: _____

Employee signature _____

Date: _____
    (Signature does not necessarily
     mean agreement)

(2)

Figure 14-1, cont'd   Sample performance review.

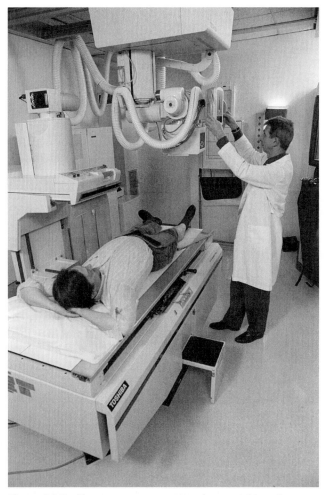

Figure 14-2 You can count on many changes taking place during your health care career. Staying up-to-date will be an ongoing process.

are a variety of ways to earn these credits, including the following:

- ☐ Classes at local colleges and universities
- ☐ Workshops sponsored by your employer, another health care facility, or your professional organization
- ☐ Written assignments offered through correspondence courses or offered in your professional journal
- ☐ Distance education classes and workshops offered over the Internet

The agency or organization that requires the units, not the education provider, determines which units will be accepted. Before participating in any learning activity for credit, make sure it will be accepted by the appropriate agency. Request documentation showing that you attended and/or completed the work necessary to earn the credits. You may be required to submit proof along with your certification renewal application. Some employers

provide training allowances and pay for classes to help their employees stay current.

An important source of learning throughout your career is your own experience. As you repeat the tasks of your profession, make decisions, and solve problems, you will gain confidence and the "knowing" that comes with practice.

 Go to page 378 to complete Prescription for Success 14-2

STAYING CONNECTED

Once you are employed, maintain and expand your network. Stay in touch with your instructors, career services staff, classmates, mentors, and any professionals who assisted you during your training or job search. There are a number of reasons for staying connected. Other professionals can help you keep up-to-date in your field by sharing knowledge, ideas, and sources of information. If you want to change jobs in the future, they can be good sources of information. And networking is a two-way street: others may need your assistance. Finally, it's fun to have friends in the profession. Seeing them at meetings, workshops, and conferences adds to the enjoyment of having a career.

BECOMING A LEADER IN YOUR PROFESSION

Achieving excellence on the job is the first step toward becoming a leader in your profession. As you gain experience, there are other actions you can take to both enhance your career and increase your contributions to your employer, profession, and the general health care field.

- ☐ Participate actively in your professional organization. Join committees, run for office, give presentations, and attend the annual conference.
- ☐ Help new employees get started. Volunteer to orient, train, and act as a mentor.
- ☐ Become a clinical supervisor at your facility. Help students acquire the on-site experience they need to complete their education.
- ☐ Teach seminars and workshops for your professional organization, facility, or local schools and colleges.
- ☐ Write articles for professional journals.
- ☐ Support legislation that promotes health care issues.
- ☐ Promote wellness and public access to health care.

EARNING A PROMOTION

"Recognize opportunities and go through the door when it's open."

—*Rick Baird*

Earning a promotion is a satisfying reward for your hard work. Did you notice the use of the word "earning"? You must demonstrate that you have what it takes to be given more responsibility, earning the confidence of those doing the promoting. If earning promotions is on your list of career goals, there are a number of ways to increase your chances, including the following:

☐ **Be 100% dependable.** Develop a reputation for being on time, being on task, and following through on all assigned duties.

☐ **Demonstrate leadership skills.** Help and encourage others, be a productive and cooperative team member, and develop excellent communication skills.

☐ **Strive for excellence.** Set high personal and professional standards. Continually develop your skills and acquire new ones.

☐ **Increase your value to the organization.** Take on additional responsibilities, and volunteer for committees and special projects. Look for ways to make positive contributions.

☐ **Advertise your interest.** Let your supervisor know you are interested in a promotion. Find out about the necessary qualifications, and develop a plan for acquiring any you don't have.

☐ **Sell yourself.** If you must formally apply for the new position, be prepared. Review your accomplishments and select examples of work that demonstrate why you are qualified for the new position. Don't assume that the interviewer—even if it is your own supervisor—is aware of all your qualifications.

 Go to page 379 to complete Prescription for Success 14-3

Becoming the Supervisor

"The purpose of management is to maximize people's strengths and make their weaknesses irrelevant."

—*Peter Drucker*

Receiving a promotion is something you can be proud of. Enjoy the good feelings that come with having attained a significant accomplishment. At the same time, recognize and be willing to accept the increased responsibilities that are almost certainly included. If you are promoted to a supervisory position, you are now accountable not only for your own work, but that of others as well. A special challenge occurs if former co-workers now report to you. This is sometimes an awkward situation, especially if you are friends outside the workplace. You may feel uncomfortable telling them what to do. On the other hand, you can build on these positive relationships to develop a team that pulls together to accomplish group goals. Your priority now must be to ensure that assigned work is completed satisfactorily. True friends will understand and support these efforts. Do take care that all employees are treated equally and fairly, regardless of previous relationships.

Being a successful supervisor may mean adding some new skills to the ones that helped you earn the new position. For example, building productive teams, organizing work schedules, and running effective meetings require skills that are different from those needed to be a good dental assistant, medical transcriptionist, or laboratory technician. The information in this section is only a brief introduction to supervision, intended to stimulate further study. If your future goals include becoming a supervisor, prepare ahead by acquiring the necessary knowledge through taking classes and/or self-study on topics such as personnel management, motivation, public speaking, budgeting, evaluation techniques, and long-range planning. Successful supervisors have good people skills. An important part of their job is to inspire others to do their best. There are many ways to accomplish this, including the following:

☐ Set a positive tone for the group. Promote the mission of the organization. Emphasize the value of the work. Be enthusiastic and share your enthusiasm with others.

☐ Keep the group focused on accomplishing worthy goals: delivering high-quality patient care, performing work accurately, and supporting the efforts of the organization.

☐ Give continuous, appropriate feedback. Encourage the employees' best efforts with public praise. Help them improve by giving constructive criticism in private. Employees deserve the opportunity to make needed changes, and this is possible only if they know what the problems are.

☐ Recognize and build on each employee's strengths and weakness, whenever possible, by assigning appropriate tasks.

☐ Clearly communicate your expectations. Assumptions are dangerous: what is obvious to you may be "clear as mud" to others.

☐ Delegate appropriately. Too much and employees will resent you. Too little and you will find yourself worn out and/or unable to complete your work.

PERSONAL REFLECTION

Think about supervisors you have worked for in the past. Would you describe any of them as excellent supervisors? (If this is a written assignment to be turned in, don't use names.)

_____

If yes, describe what made them excellent. If not, why or why not.

_____

_____

_____

_____

List the qualities you consider most important in a supervisor.

_____

_____

_____

_____

What are some ways you can learn more about the duties of a supervisor?

_____

_____

_____

_____

 with a Health Care Professional
Rick Baird

Rick Baird, Chief Human Resources Officer at Bend Memorial Clinic in Bend, Oregon, discusses how to succeed in the workplace and shares how his clinic evaluates employees.

Q How can health care employees increase their value to their employers?

A Customer service is the focus of today's health care environment—at least for our clinic. I want employees who will help make my business better. A major way they can do this is by increasing customer satisfaction—making patients feel important. Empathy is key to accomplishing this.

Showing appreciation for co-workers and being courteous with everyone may seem obvious but are sometimes overlooked. The ability to flourish in a social environment makes work satisfying and helps employees get ahead.

Q Do you have other suggestions for getting along with others?

A Yes. Demonstrate a positive, can-do attitude. Go with the flow. Be curious and seek out opportunities to learn. At the same time, be careful about not being a know-it-all. This can get you ostracized at work.

Q How do you measure employee performance?

A We do performance reviews annually. The ratings are based on objective performance standards written in concrete terms instead of them being very general. For example, we include the number of times a person was absent. We also have specific criteria that pertain to the job—for example, giving appropriate treatments to patients.

We always assign goals as part of performance reviews—two or three for each employee. We work with them to establish SMART goals.

Q What exactly are SMART goals?

A *S* stands for simple; *M* for measurable; *A* for attainable; *R* for reasonable; and *T* for time constrained—that is, it can be achieved in the time available.

At our clinic, we do focal reviews.

Q What are these?

A It means we do all employee reviews at the same time—during the month of October. This is instead of doing reviews based on each person's hire date. We plan in-house education and other activities to focus on self-improvement during the whole month.

DECIDING TO LEAVE A JOB

Making the decision to leave a job should be done thoughtfully. It is important that you are clear about why you want to leave. Take time to review the situation carefully and identify the real problems. If you are unhappy at work, changing jobs may not be the answer. For example, if your own work habits are at the root of your dissatisfaction, working elsewhere will not necessarily be an improvement. Our personal baggage, consisting of our attitudes, habits, and abilities, goes along with us. Some people spend years jumping from one job to another, yet never find the right one. They fail to realize that the changes need to come from within themselves.

Review your current job by answering the following questions as honestly as possible:
1. How might I be contributing to my own dissatisfaction?
2. Do I have difficulty communicating effectively?
3. Does it take me longer than others to complete assigned tasks?
4. What can I do to improve my performance?
5. Have I asked for help?
6. Have I spoken with my supervisor about my dissatisfaction?
7. Do I need additional skills?
8. Are my expectations about work realistic?
9. Would requesting a transfer or promotion resolve the problem?
10. Do I have the experience and training for the job I really want?

You may discover that you can transform your current job into one that is more acceptable. Once you have identified the problems, you may be able to solve them by changing your attitude, developing a plan, seeking help, and applying your best efforts. On the other hand, some factors are simply out of your control. Your best efforts may not be enough to overcome poor management, disorganization, lack of adequate resources, and low integrity. An example is being repeatedly told to perform tasks beyond your level of training and experience or outside your scope of practice. Before making the decision to leave a job, consider filing a grievance, described in Chapter 13, if you feel you are being treated unfairly or illegally. When all efforts at resolution fail or if the facility is simply unable to accommodate your needs, finding employment elsewhere may be in your best professional interest.

Seeking New Opportunities

You may like your job but still feel the need to make a change. This can happen as you gain work experience, discover areas of particular interest, and/or want more opportunities for professional growth. Changes can be necessary steps on the road to achieving your long-term personal and career goals such as in the following situations:
- ☐ You are ready—and qualified—for more challenge and responsibility, but opportunities are limited because of the size or organizational structure of your place of employment
- ☐ You want to spend more time working in a particular occupational area
- ☐ You need assistance paying for additional training, but your employer's budget does not include funding for this purpose
- ☐ You want to spend more time with your family, but the required work schedules do not permit this
- ☐ Your duties are limited, and you want a chance to apply more of your training
- ☐ You would like to work with a different patient population or health care specialty

Sometimes opportunities simply present themselves. For example, a friend tells you about an opening in the clinic where she "just loves working." Or a facility with an excellent reputation in your field announces a promising position. You may find yourself in the position of having to make a choice between the known—your current job—and the unknown—a new job that might be better.

Using a Decision Matrix

When you are faced with choosing among alternatives, a **decision matrix** helps you compare how they meet your requirements. The matrix is a table consisting of squares in which you record ratings and scores for each alternative. Here are the steps for putting together this handy tool:
1. List all the features of work that apply to the jobs you are considering. Review the list you created in Prescription for Success 9-2 and the examples in Table 14-1. Add any others that apply to you.
2. On a piece of paper, prepare a table using Table 14-1 as an example.
3. Rate each feature with a number:
   1 = Not important to me (no preference)
   2 = Somewhat important to me
   3 = Very important to me
   Write the corresponding number next to each feature in the ratings' column.
4. Rank each job as you believe it will meet your needs:
   1 = Unlikely or unknown
   2 = Very likely
   Write the numbers in the top right section of the corresponding squares.

TABLE 14-1	Sample Decision Matrix for Choosing a Job		
Feature	**Ratings (1, 2, 3)**	**Current Job**	**Proposed Job**
Population served	2	1 2× 1 = 2	2 2× 2 = 4
Geographic location	1	2 1× 2 = 2	1 1× 1 = 1
Specialty	1	2 1× 2 = 2	2 1× 2 = 2
Independence given employees	3	1 3× 1 = 3	2 3× 2 = 6
Work pace	1	2 1× 2 = 2	2 1× 2 = 2
Variety of duties	2	1 2× 1 = 2	2 2× 2 = 4
Training opportunities	3	1 3× 1 = 3	2 3× 2 = 6
Reputation of facility	3	2 3× 2 = 6	2 3× 2 = 6
Opportunities for advancement	2	1 2× 1 = 2	2 2× 2 = 4
Challenge	2	1 2× 1 = 2	2 2× 2 = 4
Responsibility	2	1 2× 1 = 2	2 2× 2 = 4
Cooperativeness of co-workers	2	2 2× 2 = 4	2 2× 2 = 4
Work and mission align with your values	3	2 3× 2 = 6	2 3× 2 = 6
Orientation to health care (emphasis on wellness, acceptance of alternative therapies)	3	1 3× 1 = 3	1 3× 1 = 3
Pay	2	1 2× 1 = 2	2 2× 2 = 4
Benefits (insurance, vacation, etc.)	2	2 2× 2 = 4	2 2× 2 = 4
Work schedule	1	2 1× 2 = 2	1 1× 1 = 1
Contribution to society	2	2 2× 2 = 4	2 2× 2 = 4
Total Scores		53	69

Note: This may require some research: good interview questions, talking with people who work at the facility, and reviewing the organization's website and published information.

5. Multiply the number assigned to each feature by the ranking number for each job (1 or 2). Write the result in the center of the intersecting square.

6. Add the results of your calculations. The job with the highest score is most likely to meet your needs.

You can create a decision matrix that includes your list of features before you interview for a new job. This provides a method for planning questions to get the exact information you'll need to make an informed decision.

If going through this process seems like too much trouble, consider the trouble that can result from making poor career decisions. Where you spend the majority of your waking hours affects the quality of your life. Taking sufficient time to research, review, and properly manage your career will pay off. Using a decision matrix enables you to identify what matters most to you and to measure to what degree your professional needs are being met.

The decision matrix is also a useful tool for periodically reviewing your level of job satisfaction. Instead of comparing two or more jobs, rate the one you have every few months and compare the results over time. How well does it continue to meet your needs? Have your preferences changed over time? Clearly identifying sources of dissatisfaction makes it much easier to seek solutions, whether that means making changes in the job you have or looking for another one. Saying "I'm bored here" is not very informative. Saying "I perform only three tasks over and over each day" is more useful information. You can request more assignments at your present job or look for a job that offers a wider variety of tasks.

Finally, using the matrix allows you to see whether your preferences align with your personal qualities and abilities. For example, if you rate "opportunities for advancement" as "very important" and "independence," "challenge," and "responsibility" as "not important," your goals are not realistic. Desires must be balanced with willingness to perform.

You can use a decision matrix in other areas of your life. Some examples include choosing the most practical car to buy, most appropriate medical insurance plan for your family, best school to attend for your advanced training, and most desirable house to buy or rent. Try using a decision matrix next time you must choose between alternatives. Use the left column to list the features most important to you. Then assign rating numbers and compare the alternatives.

 Go to page 379 to complete Prescription for Success 14-4

Preparing to Change Jobs

Most employment experts recommend that you not resign from a job until you have a firm offer for another one. It is generally believed that individuals are more employable if they are currently working. Perhaps more important, you are in a better position financially to look around and find a suitable position. This is especially true if the job market is tight and not many positions are available.

You may decide, however, that you need time to reenergize and reorganize. Difficulties at work can take all your attention and leave you with little energy to look for another job. In this case, plan to have at least 6 months of living expenses put aside. (Actually, it is good personal management to always have at least 6 months of living expenses available in case of an emergency, even if you aren't planning to leave your job.)

Develop a network of support among friends and family members. Even leaving a job voluntarily can be stressful. Call on people who endorse your decision and can offer encouragement during your job search and transition.

Long-term career success requires that you establish a stable work record. A pattern of frequent job changes can discourage employers from hiring you. They want employees to stay for a reasonable period of time because hiring and training expenses represent a substantial investment of time and money. On the other hand, remaining too long in a position that drains your enthusiasm and stifles your progress is not a sound career decision. Consider your mission, personal values, and long-term goals when deciding whether to change jobs.

Leaving on a Positive Note

Regardless of the circumstances, make your departure as gracious as possible. "It's a small world" certainly applies to employment, including health care. Employers meet at professional meetings, seminars, and country clubs. Even if you didn't like your last supervisor, he or she may play golf with someone you would love to work for. Here are some suggestions for keeping the relationship as positive as possible:

☐ Give sufficient notice. Two weeks is considered the minimum.
☐ Write a letter of resignation in which you thank the employer for the opportunities extended.
☐ It is not necessary to state the reason you are resigning, although in some cases it is appropriate.
☐ It's not a good idea to include complaints in the letter. See Figure 14-3 for a sample letter of resignation.
☐ Submit your resignation to your supervisor before discussing it with anyone else at work.
☐ Pursue job leads and attend interviews on your own time, not that of your current employer.
☐ Be willing to help train your replacement.
☐ Refrain from complaining and informing your employer and co-workers about everything you find wrong with the workplace.
☐ Put forth your best efforts through your last day. Finish all tasks and leave your work area, equipment, and files in order.

During your last days on the job, you may find it difficult to focus fully and maintain a positive attitude. Situations like these are true tests of professionalism. Doing your best and completing your obligations under any circumstances will help you build your reputation as a dependable health care professional. You are, in a sense, buying insurance for a successful future.

1642 Windhill Way
San Antonio, TX 78220
February 16, 2010

Nancy Henderson, Office Manager
Craigmore Pediatric Clinic
4979 Coffee Road
San Antonio, TX 78229

Dear Ms. Henderson:

I am writing this letter as my official resignation from Craigmore Pediatric Clinic effective March 16, 2010. I have accepted a position at Cooke Children's Hospital.

The decision to leave Craigmore was not an easy one to make. I have enjoyed my work over the past two years and feel very fortunate to have had the opportunity to begin my health care career here.

Please accept my sincere thanks for all your help. A constant source of encouragement, you are a true example of professionalism and caring. You always inspired me to aim for excellence in my work.

I wish you and Craigmore Pediatric continuing success in the future.

Sincerely,

Karen Gonzalez

Karen Gonzalez

Figure 14-3 Sample letter of resignation.

If you have enjoyed working with your supervisor, let him or her know. A thank-you note, separate from the letter of resignation, is a nice gesture. Express your appreciation for the supervisor's help. You may work with this person in the future. Add him or her to your network of contacts and stay in touch. If you are leaving on a positive note, ask for a letter of recommendation for possible future use.

Go to page 380 to complete Prescription for Success 14-5

HITTING ROUGH WATERS: WHAT TO DO IF YOU'RE FIRED

"Men's best successes come after their disappointments."

—*Henry Ward Beecher*

Being fired from a job can be like being tossed off a ship into high seas. The water is cold, and the waves are scary. You may wonder if you'll survive. Not only can you survive being fired, but you can also use the experience to grow personally and professionally.

Your first concern, however, is to stay afloat. Thrashing about by becoming angry and defensive and lashing out at your supervisor will only make matters worse and put your career in danger of drowning. When you receive the news that you are being fired, it is recommended that you do the following:

☐ Understand that firing an employee is difficult and uncomfortable for most supervisors.
☐ Ask for an explanation of the reasons for the decision. It is likely that you've already been advised about problems regarding your performance. Ask about anything you don't understand or believe had been corrected.
☐ Listen carefully and ask for feedback when necessary. This may be difficult under the circumstances, but it is critical that the communication be as clear as possible.
☐ Request an opportunity to explain your side of the situation if you believe there has been a misunderstanding. Don't insist, however, if you are told that the decision is final. It will only hurt your case to argue, yell, or use abusive language.
☐ Ask your supervisor for suggestions about what you can do to prevent this from happening at a future job.
☐ Don't bring out your list of what is wrong with the workplace, supervisor, co-workers, and so on. This gives the appearance of making excuses and acting defensively. Keep focused on learning why this decision was made about you.

Be aware that in today's legal climate, many employers have dismissal policies that may seem harsh. For example, your supervisor may not be allowed to give you details about how the decision to dismiss you was made. You may be asked to gather your things, under supervision, and leave the workplace immediately. Keep in mind that these policies apply to all employees who are dismissed, not just you. Don't feel that you have been targeted or are necessarily considered to be dishonest. Do your best to maintain your composure and not make an already difficult situation worse.

Downsizing

Downsizing means reducing the number of employees. Companies sometimes let some employees go to control costs or to survive as a business. For example, a medical laboratory may be losing money because of competition and may not be able to afford the cost of its current staff. Or an economic slowdown can reduce the amount of business. Downsizing also can occur when companies merge. If two clinics are combined as a result of one company buying another, there may be duplications in the staff.

The decision about who to keep and who to let go is not easy for managers. Frequently, downsizing requires that cuts be made at all levels, so the managers themselves may lose their jobs. If you are ever let go because of downsizing, try your best not to take it personally. You are not being fired for poor performance; rather, you are a victim of circumstances beyond your control. Future potential employers are likely to understand your situation.

Getting to Shore

"Success seems to be largely a matter of hanging on after others have let go."

—*William Feather*

Life preservers come in many forms: friends, family, mentors, instructors, and other school personnel. Use them wisely. Their role is to provide encouragement, emotional support, and honest feedback; it is not to listen to endless complaints and harrowing stories about the job and how you were mistreated.

Bring your personal resources to the rescue efforts. Rebuild your confidence by reviewing your strengths, achievements, and positive traits. Losing a job need not drown your chances for long-term success. You can get to shore by deciding to learn from the experience and by taking the actions necessary to move on with your career.

Start the process by looking at yourself honestly. Recognizing the need for self-improvement is empowering because you can take responsibility for making changes to improve your future. Blaming others, or denying that you are at fault in any way, puts change out of your control. It's like saying, "I'm doomed, because I have to depend on others to save me. There's nothing I can do."

Accepting responsibility means asking some hard questions to help you learn from the experience of being fired. This is the first step to prevent it from happening again. Whatever the problems,

TABLE 14-2	Learning from Experience	
Reason Given for Dismissal	**Types of Questions to Ask Yourself**	**Suggested Actions**
Poor work performance	Do I lack the skills? Am I simply careless? Do I work too quickly? Do I care about the quality of my work? Am I aware of my poor performance? Do I ask for help when I'm not sure about something? Am I willing to work on improving my skills?	Contact your school for refresher training. Review textbooks, notes, and tests. In the future, ask your supervisor for help when you are having difficulty. Don't ignore problems. Never try to cover up poor performance. It will become obvious and is not fair to those who depend on your work.
Excessive absences	Am I failing to make work a top priority? Am I practicing good health habits? Getting enough rest? Are there health problems I need to take care of? Do I need to improve my personal organization skills to prevent frequent personal "emergencies"?	Commit to making work a top priority. Develop good health habits and seek professional help if necessary. Develop backup plans for childcare, transportation, etc. Redefine "emergency." Work to become accident-proof rather than accident-prone. Seek help in resolving personal and/or family problems.
Violation of facility rules and/or failure to follow directions	Do I know the rules but choose to disregard them? Why? Do I misunderstand directions? How can I learn what rules are in force?	Review the importance of following rules for maintaining personal and patient safety and fulfilling legal and regulatory requirements. Ask for explanations of rules or directions you don't understand. Read policy and procedure manuals and any other sources of facility rules.
Inability to get along with others; poor interpersonal skills	Is there a pattern to my relationships with others? Do I fail to listen? Do I insist on being right and/or having my own way? Am I willing to do my share of the work? Do I gossip at work and talk about people behind their backs? Do I get involved in disputes and take sides?	Review the principles of good communication. Take a communications and/or interpersonal relations class. Request honest feedback from someone you trust. Seek counseling to help you examine and improve your relationships with others.
Poor attitude, lack of professionalism	In what ways is my behavior unprofessional? Is my concept of "professionalism" different from the employer's? Am I willing to change? Can I put patient and employer needs before my own preferences? What contributes to my poor attitude? Am I willing to change? What can I do to change?	Think about your reasons for choosing a career in health care to see whether your conduct is in alignment with them. Review the purpose and components of professionalism. Observe successful health care professionals. Seek help from a mentor.
Failure to follow safe techniques	Do I know the proper techniques? Do I understand the importance of using safe techniques? Do I understand the negative consequences of using improper techniques?	Review textbooks and notes from class and skills lab. Take refresher courses that include skills training.

you must be willing to face them and commit to finding solutions. Table 14-2 contains examples of questions and actions for dealing with specific problems.

Note: If, after conducting your self-evaluation, you sincerely believe that your dismissal was unjust, unfair, and/or based on factors that were not related to your job performance (discrimination), you may decide to seek legal advice. You must be prepared to demonstrate and document that your performance was satisfactory and to show how you were treated unfairly.

Getting Back on Course

"Turn your stumbling blocks into stepping stones."

—*Anonymous*

When looking for another job, you may worry about telling potential employers you were fired from your last one. First of all, you don't have to volunteer this information if you are not asked. But if you are, be truthful. State that it didn't work out and that you were let go. It's not necessary to explain the situation in detail. Do not blame or criticize your previous employer. Do explain what you have learned from the situation and what you have done to ensure that it won't happen again. This demonstrates your honesty and ability to learn from mistakes, important qualities in the workplace. Let the employer know you are committed to getting your career back on course and want to begin by making a positive contribution to his or her organization. Once you are reemployed, there are ways you can avoid getting back into rough waters, such as the following:

- Do your best to keep communication lines open with your new supervisor.
- Learn to recognize warning signs and address problems immediately. Don't try to deny or cover them up. This only makes the situation worse.
- Ask for help before you get into trouble.
- Request regular feedback from your supervisor about your performance.
- Be conscientious about performing regular self-evaluations.

Many people who lose their jobs manage to bounce back and achieve career success. You can, too, if you use the experience as an opportunity to learn and grow, not as an excuse for future failure.

ENRICHING YOUR CAREER

The health care field offers many employment opportunities. There are dozens of ways to add interest and variety to your career. Your training may qualify you to work in a variety of settings. For example, the following are just some of the environments in which health care professionals work:

1. Hospitals
2. Long-term care facilities
3. Schools
4. Prisons
5. Homeless shelters
6. Mobile vans that provide medical care to migrant farm workers
7. Private homes
8. International settings, such as the Peace Corps or religious missions

Some professions offer great flexibility in locations and schedules. Certain occupational areas allow you to choose between working for one employer or for an agency that sends you on a variety of assignments that range from 1 day to 6 months or longer. If you enjoy a change of scenery and even a bit of adventure, you can look for short-term assignments at locations around the country—or even around the world.

The nature of health care delivery today enables professionals to apply their skills in a variety of ways. Your profession may allow you to accept new challenges and gain enriching experiences. Let's look at a few types of jobs available for health care professionals who have the necessary qualifications:

- Direct patient care in many specialty areas
- Education of both patients and other health care personnel
- Management and administration
- Quality review (checking patient records for accuracy and completeness of documentation and treatment outcomes)
- Oversight of performance improvement (comparing a facility's performance in specific areas, such as infection control, with health care industry standards)

 Go to page 380 to complete Prescription for Success 14-6

Career Laddering

The concept of career laddering was introduced in Chapter 1. A career ladder consists of all the job titles within an occupational area that require various levels of education, skills, and responsibility. Figure 14-4 contains three health care examples.

Being successful does not necessarily mean climbing the ladder. In fact, aiming to do your best at your chosen level is a worthy goal. Gaining experience, perfecting your skills, and staying current are activities that can provide long-term satisfaction.

It is important to understand that the nature of the work varies among the levels. What is most appealing to you may not be found at higher-level jobs. For example, in the field of occupational therapy, the certified occupational therapist assistant generally spends more time working with patients than does the therapist, who often spends more time performing patient assessments, writing treatment plans, and performing administrative tasks. The conditions under which you work and the nature of the tasks may be different as well. In another example, the dental assistant works closely with the dentist, helping with a variety of procedures. The hygienist, on the other hand, primarily works alone with patients and performs similar work with each.

Positions that have more supervisory responsibilities may limit the time spent performing lab tests, getting to know patients, giving treatments, or doing other tasks you enjoy. Before deciding to pursue additional training to move up the ladder, thoroughly investigate the job title that interests you by doing the following:

☐ Observe people at work who have the position.
☐ Interview them about their duties and responsibilities.

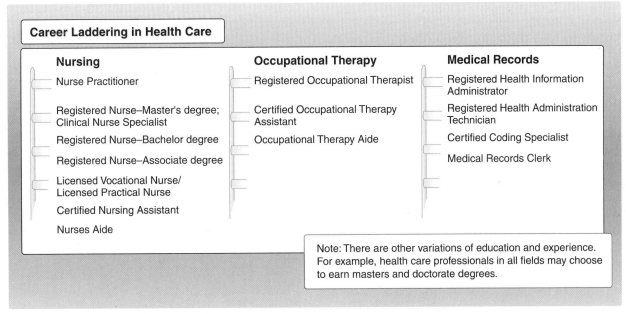

Figure 14-4   Examples of career laddering in health care.

□ If you are not working closely with professionals at the targeted level, ask permission to **job shadow** in another department or facility.

□ Read about the job title (see To Learn More at the end of the chapter).

□ Request information from the appropriate professional organization.

□ Review a sample curriculum and course descriptions.

□ Obtain job descriptions.

Some schools have **step-up programs** so students can apply the courses they took for one occupational level to the next level. For example, there are programs that grant academic credits and waive certain courses for licensed practical nurses and licensed vocational nurses who enroll in registered nurse programs. Step-up programs are not available at all schools. They may also be selective about the schools from which they accept credits. Be sure to inquire about the transfer of credit policy when deciding where to pursue advanced training.

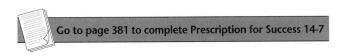

Go to page 381 to complete Prescription for Success 14-7

Developing a New Career

Many health care professionals have skills they can transfer from one occupational area to another. After acquiring work experience, you may decide to choose another type of work in which you use your health care background. Additional training or self-directed learning may be necessary to supplement your knowledge and skills.

The following examples illustrate careers open to people with health care backgrounds:

• **Sales**: Medical and pharmaceutical products

• **Instructor or program director**: Vocational schools, colleges, and universities

• **Legal assistant**: For attorneys who specialize in health care cases

• **Consultant**: Providing advice to individuals and organizations in your areas of expertise

• **Writer**: Reports, articles, proposals, textbooks, and patient education materials

The Health Care Entrepreneur

An **entrepreneur** is someone who organizes and manages a business. Starting a business or working on your own may appeal to you. Being the boss is an attractive idea: setting your own schedule, being accountable only to yourself, and enjoying the benefits of your work. There is another side, of course: having to work many hours, doing all the work yourself, and assuming responsibility for any financial losses. Not everyone is cut out for self-employment. Certain characteristics have been identified as desirable for successful entrepreneurs. Ask yourself if you have the following qualities:

□ **Competitive**. Do you see yourself as a winner? Are you willing to put in the necessary effort to be one?

□ **Professionally competent**. Are you skilled and experienced in the area you wish to pursue? Are your skills up-to-date?

☐ **Persistent.** Can you keep trying, even after experiencing failure?

☐ **Willing to take risks.** Are you comfortable taking a chance with your time? Your income?

☐ **Self-disciplined.** Do you stay with tasks until they are completed? Meet deadlines? Can you stay focused on work when there is something else you want to do?

☐ **Self-confident.** Do you believe in yourself and your ability to succeed?

☐ **A problem solver and decision maker.** Are you comfortable making decisions on your own? Do you follow through with action once decisions have been made?

☐ **Financially prepared.** Do you have enough money to support yourself until you develop an income?

☐ **Organized.** Do you organize your time well? Can you attend to more than one thing at a time?

☐ **Informed about laws and regulations.** Are you familiar with the laws that affect the area of health care in which you work? Do you understand the tax implications for people who work for themselves?

Health care lends itself to a number of home-based and small businesses. The following are just a few examples:

- Health care and nutritional product sales
- Medical report transcription
- Coding and billing services
- Consulting
- Provision of residential care

A key success factor is choosing a product or service for which there is a market. Even a good idea will fail if there aren't enough customers. Conducting market research is the first step when considering a business idea.

There are many sources of assistance for those who are interested in starting a small business or working on their own. Local chambers of commerce, the Small Business Administration, local government agencies, and SCORE, a volunteer group of retired business people, offer a variety of services ranging from free advice to reasonably priced classes to market research data. Colleges, universities, and adult education programs offer useful classes. Learn all you can before making the decision to venture out on your own.

SMOOTH SAILING

Managed wisely, your career can be a continual source of satisfaction. Choosing to work in health care ensures that what you do each day will benefit others. Monitor your performance, watch for opportunities, and enjoy the gratification that comes from staying on course and arriving at your planned career destination.

SUMMARY OF KEY IDEAS

1. Careers must be managed to stay on course.
2. Take responsibility for your performance evaluations.
3. Staying connected and current increases both your career success and your enjoyment of work.
4. Promotions are not given; they are earned.
5. Getting fired from a job is not the end of a career.
6. Never burn your bridges when leaving a job.
7. There are many opportunities to keep your career interesting and engaging.

Positive Self-Talk for This Chapter

1. I am successfully managing my career.
2. I continually strive to improve my work and stay on course.
3. I am able to make wise decisions about the direction of my career.
4. I effectively use self-management tools like performance evaluations, decision matrices, and self-questioning.
5. I get great satisfaction from my work.

To Learn More

Mind Tools

www.mindtools.com

This career-success web site has articles on many topics including leadership and decision-making.

Monster

www.monster.com

In addition to job leads and job-search tips, the Monster web site has a section filled with articles about career development and changes. At the bottom of the web page, click on "For Your Career" and then on "Develop Your Career."

Occupational Outlook Handbook

U.S. Department of Labor

www.bls.gov/OCO/

This is a source of detailed information about hundreds of careers, including typical job descriptions, educational requirements, and average salaries. It is updated every two years. It is a good source to explore career laddering, careers that are related, and possible work settings for various occupations.

Quintessential Careers

www.quintcareers.com/workplace_resources.html

The "Workplace Resources for Dealing With Your Current Job/Employer" page has links to dozens of helpful articles.

INTERNET ACTIVITIES

For active web links to the web sites needed to complete these activities, visit **http://evolve.elsevier.com/Haroun/career/**.

1. Monster provides career development advice. Choose an article from their Career Library and write a short summary.
2. Quintessential Careers contains many career tools, including short articles on job-related issues. Read at least five of the articles and prepare a list of 10 recommendations for achieving workplace success.

3. *The Wall Street Journal's* career web site has articles and corresponding quizzes to help readers achieve career success. Choose an article to read and write a paragraph describing what you learned.
4. *U.S. News and World Report* can help you keep up on trends in health care. Choose two articles to read and report on.

Prescription for Success 14-1
Make Reviews Work for You

Role-play the following situations with a classmate who takes the role of your supervisor.

1. Explain that you failed to follow certain safety procedures because you weren't told about them when you were hired.
2. Discuss three goals you want to achieve by your next formal evaluation.

Prescription for Success 14-2
Getting Those Units

Identify ways you can earn the continuing education units (CEUs) necessary for your profession. Create a table to organize the information.

Learning Activity	Sponsor	Requirements	Units and Cost
Workshops	_____	_____	_____
College classes	_____	_____	_____
Distance learning	_____	_____	_____
Reading assignments	_____	_____	_____
Hands-on activities	_____	_____	_____
Professional conferences	_____	_____	_____
Other	_____	_____	_____

_____

_____

_____

_____

_____

_____

_____

_____

Prescription for Success 14-3
Getting Ahead

Research the promotional opportunities that are available in your field.

1. Is additional training necessary? If so, describe it.

_____

_____

_____

2. Do these promotions usually include supervisory responsibilities? _____

3. Is being promoted a goal for you? _____

4. If yes, what can you do in your first job to start working toward this goal? _____

_____

_____

_____

_____

Prescription for Success 14-4
What's Important to Me?

Create and use a decision matrix to assist in making a decision in your personal life.

1. Describe the results.

_____

_____

_____

_____

2. If you found the process helpful, explain how.

_____

_____

_____

_____

Prescription for Success 14-5
Put It in Words

Write a letter of resignation for a job that you have enjoyed. You are leaving to work in a larger facility where you have been offered a position with more responsibilities at higher pay.

Prescription for Success 14-6
Find Out More

Research the work settings and types of jobs available in your occupational area.

1. How many can you find? List five here.

_____

_____

_____

_____

_____

_____

2. What qualifications are necessary for each?

_____

_____

_____

_____

_____

_____

3. Which ones seem most interesting to you?

_____

_____

_____

_____

Investigate the career ladder(s) in your occupational field.

1. What are the specific job titles on each rung of the ladder?

_____

_____

_____

_____

2. What are the educational requirements for each?

_____

_____

_____

_____

3. What are the licensing requirements for each?

_____

_____

_____

_____

4. Describe the differences in skill level and responsibility among the levels.

_____

_____

_____

_____

5. How are the tasks different?

_____

_____

_____

_____

Appendix

Professional Organizations for Health Care Occupations

Occupation	Organization	Contact Information
Cardiovascular Technologist	Alliance of Cardiovascular Professionals	P.O. Box 2007 Midlothian, VA 23113 (804) 632-0078 www.acp-online.org
Dental Assistant	American Dental Assistants Association	35 E. Wacker Drive Suite 1730 Chicago, IL 60601 (312) 541-1550 www.dentalassistant.org
Dental Hygienist	American Dental Hygienists' Association	444 N. Michigan Avenue, Suite 3400 Chicago, IL 60611 www.adha.org
Dental Laboratory Technician	National Association of Dental Laboratories	325 John Knox Road L103 Tallahassee, FL 32303 (850) 205-5626 (850) 222-0053 www.nadl.org
Diagnostic Medical Sonographer	Society of Diagnostic Medical Sonographers	2745 Dallas Parkway Suite 350 Plano, TX 75093 (800) 229-9506 (214) 473-8057 www.sdms.org
Dietary Technician	American Dietetic Association	120 South Riverside Plaza, Suite 2000 Chicago, IL 60606 (800) 877-1600 www.eatright.org
	Society for Nutrition Education	9100 Purdue Road Indianapolis, IN 46268 (800) 235-6690 (317) 328-4627 www.sne.org
ECG Technician (Electrocardiographic Technician)	Alliance of Cardiovascular Professionals	P.O. Box 2007 Midlothian, VA 23113 (804) 632-0078 www.acp-online.org

Continued

Occupation	Organization	Contact Information
EEG Technician (Electroneurodiagnostic Technician or Technologist)	American Society of Electroneurodiagnostic Technologists	6501 East Commerce Avenue Suite 120 Kansas City, MO 64120 (816) 931-1120 www.aset.org
Emergency Medical Technician	National Association of Emergency Medical Technicians	P.O. Box 1400 Clinton, MS 39060 (800) 346-2368 www.naemt.org
Health Information Technician	American Health Information Management Association	233 N. Michigan Avenue 21st Floor Chicago, IL 60601 www.ahima.org
Home Health Aide	National Network of Career Nursing Assistants	3577 Easton Road Norton, OH 44203 (330) 825-9342 www.cna-network.org
Massage Therapist	American Massage Therapy Association	500 Davis Street Suite 900 Evanston, IL 60201 (877) 905-2700 www.amtamassage.org
	Associated Bodywork and Massage Professionals	25188 Genesee Trail Road Golden, CO 80401 (800) 458-2267 www.abmp.com
Medical Assistant	American Association of Medical Assistants	20 N. Wacker Drive Suite 1575 Chicago, IL 60606 (312) 899-1500 www.aama-ntl.org
	American Medical Technologists	10700 West Higgins Road Suite 150 Rosemont, IL 60018 (847) 823-5169 (800) 275-1268 www.amt1.com
Medical Biller	Medical Association of Billers	2620 Regatta Drive Suite 102 Las Vegas, NV 89128 (702) 240-8519 www.physicianswebsites.com
Medical Insurance Coder	American Academy of Procedural Coders	2480 South 3850 West Suite B Salt Lake City, UT 84120 (800) 626-2633 www.aapc.com
	American Health Information Management Association	233 N. Michigan Avenue, 21st Floor Chicago, IL 60601 (312) 233-1100 www.ahima.org
Medical Laboratory Assistant or Medical Laboratory Technician	American Medical Technologists	10700 West Higgins Road Suite 150 Rosemont, IL 60018 (847) 823-5169 (800) 275-1268 www.amt1.com
	American Society for Clinical Laboratory Science	6701 Democracy Boulevard, suite 300 Bethesda, MD 20817 (301) 657-2768 www.ascls.org

Occupation	Organization	Contact Information
Medical Transcriptionist	American Association for Healthcare Documentation Integrity	4230 Kiernan Avenue Suite 130 Modesto, CA 95356 (800) 982-2182 www.ahdionline.org
Nursing Assistant	National Network of Career Nursing Assistants	3577 Easton Road Norton, OH 44203 (330) 825-9342 www.cna-network.org
Occupational Therapy Assistant	American Occupational Therapy Association	4720 Montgomery Lane PO Box 31220 Bethesda, MD 20824 (301) 652-2682 www.aota.org
Ophthalmic Laboratory Technician	Opticians Association of America	441 Carlisle Drive Herdon, VA 20170 (800) 433-8997 www.oaa.org
Ophthalmic Medical Assistant	Association of Technical Personnel in Ophthalmology	2025 Woodlane Drive St Paul, MN 55125 (800) 482-4858 www.atpo.com
Optician	Opticians Association of America	441 Carlisle Drive Herndon, VA 20170 (703) 437-8780 (800) 433-8997 www.oaa.org
	National Academy of Opticianry	8401 Corporate Drive Suite 605 Landover, MD 20785 (800) 229-4828 www.nao.org
Optometric Technician	American Optometric Association	1505 Prince Street Suite 300 Alexandria, VA 22314 and 243 North Lindbergh Boulevard St Louis, MO 63141 (800) 365-2219 www.aoanet.org
Pharmacy Assistant or Technician	National Pharmacy Technician Association	P.O. Box 683148 Houston, TX 77268 (888) 247-8700 www.pharmacytechnician.org
	American Pharmacists Association	2215 Constitution Avenue NW Washington, DC 20037 (202) 628-4410 www.pharmacist.com
Phlebotomist	American Medical Technologists	10700 West Higgins Road Suite 150 Rosemont, IL 60018 (847) 823-5169 (800) 275-1268 www.amt1.com
Physical Therapist Assistant	American Physical Therapy Association	1111 North Fairfax Street Alexandria, VA 22314 (703) 684-2782 (800) 999-2782 www.apta.org
Physician Assistant	American Academy of Physician Assistants	950 N. Washington Street Alexandria, VA 22314 (703) 836-2272 www.aapa.org

Continued

Occupation	Organization	Contact Information
Practical or Vocational Nurse	National Association for Practical Nurse Education and Service	1940 Duke Street Suite 200 Alexandria, VA 22314 (703) 933-1003 www.napnes.org
Psychiatric or Mental Health Technician	American Association of Psychiatric Technicians	1220 S Street Suite 100 Sacramento, CA 95811 (800) 391-7589 www.psychtechs.org
Radiographer or Radiologic Technologist	American Society of Radiologic Technologists	15000 Central Avenue SE Albuquerque, NM 87123 (800) 444-2778, press 5 (505) 298-4500 www.asrt.org
Registered Nurse	National League for Nursing	61 Broadway, 33rd Floor New York, NY 10006 (212) 363-5555 www.nln.org
	American Nurses Association	8515 Georgia Avenue Suite 400 Silver Spring, MD 20910 (800) 274-4262 www.nursingworld.org
Respiratory Therapist	American Association for Respiratory Care	9425 N. MacArthur Boulevard Suite 100 Irving, TX 75063 (972) 243-2272 www.aarc.org
Surgical Technologist	Association of Surgical Technologists	6 West Dry Creek Circle Suite 200 Littleton, CO 80120 (800) 637-7433 www.ast.org
Veterinary Technician	National Association of Veterinary Technicians in America	50 S. Pickett Street Suite 110 Alexandria, VA 22304 (703) 740-8737 www.navta.net

Appendix

Useful Spanish Phrases

GENERAL SPANISH PHRASES

English	Spanish
Hello, hi.	Hola. (OH-lah)
Good morning.	Buenos días. (bway-nohs DEE-ahs)
Good afternoon.	Buenas tardes. (bway-nahs TAR-dace)
Good evening, good night.	Buenas noches. (bway-nahs NO-chase)
Please.	Por favor. (por fah-VOR)
Thank you.	Gracias. (GRAH-see-ahs)
You're welcome.	De nada. (day NAH-dah)
Yes.	Sí. (see)
No.	No (no)
My name is _____.	Me llamo _____ (may YAH-mo) *or* Mi nombre es_____ (me NOHM-bray ace)
What is your name?	¿Cómo se llama usted? (COH-moh say YA-mah oo-sted)
Nice to meet you.	Mucho gusto. (MOO-choh GOO-stoh)
Do you speak English?	¿Habla usted inglés? (AH-blah oo-STED eeng-GLACE)
Do you understand English?	¿Comprende usted inglés? (comb-PREN-day oo-STED eeng-GLACE)
Do you understand me?	¿Me comprende usted? (may comb-PREN-day oo-STED)
Repeat, please.	Repita usted, por favor. (ray-PEE-tah oo-STED por fah-VOR)
I don't understand Spanish very well.	No comprendo el español muy bien. (no comb-PREN-doh el es-pahn-NYOL moo-ee bee-EN)
How do you feel?	¿Cómo se siente? (COMB-moh say see-EN-tay)
Good.	Bien. (bee-EN)
Fair.	Así, así (ah-SEE, ah-SEE) *or* Regular (ray-goo-LAHR)
Bad.	Mal. (mahl)
What is wrong?	¿Cuál es el problema? (kwal es el pro-BLAY-mah) *or* ¿Qué le pasa? (kay lay pah-sah)
Do you have pain?	¿Siente usted dolor? (see-EN-tay oo-STED doh-LOR)
Where?	¿Dónde? (DOHN-day)
Show me.	Enséñeme. (en-SEN-yay-may)
Are you comfortable?	¿Está usted cómodo? (es-TAH oo-STED COH-moh-doh)
It is important.	Es importante. (es eem-por-TAHN-tay)
Be calm, please.	Cálmese usted, por favor. (CALL-may-say oo-STED, por fah-VOR)

Continued

English	Spanish
Don't be frightened.	No tenga usted miedo. (no TAYNG-gah oo-STED mee-AY-doh)
We are here to help you.	Estamos aquí para ayudarle.(eh-STAH-mohs ah-KEY pah-rah ah-you-DAR-lay)
Please come with me.	Acompáñeme, por favor. (ah-comb-PAN-yay-may por fah-VOR) or Por favor, venga conmigo. (por fahVOR VEN-gah cone-MEEgo)
Go to the hospital.	Vaya usted al hospital. (VAI-yah oo-STED ahl oh-spee-TAHL)

BASIC EMERGENCY ADMISSION QUESTIONS

Allergies	Alergias (ah-LAIR-hee-ahs)
Antibiotics? Which ones?	¿Antibióticas? ¿Cuáles? (ahn-tee-bee-O-tee-cahs KWAH-lace)
Aspirin?	¿Aspirina? (Ah-spee-REE-nah)
Sulfa drugs?	¿Drogas de azufre? (DROO-gahs day ah-SOO fray)
Pain medications? Which ones?	¿Pastillas para dolor? ¿Cuáles? (paw-STEE-yahs paw-rah doe-lore. KWAH-lace)
Others?	¿Otras? (OH-trahs)
Required medications	Medicinas requiridas (meh-dee-SEE-nahs ray-care-EE-dahs)
Medical problems	Problemas médicos (pro-BLAY-mahs MEH-dee-cohs)
Blood type	Grupo sanguineo (GROO-poh sahn-GEE-nay-oh)
Religion	Religión (ray-lee-hee-OHN)
Referral physician	Médico que le mandó (MEH-dee-coh kay lay mahn-DOE)
What type of medical insurance do you have?	¿Qué tipo de seguro médico tiene used? (kay tee-poh day say-GOO-roh tee-EN-ay oo-STED)
What is your Blue Cross number? Kaiser?	¿Cuál es su número de Blue Cross? ¿De Kaiser? (kwal es sue NEW-mehr-o day Blue Cross? Day Kaiser?)
Do you have a Medicare card?	¿Tiene usted tarjeta de Medicare? (tee-EN-ay oo-STED tar-HEY-tah day Medicare)
Fill out this form, please.	Llene esta forma (or planilla), por favor. (Yeah-nay ES-ta FOR-mah, por fah-VOR)
Sign here, please.	Firme aquí, por favor. (Fear-may ah-KEY, por fah-VOR)
This is an authorization form. Please read it and sign here.	Esta es una forma de autorización (or forma de permiso). Favor de leerla y firmarla aquí. (ES-tah es OO-nah FOR-mah day ow-tore-ee-sah-see-OWN (FOR-mah day pair-MEE-so). Fah-VOR day lay-err-lah ee fear-mar-lah ah-KEY.

HOW TO USE THE PRONUNCIATION GUIDES

1. Stress the syllables (parts of words) that are in capital letters.
2. "oh" is pronounced as in "toe."
3. "ah" is pronounced as in "father."
4. "ay" is pronounced as in "say."
5. "oo" is pronounced as in "moon."
6. "s" is always pronounced as in "set."
7. When there is an English word given as a syllable, pronounce it as you would the word by itself. If letters in the word are silent in English, do not pronounce them. In "comb," for example, don't pronounce the "b." Just say the word.

    Here are the words used to show the pronunciation of Spanish syllables: chase, see, us, no, day, moo, goo, blah, comb, may, ray, pee, bee, say, call, you, lay, yeah.
8. The "h" in Spanish is always silent.

    Note: The "official" phonetic alphabet is not used here because many people who have not studied languages are not familiar with the special markings.

Index

Page numbers followed by f indicate figures; t, tables, b, boxes.

Employer meetings
as source of employment leads, 248–250
Employers
goal alignment with first, 13–14
needs of, 289, 301t
sources, 289
Employment; *See also* job search
headquarters, 240–243, 241b
job-selection process, 319–321, 319b
offers
accepting, 321–323
considering, 319–321, 320f
turning down, 323, 324f
search (*See* job search)
short and long-term goals, 239
sources of leads
direct employer contacts, 246–247
government resource centers, 246
job fairs, 248
leads, 238, 241–242, 244, 245f
networking, 247, 247b
school career services, 245, 247b
websites and employer meetings, 248–250
Employment ads
responding to, 251, 253f
where to find, 244, 245f
English language
exercises to evaluate, 113b–115b
steps to improve, 93–100, 93t
English-as-a-second language students
exercises to evaluate skills, 113b–115b
grammar, 97–100
idiomatic expressions, 84, 95
improving pronunciation, 95–96
increasing your vocabulary, 93t, 94–95
informational resources for, 108
medical words in everyday Spanish, 93t
for non-native speakers, 92–93
reading comprehension, 96
spelling, 97–98
steps to improve English, 93–100, 93t
using verbs correctly, 98–99
Entrepreneurs, 361, 375–376
Equal Pay Act, 345
E-resumes, 271–272
Essay questions, 171
Essays, 146, 171
Ethical behavior
behavioral interview questions regarding, 291t
defining, 1, 337–339
exercise to assess, 19b–20b
versus cheating, 173, 173b
Ethics
admitting mistakes, 337–339
Code of Ethics, 332, 337, 337b, 352b
developing competencies in, 332, 337, 337b, 352b
Ethnic
definition of, 1
Evaluation
definition of, 180, 185–186
Experience
clinical, 34–35
resume tips concerning, 33–35
Eye contact
cultural beliefs concerning, 213t
Eye-level reading ruler, 83

F

Family
Family Medical Leave Act (FMLA), 345
and time management, 86–92, 87f–88f
Family Medical Leave Act (FMLA), 345
Fax machine, 238, 243

Fear
irrational, 85, 85t
versus understanding and appreciating diversity, 211–214
Federal Age Discrimination Act, 346
Feedback
following job loss, 372–374, 373t
in interviews, 289, 296–297
in oral communication, 208, 217, 219t
Fill-in-the-blank questions, 170
Final impressions
in interviews, 303–305
Financial planning
budgeting
personal expenses, 53b–54b
Q&A on, 37b
First drafts
in writing, 152–154
First impressions
in interviews, 289–290, 294–296
resumes and cover letters giving, 283b
in workplace, 334
Five "Ps" of marketing
packaging
as the third "P" of marketing yourself, 30–32
planning
as the first "P" of marketing yourself, 8–14
presentation
as the fourth "P" of marketing yourself, 32–37
production
as the second "P" of marketing yourself, 30
promotion
as the fifth "P" of marketing yourself, 37–38
Flash cards
as learning tool, 70t
to practice math, 186
Flexibility
behavioral interview questions regarding, 291t
Focus
on goals in workplace, 347–348
shifting in workplace, 333–334
strategies for students with learning disabilities, 102t
Form
and details, 154–158
in writing, 152–154, 173
401(k) retirement plans, 315
Fraud, 146, 173
Freewriting, 146, 152–154
Functional resumes, 265, 267f, 273f

G

Gender
cultural beliefs concerning, 213t
Equal Pay Act, 345
Gerunds, 83, 98–99
Global learning styles
examples of, 70t
versus linear learning, 68t
suggestions when reviewing textbook, 135
when studying from notes, 129
Glossary
definition of, 117, 132
Goals
characteristics of effective, 57–59
employment, 239
exercise to practice, 74b–75b
focus in workplace, 347–348
short and long term, 58–59

Goals (*Continued*)
SMART goals, 367b
study skill, 2–5, 3t
success tips for achieving, 59
supporting, 58–59
using on the job, 59b
Goal-setting
purpose of, 57–59
Gossip
as nonrespectful behavior, 209–210
Government resource centers, 246
Grammar
basics in English language, 97–100
defining system for writing, 146, 154–158
exercise for evaluating your own, 177b
and spelling in writing, 154–158, 156t, 158t, 160t–165t
Grievances
in workplace, 332, 348
Guided imagery, 83, 102b

H

Habits
for success, 1–5
"Hands on" learning style, 67–68, 68t
Health care
cultural beliefs concerning, 213t
skills to emphasize on resume, 33–34
time management, 62b
Health care research
websites, 117, 137–139. *See also* Appendix A
Health Common Procedure Coding System (HCPCS), 332
Health Insurance Portability and Accountability Act (HIPAA), 338–339
Healthcare entrepreneurs, 361, 375–376
Helping verbs, 83, 98–99
Honesty
developing competencies in, 332, 337–339, 352b
exercise to assess, 19b–20b
Honors and awards
exercises, 46b, 285b
resume tips concerning, 35, 263
Human resources departments, 246–247
Hygiene
importance of, 29, 31–32
personal reflection concerning, 32b
Hyperactivity
with learning disabilities, 102t

I

Idiomatic expressions, 84, 95
Illegal questions
in interviews, 288, 299–301, 300t
Indexes
in textbooks, 132
Individual learning
examples of, 70t
versus interactive, 68t
Inductive learning
versus deductive, 68t
examples of, 70t
suggestions when reviewing textbook, 135
Infinitives, 84, 98–99
Informal outlines
note-taking, 122, 124f
Information; *See also* informational resources; research
gathering for problem-solving, 200–201
gathering for writing, 148–149
Informational interviews, 2, 25b–26b